Urologic Reconstructive Surgery

Editor

JILL C. BUCKLEY

UROLOGIC CLINICS
OF NORTH AMERICA

www.urologic.theclinics.com

Consulting Editor
KEVIN R. LOUGHLIN

August 2022 • Volume 49 • Number 3

ELSEVIER

1600 John F. Kennedy Boulevard • Suite 1800 • Philadelphia, Pennsylvania, 19103-2899

http://www.theclinics.com

UROLOGIC CLINICS OF NORTH AMERICA Volume 49, Number 3
August 2022 ISSN 0094-0143, ISBN-13: 978-0-323-98793-6

Editor: Kerry Holland
Developmental Editor: Diana Ang

Urologic Clinics of North America (ISSN 0094-0143) is published quarterly by Elsevier Inc., 360 Park Avenue South, New York, NY 10010-1710. Months of issue are February, May, August, and November. Business and Editorial Offices: 1600 John F. Kennedy Blvd., Suite 1800, Philadelphia, PA 19103-2899. Periodicals postage paid at New York, NY and additional mailing offices. Subscription prices are $403.00 per year (US individuals), $1054.00 per year (US institutions), $100.00 per year (US students and residents), $459.00 per year (Canadian individuals), $1075.00 per year (Canadian institutions), $100.00 per year (Canadian students/residents), $530.00 per year (foreign individuals), $1075.00 per year (foreign institutions), and $240.00 per year (foreign students/residents). Foreign air speed delivery is included in all *Clinics* subscription prices. All prices are subject to change without notice. **POSTMASTER:** Send address changes to *Urologic Clinics of North America*, Elsevier Health Sciences Division, Subscription Customer Service, 3251 Riverport Lane, Maryland Heights, MO 63043. **Customer Service: 1-800-654-2452 (US). From outside the United States, call 1-314-447-8871. Fax: 1-314-447-8029. E-mail: JournalsCustomerServiceusa@elsevier.com (for print support)** and **JournalsOnlineSupport-usa@elsevier.com (for online support)**.

Reprints. For copies of 100 or more, of articles in this publication, please contact the Commercial Reprints Department, Elsevier Inc., 360 Park Avenue South, New York, New York 10010-1710. Tel.: 212-633-3874; Fax: 212-633-3820; E-mail: reprints@elsevier.com.

Urologic Clinics of North America is covered in MEDLINE/PubMed (*Index Medicus*), *Excerpta Medica, Current Contents/Clinical Medicine, Science Citation Index,* and *ISI/BIOMED*.

Contributors

CONSULTING EDITOR

KEVIN R. LOUGHLIN, MD, MBA
Emeritus Professor of Surgery (Urology),
Harvard Medical School, Visiting Scientist,
Vascular Biology Research Program at Boston
Children's Hospital, Boston, Massachusetts,
USA

EDITOR

JILL C. BUCKLEY, MD, FACS
Professor of Urology, Reconstructive Urology,
Robotic Surgery, Cancer Survivorship,
Director, Urology Residency Program,
Director, Reconstructive Urology Fellowship
(GURS), UC San Diego Health, La Jolla,
California, USA; Professor of Urology,
University of California, San Diego, San Diego,
California, USA

AUTHORS

IGNACIO ALVAREZ DE TOLEDO, MD
Department of Urology, Eastern Virginia
Medical School, Norfolk, Virginia,
USA

MARCO BANDINI, MD
Kulkarni Reconstructive Urology Center, Pune,
India

BENJAMIN N. BREYER, MD, MAS
Professor, Department of Urology, University
of California, San Francisco, San Francisco,
California, USA

JILL C. BUCKLEY, MD, FACS
Professor of Urology, Reconstructive Urology,
Robotic Surgery, Cancer Survivorship,
Director, Urology Residency Program,
Director, Reconstructive Urology Fellowship
(GURS), UC San Diego Health, La Jolla,
California, USA; Professor of Urology,
University of California, San Diego, San Diego,
California, USA

JACK G. CAMPBELL, MD
Division of Urology, Lahey Hospital and
Medical Center, Burlington, Massachusetts,
USA

**A. NIM CHRISTOPHER, MBBS, MPhil, FRCS
(Urol)**
University College London Hospitals NHS
Foundation Trust, St Peter's Andrology Centre,
London, United Kingdom

ADAM M. DAILY, MD, MS
Virginia Mason Franciscan Health, Seattle,
Washington, USA

JESSICA DELONG, MD, FACS
Associate Professor, Department of Urology,
Eastern Virginia Medical School, Norfolk,
Virginia, USA

MOLLY E. DEWITT-FOY, MD
Genitourinary Reconstructive Fellow,
University of Minnesota, Minneapolis,
Minnesota, USA

JASON ELYAGUOV, MD
Department of Urology, Westchester Medical
Center-New York Medical College, Valhalla,
New York, USA

SEAN P. ELLIOTT, MD, MS
Professor and Vice Chair of Urology, Director of
Reconstructive Urology, University of
Minnesota, Minneapolis, Minnesota,
USA

BRADLEY A. ERICKSON, MD, MS
Professor, Department of Urology, University
of Iowa, Carver College of Medicine, Iowa City,
Iowa, USA

KEVIN J. FLYNN, MD
Fellow, Genitourinary Reconstruction,
Department of Urology, Carver College of
Medicine, University of Iowa, Iowa City, Iowa,
USA

THOMAS W. FULLER, MD
Virginia Mason Franciscan Health, Seattle,
Washington, USA

WAI GIN LEE, MBChB, PhD, FRACS (Urol)
University College London Hospitals NHS
Foundation Trust, St Peter's Andrology Centre,
London, United Kingdom

KEVIN J. HEBERT, MD
Division of Urology, University of Utah, Salt
Lake City, Utah, USA

PANKAJ M. JOSHI, MD
Kulkarni Reconstructive Urology Center, Pune,
India

MELISSA R. KAUFMAN, MD, PhD
Department of Urology, Vanderbilt University
Medical Center, Nashville, Tennessee, USA

GEORGE E. KOCH, MD
Department of Urology, Vanderbilt University
Medical Center, Nashville, Tennessee, USA

KEVIN KRUGHOFF, MD
Division of Urology, Genitourinary Cancer
Survivorship Program, Duke University
Medical Center, Durham, North Carolina,
USA

SANJAY B. KULKARNI, MD
Kulkarni Reconstructive Urology Center, Pune,
India

YEONSOO S. LEE, BS
Mayo Clinic Alix School of Medicine,
Rochester, Minnesota, USA

ZIHO LEE, MD
Department of Urology, Northwestern
University, Feinberg School of Medicine,
Chicago, Illinois, USA

RANO MATTA, MD, MSc, MASc
Division of Urology, University of Utah, Salt
Lake City, Utah, USA

KIRTISHRI MISHRA, MD
NYU Langone Health, Department of Urology,
New York, New York, USA

JEREMY B. MYERS, MD, FACS
Professor and Chief of Urology, Genitourinary
Injury and Reconstructive Surgery, Department
of Surgery (Urology), University of Utah, Salt
Lake City, Utah, USA

ELIZABETH NAUD, MD, FRCSC
Reconstructive Urology, Fellow, Division
of Urology, Department of Surgery,
University of Alberta, Edmonton, Alberta,
Canada

DMITRIY NIKOLAVSKY, MD
Department of Urology, SUNY Upstate Medical
University, Department of Urology, Upstate
University Hospital, Syracuse, New York,
USA

ANDREW C. PETERSON, MD, MPH, FACS
Division of Urology, Genitourinary Cancer
Survivorship Program, Duke University Medical
Center, Durham, North Carolina, USA

DAVID J. RALPH, MBBS, MS, FRCS (Urol)
University College London Hospitals NHS
Foundation Trust, St Peter's Andrology Centre,
London, United Kingdom

KEITH ROURKE, MD, FRCSC
Professor, Division of Urology, Department of
Surgery, University of Alberta, Kipnes Urology
Centre, Edmonton, Alberta, Canada

JESSICA N. SCHARDEIN, MD
Department of Urology, SUNY Upstate Medical
University, Department of Urology, Upstate
University Hospital, Syracuse, New York,
USA

JOSHUA SHAPIRO, MD
Department of Orthopaedics, The University of North Carolina at Chapel Hill, Chapel Hill, North Carolina, USA

JOLIE SHEN, MD
Department of Urology, University of Washington School of Medicine, Seattle, Washington, USA

JOSHUA STERLING, MD
Department of Urology, SUNY Upstate Medical University, Syracuse, New York, USA; Department of Urology, Yale School of Medicine, New Haven, Connecticut, USA

ALEX J. VANNI, MD
Associate Professor, Department of Urology, Division of Urology, Tuft University School of Medicine, Lahey Hospital and Medical Center, Burlington, Massachusetts, USA

HUNTER WESSELLS, MD, FACS
Department of Urology, University of Washington School of Medicine, Seattle, Washington, USA

ALEX J. XU, MD
Department of Urology, NYU Langone Health, New York, New York, USA

LEE CHENG ZHAO, MD
NYU Langone Health, Department of Urology, New York, New York, USA

Contents

 Video content accompanies this article at http://www.urologic.theclinics.com.

Urethroplasty has evolved over time. The twentieth century saw management of urethral strictures and hypospadias with flaps. Things changed in the late 1990s with reintroduction of grafts. Buccal mucosa grafts gained popularity. There are failed urethroplasties and obliterative strictures, mostly iatrogenic, after urologic endosurgery. Such strictures need vascularized augmentation or substitution with flaps. Reconstructive urologists should be well versed in management of all types of complex cases. This article discusses the commonly used flaps in genitourinary reconstruction. Penile flaps are the commonest. Overall, the winner is the dartos. All penile flaps are based on the excellent vascularity of dartos.

 Video content accompanies this article at http://www.urologic.theclinics.com.

While patient preference often helps guide treatment decisions, poor long-term success combined with cumulative risk of repeat endoscopic treatments and the complications innately associated with urethral stricture emphasize that urethroplasty is most often the best choice for successful treatment in the long-term. This has led to the need to better refine urethroplasty techniques and optimize patient outcomes. Urethroplasty has now largely transitioned to a day-surgery procedure in the majority of centers. Some evidence suggests that avoiding urethral transection and/or avoiding overzealous urethral mobilization may lead to a reduction in postoperative sexual dysfunction. The trend toward single stage penile urethroplasty with buccal mucosal grafts likely minimizes patient morbidity without compromising urethroplasty success. For urethroplasty success to further improve particularly in patients at high risk for stricture recurrence, the synergistic potential of combining wound healing enhancing agents with evolving tissue-engineering represents an exciting future opportunity in the quest to perfect urethroplasty outcomes.

plication, grafting, and implants to achieve satisfactory outcomes across the full range of etiology and degree of surgical complexity.

Video content accompanies this article at http://www.urologic.theclinics.com.

It is generally accepted that robotic ureteral reconstruction provides equivalent results to open and laparoscopic approaches while decreasing pain and length of
stay. There is a rapid expansion of robotic ureteral reconstructive techniques, platforms, and adjunctive technologies, enabling more efficient, safer, and novel surgical approaches that could not be done in the past. For instance, indocyanine green
use allows rapid, precise location of ureteral stenosis and determination of tissue
perfusion. Multi-image display allows the surgeon to integrate the robotic field and
ureteroscopic images. Novel robotic surgical techniques, such as buccal mucosa
ureteroplasty, are changing the treatment algorithm for ureteral strictures.

With the widespread dissemination of robotic surgical platforms, pathologies that
were previously deemed challenging can now be treated more reliably with minimally invasive procedures via the robot. The advantages of precise articulation for
dissection and suturing, tremor reduction, three-dimensional magnified visualization, and small incisions allow for the management of diverse lower urinary tract
(LUT) disease. These may include recurrent or refractory bladder neck stenoses or
intracorporeal urinary diversion with excellent perioperative and functional outcomes. Here, we review the recent literature comprising of developments in
robotic-assisted LUT genitourinary reconstruction, with a view toward emerging
technologies and future trends in techniques.

We present a phenotype-based approach to neurogenic bladder (NGB) by
describing prototypical patients with spinal cord injury (SCI), spina bifida (SB), cerebral palsy (CP), and multiple sclerosis (MS). Surgical management is categorized by
failure to store and failure to empty, with a focus on catheterizable channels, bladder
augmentation, and bladder outlet procedures. Mitigation and management of common complications are reviewed. Specific attention is paid to social support, body
habitus, and extremity function, as we believe a holistic approach is necessary for
appropriate surgical selection.

Urinary diversion selection depends highly on surgeon experience, patient comorbidities, operative indication, and preoperative risk assessment. Navigating this process in the setting of emerging surgical approaches, new operative technology, and
evolving perioperative care plans can be difficult for general and reconstructive urologists alike. In this article, we highlight considerations for urinary diversion selection
and review new updates in the literature regarding preoperative patient assessment
and nutrition optimization. In addition, we review unique perioperative considerations including role of preoperative bowel prep and intraoperative maneuvers in
the setting of obesity and prior radiation. Last, we examine postoperative

expectations, long-term outcomes, and emerging technology to mitigate postoperative risk associated with urinary diversions.

Rectourethral fistula (RUF) and puboprostatic fistula (PPF) are potentially devastating complications that can develop after various pelvic insults, most notable treatment of prostate cancer. Both entities represent surgical challenges given the complex anatomy, risk of injury to adjacent structures, and poor tissue quality and wound healing. While extirpative surgery may be necessary for some patients, meticulous surgical dissection and interposition of healthy muscle allow for fistula repair in a high proportion of appropriately selected patients, especially in RUF. Herein the authors describe the nature, management, and outcomes of RUF and PPF with a full review of the literature.

UROLOGIC CLINICS OF NORTH AMERICA

SERIES OF RELATED INTEREST
Surgical Clinics of North America
https://www.surgical.theclinics.com/

Foreword

Reconstructive Urology: Michelangelo Buonaroti, Andreas Vesalius, and the Marriage of Surgery and Art

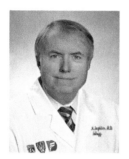

Kevin R. Loughlin, MD, MBA
Consulting Editor

"I saw an angel in the marble and carved until I set him free."[1] These words were spoken by Michelangelo Buonaroti about 500 years ago. He is part of the long-shared tradition of artists and surgeons in the study of anatomy. When he was only seventeen, Michelangelo started his dissections of cadavers from the hospital of the Monastery of Santo Spirito after the death of his mentor, Lorenzo de Medici.[2]

Living at the same time as Michelangelo was a physician, Andreas Vesalius, who, after completing his studies at the University of Louvan, arrived at the University of Paris in 1533 and transformed the way anatomy was taught.[3] He was aided by the fact that, in 1537, Pope Clement VII accepted the teaching of anatomy by dissection. Vesalius was so convinced of the necessity of human dissection that it was reported that he performed a dissection on a Spanish aristocrat while the heart was still beating.[4]

The quest for human dissection to aid in the study of human anatomy continued for several centuries. In 1770, John Warren and several other Harvard Medical School students formed what was known as the "Spunker Club" to raid cemeteries to harvest bodies for anatomic dissection.[3]

Nowhere is the shared tradition of art and surgery more apparent than in the field of reconstructive urology. Dr Buckley has assembled a group of this era's best reconstructive urologists, who review a panoply of topics, including flaps, urethroplasties, penile surgery, gender-affirmation surgery, robotic reconstruction, and fistula repair, just to enumerate a partial list of the techniques covered in this issue.

It is not hyperbole to assert that this is a "state-of-the-art" issue that will be referenced by this and the next generation of reconstructive surgeons for years to come. Urologic surgery can be divided into three areas: diagnostic, extirpative, and reconstructive. It can be argued, that of the three, reconstructive is the most challenging because, like Michelangelo, it requires not only the manual performance of the procedure but also the ability to envision the final reconstructed result. When Dr Buckley and her colleagues enter the operating room, their goal is nothing less

Urol Clin N Am 49 (2022) xiii–xiv
https://doi.org/10.1016/j.ucl.2022.06.002
0094-0143/22/© 2022 Published by Elsevier Inc.

urologic.theclinics.com

than, like Michelangelo, to uncover the anatomic angel within the human tissue that they see.

Kevin R. Loughlin, MD, MBA
Vascular Biology Program at
Boston Children's Hospital
300 Longwood Avenue
Boston, MA 02115, USA

E-mail address:
kloughlin@partners.org

REFERENCES

1. Brainy quote. Available at: Brainyquote.com/quotes. michelangelo.161309. Accessed May 26, 2022.
2. Pearce JMS. The anatomy of Michelangelo (1475-1564). Hektoen Int J 2019;11(2). Spring 2019.
3. Loughlin KR. Harvard Medical School and the body snatchers. Hektoen Int J 2019;11(3). Summer 2019.
4. Persaud TV. Early history of human anatomy: from antiquity to the beginning of the modern era. Springfield (IL): Charles C. Thomas; 1984.

Preface
Reconstructive Urology

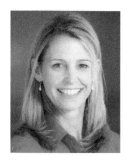

Jill C. Buckley, MD, FACS
Editor

Reconstructive Urology is broad, expanding, and ever changing. The field is rooted in plastic surgery principles focused on tissue transfer techniques, blood supply, wound healing, flaps, and grafts and is focused on both functional and cosmetic outcomes. In this dedicated *Urologic Clinics of North America*, we have experts from around the world who put together state-of-the-art articles on the vast array of conditions we treat as reconstructive urologists. Topics range from common flaps and grafts used in the urinary system, anterior and posterior urethral reconstruction, neurogenic bladder management and common operative solutions, common types of bowel diversion, upper and lower tract robotic reconstruction, fistula repair, gender-affirmation surgery, to genital reconstruction, and more. The authors offer keen insight into the many challenging and highly surgical conditions we treat.

It has been exciting to see the field grow and transform especially in the last couple of decades with new techniques (vessel-sparing urethral and ureteral reconstruction), new technology (wound vacs to help close complex perineal wounds and the adoption of robotics), and a growing focus on antifibrotic agents that alter the wound's local environment to assist in more regenerative healing. The future of our relatively young subspecialty is indeed bright. Who knows what the next two decades will hold? My sense is that it will be focused on more minimally invasive techniques, more robotic-assisted reconstructive surgery, use of off-the-shelf matrixes for urethral and ureteral repair, improved wound healing agents that halt excessive fibrosis and hasten regenerative healing, organ replacement with tissue engineering, and improved prosthetic technology, to name just a few.

To the readers, I hope you enjoy this collection of articles focused on all aspects of Reconstructive Urology. To my colleagues, a very sincere *Thank You* for taking the time as leaders in our field to share your knowledge and insight.

With warm regards,

Jill C. Buckley, MD, FACS
Reconstructive Urology, Robotic
Surgery, Cancer Survivorship
UC San Diego Health
9444 Medical Center Drive
La Jolla, CA 92037-7897, USA

E-mail address:
jcbuckley@health.ucsd.edu

Urol Clin N Am 49 (2022) xv
https://doi.org/10.1016/j.ucl.2022.06.001
0094-0143/22/© 2022 Published by Elsevier Inc.

Common Flaps in Genitourinary Reconstruction

Pankaj M. Joshi, MD*, Marco Bandini, MD, Sanjay B. Kulkarni, MD

KEYWORDS

- Fasciocutaneous flap • Augmentation • Urethroplasty • Reconstructive urology
- Enterourethroplasty • Flaps • BMG

KEY POINTS

- BMG is still the commonest choice of material used for augmentation urethroplasty.
- Flaps are required for redo and complex cases.
- Preputial /penile fasciocutaneous flaps are best suited for urethral reconstruction.
- They are easy to harvest and have good Long term success.
- Flaps should be performed by experienced reconstructive urologists.

 Video content accompanies this article at http://www.urologic.theclinics.com.

INTRODUCTION

Urethroplasty is a very antique technique, and its origin is from ancient times.[1] Nonetheless, it is from less than a century that urethroplasty has become a common procedure in everyday practice. Anastomotic techniques have represented the cornerstone for reconstructing the strictured urethra for more than 50 years. Before the 1990s, the only alternative to anastomotic urethroplasty was the use of fasciocutaneous flaps from genital skin. However, the use of flaps was frequently associated with complications[2] such as fistulae and diverticula formation resulting in suboptimal outcomes and low patency rates.[1] Harvesting of flap was technically difficult given also the limited technologies that were used in surgery at that time: primitive electrocautery, lack of loupes, and so on. Thus, when the buccal mucosa grafts (BMGs) came back to practice in 1996 (Morey and McAninch[3]) the use of flaps rapidly decreased in favor of BMGs, which rapidly become the first option in nontraumatic strictures. For more than 25 years, the use of flaps was practically anecdotical. However, history is made of course and recourse, and it was just a matter of time that flaps were finding a new way to come back in our practice. The reconstruction of the urethra with the use of BMGs represented a great step forward; indeed, patency rate was improved compared with previous techniques. Nonetheless, BMG augmentation can also fail. Patency rates after BMG augmentation vary between 75% and 85%. It means that 15% to 25% patients will fail after surgery and they will require a re–do procedure. Here comes the major problem of grafts: the source for BMGs is limited. The need for a plan B after failed BMG urethroplasty pushed reconstructive urology to look around for alternatives in these patients. Whether the advance of bioengineering represents a valid solution for the future, at present reliable and affordable solutions in patients with failed BMG urethroplasty are few. A plea for alternative solutions again pushed reconstructive urologists to look back and reinvent the

Kulkarni Endo Surgery Institute and Reconstructive Urology Centre, 3, Rajpath Society, Paud Road, Pune, Maharashtra 411038, India
* Corresponding author: Kulkarni Endo Surgery Institute and Reconstructive Urology Centre, 3, Rajpath Society, Paud Road, Pune, Maharashtra 411038, India.
E-mail address: drpankajmjoshi@gmail.com

Urol Clin N Am 49 (2022) 361–369
https://doi.org/10.1016/j.ucl.2022.04.001

use of flap on urethral reconstruction. In the very last years, there has been a rapid increase of the use of flaps in daily practice. Differently from the past, surgery has also evolved introducing new instruments and advanced technologies, which improved outcomes and reduced complications. This has certainly contributed to lowering the morbidity associated with flap harvesting also increasing the patency rates. Nowadays, flaps are part of the armamentarium of many reconstructive urologists in referral centers. This article describes all common flaps that are commonly harvest for urethral reconstruction and also presents a practical algorithm for their use. Technical aspects, tips and tricks, and approach to manage the complications of flap harvesting are discussed.

There are many types of flaps and multiple ways in which they have been classified. Principally, flaps have their own blood supply, and this is an advantage in reconstructive urology where we need vascularized tissues.

Local Flaps or Pedicled Flaps

These flaps are rotated or moved in a manner from an adjacent area to the area of interest. So they remain attached to the body at its base.

Local flaps are further divided into.

- Advancement flaps: move directly forward with no lateral movement
- Rotation flaps: rotate around a pivot point
- Transposition flaps: move laterally
- Interpolation flaps: there is a skin bridge below which such flaps are tunneled to an adjacent area

Free flaps

These are flaps that are detached from their donor site and then surgically reconnected to vessels around the area of interest.

Most flaps used for urethral reconstruction are local flaps.

This article discusses technical aspects of harvesting local flaps.

To date, the use of flaps is common in 2 different scenarios.

Anterior urethra

1. Patients with long obliterative strictures, urethral plate is missing, and its substitution is only possible with vascularized flaps.
2. Revision of perineal urethrostomy
3. Hypospadias (beyond the scope of this article)

Posterior urethra

Bulbar urethral necrosis The most commonly harvested flaps in everyday practice are:

- Orandi and modified Orandi flap
- Pedicled preputial flap
- Distal penile skin flap
- Graft plus flap
- Q-flap
- Lotus flap
- Enterourethroplasty

Orandi Flap

Indications

Obliterative penile stricture, without lichen sclerosus Orandi[4] introduced this flap in 1968 reporting the outcomes of 21 patients treated with this technique for penile urethral stricture. The use of the Orandi flap is more suitable for penile urethral stricture given the lower thickness of the subcutaneous tissue and the vicinity between the urethra and the skin. The Orandi flap allows a reconstruction of the penile urethra in 1 stage. This flap rapidly became a valid alternative to the 2-stage BMG reconstruction of Bracka or Asopa single-stage BMG reconstruction. Head-to-head comparison between Orandi flap and BMG augmentation is still lacking. Thus, the decision to rely on one technique or another remains a surgeon's preference.

Technical aspect

A midline longitudinal incision is performed on the ventral penile surface and a skin penile island is demarked aside (usually left side from the midline). The penile urethra is opened at the level of stricture on the ventral surface. The vascularized pedicle of dartos is mobilized to allow a transition of the fasciocutaneous flap. The medial margin of the island skin is sutured to the margin of the penile urethra on the left side. The skin island is rotated over the opened urethra and sutured to the opposite urethral margin. The incision is closed in layers and a catheter is kept. Owing to the lack of support, the penile island skin flap usually evolves into a diverticulum; this frequently causes post-micturition dribbling (**Fig. 1** A, B).

Modified Orandi Flap

This flap was introduced by Barbagli and colleagues[5] and the authors' group in 2019 to improve functional outcomes and reduce diverticulum formation, which was common with the standard technique. The midline longitudinal incision and the penile island skin flap are marked on the ventral penile surface on the right side as described in the original technique. Differently from the Orandi technique, the penile urethra is mobilized circumferentially from the corpora cavernosa and 1 is opened along its dorsal surface. The skin island is transposed and sutured to the

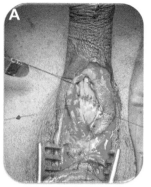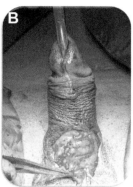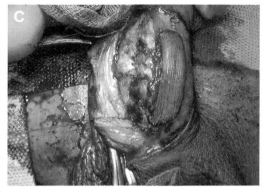

Fig. 1. (*A,B*) Orandi flap. (*C*) Modified Orandi flap.

right urethral margin over the corpora cavernosa. Second running suture between the left margin of the flap and the left urethral margin is completed over a 14 French All Silicone Foleys catheter. Given the dorsal position of the flap, which is in this technique supported by the corpora cavernosa, the risk of diverticula formation is negligible (**Fig. 1**C).

Challenges
If the harvested flap is too wide, skin closure becomes difficult and risk of fistulae increases.

Disadvantage
This is a horizontal dartos-based flap, so it cannot be swung down in the perineum and its use is limited to the reconstruction of the penile urethra.

Pedicled Preputial Flap

This flap was first described by Asopa and colleagues[6] for the surgical treatment of penile urethra in patients with hypospadias. The authors[7–11] have extended its use also for the reconstruction of the bulbar urethra in specific scenarios.

Indications
Bulbar urethral necrosis Long obliterative anterior urethral strictures as graft plus flap augmentation.[7,12]

Technical aspect
Prepuce is a unique component of the phallus. Prepuce is constituted by 2 layers of skin, both being supplied by dartos fascia that is crossed by vessels that carry its vascular supply. From this very versatile source of tissue it is possible to harvest a vascularized flap and/or a free skin graft. When the aim is to convert the prepuce into a flap, the outer or the inner skin is detached to avoid its entrapment in the tissue and consequent formation of dermoid cysts. This "discarded" graft

can be used if additional free skin is required for reconstruction.

The harvesting process starts with 2 parallel circumcision incisions on the outer and inner surfaces of the prepuce. The outer circumcision incision is deepened to the skin and superficial to the dartos fascia. This dissection is carried forward until the base of penis. The inner circumcision incision is carried deeper to the dartos but superficial to the Buck fascia. The entire prepuce is then mobilized based on its dartos pedicle. This pedicle ring of prepuce is then converted into a flap by a ventral incision. Indeed, the vascular supply of the prepuce usually comes from the dorsal side, thus the ring can be opened only along the ventral surface.

Given the great elasticity of the dartos, the harvested flap can be transposed to the perineum through an opening at the basis of the penis. To this point the flap can be used in its current form or it can be tubularized. In both these scenarios, 1 of the 2 surfaces of the prepuce has to be sacrificed. Considering the robust blood supply to the outer prepuce, the inner surface is usually detached (**Fig. 2**).

Usual length of tube
10 to 12 cm depending on the girth of penis

Use of the excised inner (or outer) part of the prepuce
Usually the detached skin is discarded. Nonetheless, there are situations in which the urethral gap is considerably long (greater than 12 cm), and it is impossible to bridge the 2 urethral ends with the tube alone. In these rare events, the discarded skin graft can be used; it can be placed as onlay graft or as a tube. In the second scenario, the free graft is wrapped around the catheter and the dartos of the pedicle tube is flapped in support of the graft. The authors have performed this

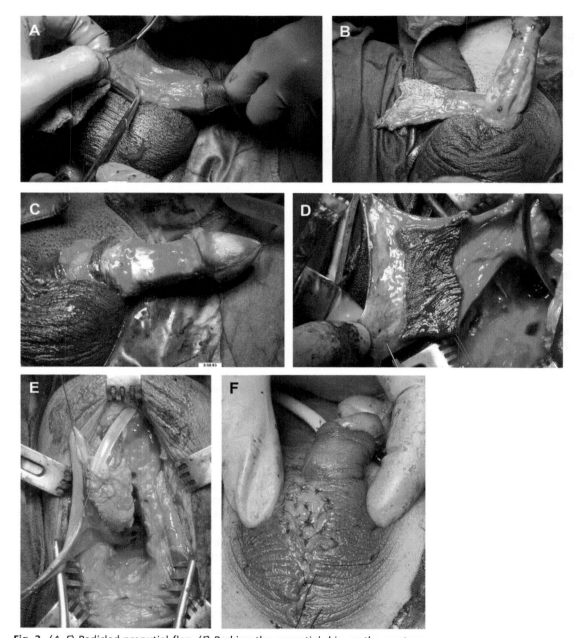

Fig. 2. (*A–E*) Pedicled preputial flap. (*F*) Parking the preputial skin on the scrotum.

modified approach in a few patients (7 for the records), where the alternative option was to leave the meatus at the penoscrotal junction. To date, all patients present a good flow and no failure has been recorded. Probably, the vascular support offered by the pedicle dartos flap helps the free graft avoiding shrinkage and necrosis.

When the inner preputial skin is not required, it can be still kept for future use instead of being discarded. To save this precious source of hairless skin, the free graft can be parked in the genitals

for future uses. The preferred parking area is the scrotum given its abundant source of dartos and its position half way between the scrotum and the penis. An incision is carried on the scrotum midline of the same length of the graft. The incision is widened laterally, and space is created for the graft. The underlying dartos represents the ideal bed for the graft. The latter is secured with quilting sutures. Postoperative dressing is important for preserving this graft. If the transplant is successful, the inner preputial skin can be used in the future as free graft of pedicle flap to reconstruct bulbar or penile urethra given its hairless nature and the new strategic position.

Complications

1. The extensive mobilization of the skin may undermine the vascularity eventually causing necrosis. Usually, this event may occur to the distal part of the skin and it is self-limiting healing on its own.
2. The preputial skin tube may form a diverticulum leading to urinary symptoms such as postmicturition dribbling and sensation of a sac in the perineum during voiding. Sometimes, the diverticulum requires revision to reduce the size.
3. Asthenic ejaculation due to the lack of the bulbospongiosus muscle.

Disadvantage

Given the need to take the dartos along with the preputial skin, the thickness of the penis and the elasticity of the remaining skin can be affected. Patients may complain of sexual discomfort such as reduced penile girth and skin friction during intercourse. These patients have preexisting ED due to pelvic fracture urethral injury. Usually, the situation stabilizes after some months. The implant of a penile prosthesis can be discussed and taken into consideration after complete healing. Given the presence of flap and reconstructed urethra, the implant is challenging and should be carried out only be expert surgeons.

Distal Penile Skin Flap: (McAninch)

In case of previous circumcision the distal penile skin can be used instead of the prepuce.[13] The approach is essentially the same as the one described previously.

The flap is demarked on the distal penile shaft below the sulcus. Care should be taken when harvesting this flap given the fact that the remaining penile skin might not be sufficient to close the circumcision incision ending in disastrous situations (**Fig. 3**).

Q-Flap

Indications: almost panurethral obliterative strictures

Pedicled preputial flap and distal penile skin flaps all have in common that the length of the flap corresponds to the girth of penis. Based on anthropomorphology, this measure varies between 8 and 12 cm according to the ethnicity. Nonetheless, the total length of anterior urethra is around 18 to 20 cm. Thus, in those patients presenting with panurethral stricture where the entire anterior urethra is affected by the disease (eg, lichen sclerosus) and requires substitution, "traditional" flaps are not sufficient. In these particular cases, the "Q" flap by Morey and colleagues[14,15] represents a valid alternative. Indeed, the length of this flap reaches up to 20 cm, according to penile length. The Q-flap presents 2 segments: the first segment comes from the skin that surrounds the distal penile shaft or the prepuce itself and measures around 8 to 12 cm; the second segment continues from the precedent on the ventral penile shaft according to the length needed (up to 8 cm). Together these segments create a "Q"-shaped structure, which gives the flap its name. A video of a Q-flap harvested at the authors' center is provided with the text (Video 1).

Drawbacks

- Owing to a large amount of skin harvested, the closure can become challenging. and it requires particular care.
- Postmicturition dribbling
- Diverticulum formation.

Because the incidence of diseases such as lichen sclerosus is increasing, the use of fasciocutaneous skin flap alone cannot stem the increasing request of alternative reconstruction techniques for the strictured urethra. The Aim of a reconstructive centre is to find innovative solution as soon the precedent has become common practice. Thus the authors have enlarged their armamentarium with a new technique that merges the advantages of having a vascular support, which is typical of flaps, and the versatility of BMG: the oral mucosa flap (OMF).

Oral Mucosa Flap

This flap was described by our group a few years ago,[9,10,16,17] and its use was conceived for 2-stage procedures. During the first stage, the urethra is opened at the level of the stricture and marsupialized to the skin. Meanwhile, a BMG is harvested from the check with length matching the stricture length. The BMG is allocated in the scrotum after creating a vascularized bed of dartos at the level of the medium raphe. The BMG is quilted, and compressing moisture dressing is kept for some days to facilitate the taking of the transplant. After 6 months, the OMF is ready to be harvested. The incision is carried on the perimeter of the graft and deepened down to the level of the scrotal raphe, which is used as pedicle of the flap. The raphe is indeed rich of vessels and represents a valid source of blood for this random flap. The edges of the OMF are trimmed to check for

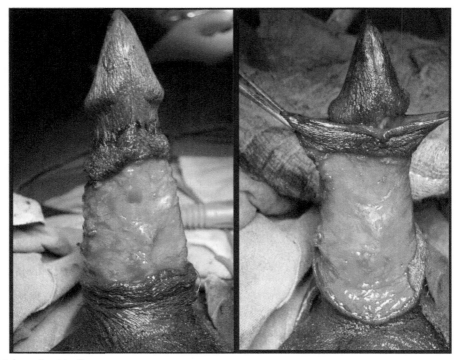

Fig. 3. Distal penile skin flap.

vascularity. The flap can be transposed to perineum and placed as dorsal onlay or ventral onlay or it can be tubularized to serve as tube in complete substitution (**Fig. 4**).

Drawbacks

This flap is a random one. The edges of flap may be ischemic so they need to be trimmed before anastomosis.

Enterourethroplasty

Since 1995, the authors have performed 5 enterourethroplasties at their tertiary referral center.

The technique for enterourethroplasty was reported in the literature only in 2010 by Mundy and Andrich.[18,19] Patient selection for these procedures is of paramount importance. The key is to evaluate which patients could benefit from urethral substitution using a bowel segment, because this is a no turning back surgery. Second, it is very important to find the best suited bowel segment for the reconstruction. Usually the segment of bowel with the highest mobility and the highest proximity to the prostate is the chosen one. Based on these characteristics, the choice usually falls on the sigmoid tract. Urethroplasty usually starts with

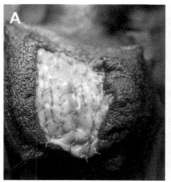
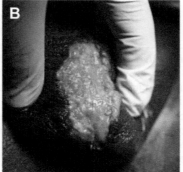
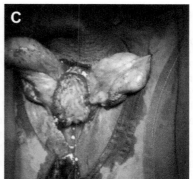

Fig. 4. (*A–C*) Oral mucosa flap.

a perineal incision. The healthy distal end of anterior urethra is identified. Crural separation and inferior pubectomy are performed based on the need to reduce the gap between the distal end and the bowel flap. Frequently, the authors approach the posterior urethra with an additional access. From a suprapubic incision the extraperitoneal space of Retzius can be reached, which allows to excise additional wedges of the pubic bones and to remove more scar tissue. The posterior urethra is incised on a bougie passed from the SPC tract through the bladder and the bladder neck. Once the posterior urethra is circumferentially mobilized, the gap between the 2 urethral ends is approached. The sigmoid colon is then disconnected from the intestine and mobilized on its mesentery. The more distal portion of the sigmoid is usually sacrificed due to its poor blood supply, whereas the upper part is swung down on its pedicle. The sigmoid is tailored on a 26F to 30F Nelaton catheter. Then, the enteric segment is transposed to the perineum and the 2 anastomoses between proximal sigmoid-end and bulbomembranous junction, as well as between the distal sigmoid-end and the anterior urethra, are performed. Finally, the omentum is mobilized and wrapped around the proximal anastomosis to offer a vascular support and to prevent from leak and fistulae. Catheter is removed after 6 weeks if pericatheter urethrogram does not show leakage (**Fig. 5**).

Drawbacks

1. Bowel anastomosis can leak and lead to peritonitis.
2. Postmicturition dribbling.
3. Bowel has convolutions making future follow-up challenging.

Use of Buccal Mucosa Graft Dorsally and Flap Ventrally

There are 3 situations when this option can be used.[20]

1. Failed hypospadias with scarred urethral plate
2. Bulbar necrosis where previous surgery did not have pubectomy (so the crura are intact in the midline allowing a BMG to be allocated)
3. Long semi or completely obliterative segments.

In few words, the BMG graft is placed as dorsal onlay over the corpora to reconstruct the dorsal plate of the neourethra. The flap instead is place ventrally to reconstruct the ventral plate of the neourethra. If present, the remaining corpus spongiosum is wrapped around the flap to offer support preventing from diverticula formation.

Lotus Petal Flap

The lotus petal flap, based on the rich network of perforating vessels of the internal and external pudendal artery, was originally described by Yii and Niranjan in 1996, and it was historically used to reconstruct vulvar defects after oncological procedure in female patients. Recently Chauhan and colleagues[21] described the use of this flap for urethral reconstruction. The shape of petal is marked on the perineum on one side. The position of perforating vessels can be confirmed using an intraoperative colour Doppler.

The skin of the flap is incised until the underlying fascia of the muscle is mobilized by elevating the flap, with a lateral to medial direction. During mobilization, the lateral perforator vessels must be sacrificed. The medial large perforator vessels can be encountered and should be spared as much as possible. Closing the donor site will give

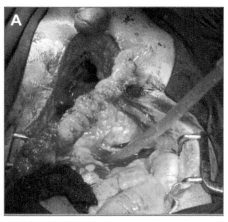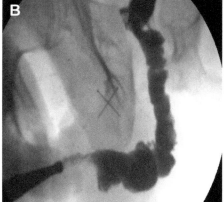

Fig. 5. (*A, B*) Enterourethroplasty.

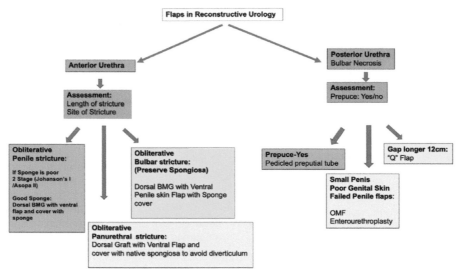

Fig. 6. Our Algorithm for using Flaps.

some extra length to the flap because the pivot point is advanced cranially. A drain is usually placed on the donor site. The flap is then rotated to the middle to match the perineal urethrostomy. The lotus petal flap is then used as dorsal onlay or it can be tubularized.

Drawbacks

This is a local flap and does not have a long pedicle, thus it cannot be used for the distal anterior urethra.

Other Flaps

There are various techniques such as Singapore flap, Hong Kong flap, "7" flap, gracillis with buccal grafts, and prelaminated flaps.[19,22] Nonetheless, the authors have rarely relied on these flaps in their practice and the description of these techniques goes beyond the scope of this article (**Fig. 6**).

SUMMARY

The use of flaps is gaining momentum in surgical practice, especially when at the time of redo surgery or complex strictures. Several flaps have been described, and for each one of them exists specific indications on how, when, and where to use it. Orandi flap is recommended for penile stricture; preputial, distal penile, OMF and Q-flaps are used for long strictures involving the penile and/or the bulbar urethra. Tubes are useful when an entire segment of urethra is lost and needs to be replaced (eg, bulbar urethral necrosis). Enterourethroplasty should be reserved as the last option available given the significant challenge in

harvesting this flap and the challenge on postoperative management of the patient, including follow-up.

Commonly used flaps for urethral reconstruction have been discussed.

Various other flaps such as gracilis, rectus flaps used for pelvic reconstruction, and flaps for penile and scrotal reconstruction are discussed in other article.

The authors hope that the readers have had the "joy of learning" technical aspects of performing flaps.

CLINICS CARE POINTS

- Clinical examination of patient should include the examination of prepuce and quality of distal penile skin.

- Patient should be counselled for need of flaps in the out patient clinic.

- Flaps may form diverticulum and patients may have post micturition dribbling. 4Flaps have good long term results.

DISCLOSURE

The authors have nothing to disclose.

SUPPLEMENTARY DATA

Supplementary data related to this article can be found online at:https://doi.org/10.1016/j.ucl.2022.04.001.

REFERENCES

1. Barbagli G, Balò S, Montorsi F, et al. History and evolution of the use of oral mucosa for urethral reconstruction. Asian J Urol 2017;4(2):96–101.
2. Bandini M, Barbagli G, Leni R, et al. Assessing in-hospital morbidity after urethroplasty using the European Association of Urology Quality Criteria for standardized reporting. World J Urol 2021 Oct; 39(10):3921–30.
3. Morey AF, McAninch JW. When and how to use buccal mucosal grafts in adult bulbar urethroplasty. Urology 1996;48(2):194–8.
4. Orandi A. One-stage urethroplasty: 4-year followup. J Urol 1972;107(6):977–80.
5. Barbagli G, Joshi PM, Kulkarni SB, et al. Penile urethroplasty using Orandi's dorsal skin flap: a new technique. BJU Int 2019;124(5):892–6.
6. Asopa HS, Elhence IP, Atri SP, et al. One stage correction of penile hypospadias using a foreskin tube. a preliminary report. Int Surg 1971;55(6): 435–40.
7. Joshi PM, Desai D, Kulkarni SB. Bulbar urethral necrosis. In: Martins FE, Kulkarni SB, Köhler TS, editors. Textbook of male genitourethral reconstruction [Internet]. Cham: Springer International Publishing; 2020. https://doi.org/10.1007/978-3-030-21447-0_28 [cited 2022 Jan 21]. p. 345–51. Available at.
8. Joshi PM, Kulkarni SB. Management of urethral injuries associated with complex pelvic fracture. In: Martins FE, Kulkarni SB, Köhler TS, editors. Textbook of male genitourethral reconstruction [Internet]. Cham: Springer International Publishing; 2020. https://doi.org/10.1007/978-3-030-21447-0_22 [cited 2022 Jan 21]. p. 267–78. Available at.
9. Kulkarni SB, Joshi PM, Hunter C, et al. Complex posterior urethral injury. Arab J Urol 2015;13(1): 43–52.
10. Joshi PM, Kulkarni SB. Management of pelvic fracture urethral injuries in the developing world. World J Urol 2020;38(12):3027–34.
11. Sreeranga YL, Joshi PM, Bandini M, et al. Comprehensive analysis of pediatric pelvic fracture urethral injury-reconstructive center experience. BJU Int 2022. https://doi.org/10.1111/bju.15686.
12. Kulkarni S, Joshi P, Surana S, et al. Pedicled preputial tube urethroplasty for bulbar urethral necrosis after failed anastomotic urethroplasty for pelvic fracture urethral distraction defects 2018.
13. McAninch JW. Reconstruction of extensive urethral strictures: circular fasciocutaneous penile flap. J Urol 1993;149(3):488–91.
14. Morey AF, Tran LK, Zinman LM. Q-flap reconstruction of panurethral strictures. BJU Int 2000;86(9): 1039–42.
15. Raffoul L, Rod J, Ravasse P, et al. Q-island flap urethroplasty: 1-stage procedure for reconstruction of Y-type urethral duplications in children. J Urol 2015;193(6):2068–72.
16. Kulkarni SB, Joglekar O, Alkandari MH, et al. Redo hypospadias surgery: current and novel techniques. Res Rep Urol 2018;10:117–26.
17. Kulkarni SB, Orabi H, Kavanagh A, et al. RE Re Do urethroplasty after multiple failed surgeries of pelvic fracture urethral injury. World J Urol 2020;38(12): 3019–25.
18. Mundy AR, Andrich DE. Entero-urethroplasty for the salvage of bulbo-membranous stricture disease or trauma. BJU Int 2010;105(12):1716–20.
19. Martins FE, Kulkarni SB, Köhler TS. Textbook of male genitourethral reconstruction. Springer Nature; 2019. p. 967.
20. Joshi PM, Bandini M, Bafna S, et al. Graft plus fasciocutaneous penile flap for nearly or completely obliterated long bulbar and penobulbar strictures. Eur Urol Open Sci 2022;35:21–8.
21. Reilly DJ, Sham EK, Chee JB, et al. A novel application of the lotus petal flap in high-risk perineal urethrostomy: principles and outcomes. Australas J Plast Surg 2018;1(1):135–9.
22. Jordan GH. Scrotal and perineal flaps for anterior urethral reconstruction. Urol Clin North Am 2002; 29(2):411–6.

Recent Trends and Advances in Anterior Urethroplasty

Elizabeth Naud, MD, FRCSC, Keith Rourke, MD, FRCSC*

KEYWORDS

- Anterior urethral strictures • Urethral reconstruction • Urethroplasty • Urethral strictures

KEY POINTS

- While patient preference often helps guide treatment decisions, poor long-term success combined with the cumulative risk of repeat endoscopic treatments and the complications innately associated with urethral stricture emphasize that urethroplasty is most often the best choice for successful treatment in the long-term.
- Urethroplasty has now largely transitioned to a day-surgery procedure in the majority of centers.
- Although sexual dysfunction after urethroplasty is uncommon, some evidence suggests that avoiding urethral transection and/or avoiding overzealous urethral mobilization may lead to a reduction in post-operative sexual dysfunction.
- The trend toward single stage penile urethroplasty with buccal mucosal grafts likely minimizes patient morbidity without compromising urethroplasty success.
- For urethroplasty success to further improve particularly in patients at high risk for stricture recurrence, the synergistic potential of combining wound healing enhancing agents with evolving tissue-engineering represents an exciting future opportunity in the quest to perfect urethroplasty outcomes.

 Video content accompanies this article at http://www.urologic.theclinics.com.

INTRODUCTION

Urethral stricture is likely the oldest urologic disease with documentation of its existence more than 4000 years ago.[1] At its simplest, "urethral stricture" refers to any abnormal narrowing of the urethral lumen within the corpus spongiosum. Thus, the term "stricture" is reserved specifically for fibrosis and coexistent narrowing within the anterior urethra from the urethral meatus to the proximal bulbar urethra.[2] Although the prevalence has likely changed over the course of human history, urethral stricture remains a burdensome and increasingly common urologic condition, which causes a broad spectrum of associated signs, symptoms, and complications.[3] Urethral stricture can occur as a result of 1 of 2 general mechanisms. Injury to the outside of the spongiosum, leading to spongiofibrosis, as a result of blunt or penetrating trauma. Alternatively, instrumentation or inflammatory disease can cause internal disruption of the urethral epithelium also leading to spongiofibrosis. The most common cause for urethral stricture in developed countries is idiopathic (41%) followed by iatrogenic (35%).[4–6] Inflammation counts for ~15% of urethral strictures usually related to lichen sclerosus (LS).[2] The bulbar urethra is the most common stricture location but some specific causes such as LS and posthypospadias repair will more frequently involve the penile urethra.[4]

Division of Urology, Department of Surgery, University of Alberta, Kipnes Urology Centre, 7th Floor, Kaye Edmonton Clinic, 11400 University Avenue, Edmonton, Alberta T6G1Z1, Canada
* Corresponding author.
E-mail address: krourke@ualberta.ca

Urol Clin N Am 49 (2022) 371–382
https://doi.org/10.1016/j.ucl.2022.04.002
0094-0143/22/© 2022 Elsevier Inc. All rights reserved.

Through the eyes of the patient, the decision on if and how to treat a urethral stricture depends on several factors, including presenting symptoms, complications related to urethral stricture, prior interventions, and the impact of the urethral stricture on health-related quality of life.[7] Most commonly, patients undergo either endoscopic treatment [urethral dilation or direct visual internal urethrotomy (DVIU)] or urethroplasty. Despite poor long-term success rates especially in the setting of recurrent stricture, patients still commonly undergo multiple endoscopic treatments.[8] Given the low rates of cure with repeat endoscopic treatment, multiple urologic association guideline statements recommend urethroplasty after failure of endoscopic treatment or in patients at high risk for stricture recurrence.[9–11] These recommendations have placed further emphasis on the need to better refine urethroplasty techniques and optimize outcomes. The main goal of this article is to highlight recent trends and future directions in anterior urethroplasty focusing on minimizing morbidity and maximizing success throughout the patient journey.

THE UNDERESTIMATED MORBIDITY OF URETHRAL STRICTURE AND THE EXPANDING ROLE OF URETHROPLASTY

When the urethral lumen progressively narrows and lower urinary tract obstruction occurs, symptoms develop both directly and indirectly. Most commonly symptoms include lower urinary tract symptoms (LUTS) both voiding and storage related.[12] However, signs and symptoms such as genitourinary pain, urinary tract infection, ejaculatory dysfunction, urethral discharge, and hematuria may also occur.[3] The spectrum of signs and symptoms is outlined in **Table 1**. The prevailing mindset has been that urethral stricture adversely affects the voiding function and quality of life but infrequently affects overall health status.[13,14] When complications occur, at least in developed nations and in the modern era, they are often thought to be infrequent and minor.[15–17] Severe complications are thought to be more common in nonindustrialized nations. For example, in a population of patients with urethral stricture in South Africa, the incidence of perineal sepsis and renal failure occurs is approximately 39% and 9%, respectively.[18,19] However, in the setting of longstanding lower urinary tract obstruction with elevated urinary tract pressures and risk of chronic infection, patients with urethral stricture have potential for adverse complications impacting overall health status. More recently, it has become clear that a substantial proportion (~40%) of patients

with anterior urethral stricture even in an "industrialized" country will present with complications directly related to urethral stricture requiring emergent urologic care including acute urinary retention (32.6%), difficult catheterization (16.0%), renal failure (3.1%), and urosepsis/urethral abscess (5.0%).[3,20] Moreover, 7.0% of patients will experience complications deemed life-threatening. Patients at highest risk for complications on multivariate analysis seem to be those with longer strictures, lack of reported LUTS, and traumatic strictures. Recent evidence suggests that urethral stricture is a relatively morbid condition independent of geography with the potential to adversely not only impact patient quality of life but also global health status.

Although patient preference often helps guide treatment decisions, poor long-term success, cumulative risk of repeat endoscopic treatments and the complications innately associated with urethral stricture further emphasize that urethroplasty is most often the best choice for treatment in the long-term.[11,21]

REDUCING PATIENT MORBIDITY AND OVERALL BURDEN OF URETHROPLASTY

Once the decision is made to pursue anterior urethroplasty, the next step is to consider the different techniques to reduce patient morbidity and the costs associated with urethroplasty. Urethroplasty involves either anastomotic or substitution techniques in either a single-stage or multistage approach. Anastomotic urethroplasty either with or without transection of the urethra is most appropriate for bulbar urethral strictures of relatively short stricture length (<2 cm). Classically, the transecting anastomotic urethroplasty also known as excision and primary anastomosis (EPA), typically has a high success rate (>90%), relatively minimal morbidity and potentially lower recurrence rate when compared with other urethroplasty techniques (Video 1).[22] The other common approach to urethroplasty involves the augmentation of the urethral lumen. This can be carried out using a variety of potential grafts (most commonly oral mucosa) as either a ventral or dorsal onlay (**Fig. 1**) or genital (penile) fasciocutaneous flaps.[22,23] There are a variety of technical considerations that go into selected an operative approach in these cases; in general, both grafts and flaps have equivalent success rates but flaps are associated with higher morbidity.[23]

Potential Complications of Urethroplasty

When performing any procedure, minimizing complications should always be an important

Table 1
Presenting, associated and presence of signs and symptoms for patients presenting with anterior urethral stricture

Patient Reported Sign or Symptom	Presenting Symptoms	N (%) Associated Symptoms	Presence of Symptoms
Lower Urinary Tract Symptoms	332 (54.3%)	234 (38.6%)	566 (92.9%)
Acute Urinary Retention	143 (23.4%)	39 (6.4%)	182 (29.8%)
Urinary Tract Infection	37 (6.1%)	87 (14.2%)	124 (20.3%)
Difficult Urinary Catheterization	29 (4.8%)	54 (8.8%)	83 (13.6%)
Gross Hematuria	19 (3.1%)	50 (8.2%)	69 (11.3%)
Genitourinary Pain	18 (2.9%)	122 (20.0%)	140 (22.9%)
Urethral Abscess	14 (2.3%)	6 (1.0%)	20 (3.3%)
Renal Failure/ Hydronephrosis	8 (1.3%)	17 (2.8%)	25 (4.1%)
Urinary Incontinence	6 (1.0%)	13 (2.1%)	19 (3.1%)
Sexual Dysfunction	5 (0.8%)	69 (11.3%)	74 (12.1%)

consideration. Even though anterior urethroplasty is generally well tolerated, serious postoperative complications (hematoma, wound abscess, urosepsis, fistula, urinary incontinence) can sometimes occur adversely impacting patient outcomes and dramatically reduce cost-effectiveness.[24,25] Other more minor complications that can arise after urethroplasty are wound-related, UTI, diverticulum, edema, scrotal paresthesia, postvoid dribbling, and urinary stream spraying as well as sexual dysfunction including erectile dysfunction (ED), ejaculatory dysfunction, chordee, and reduced penile length.[11,26,27] Sexual dysfunction after urethral surgery has recently become a subject of some interest among reconstructive urologists. Sexual dysfunction after urethroplasty can include multiple disorders in relation to sexual health such as ED, ejaculatory dysfunction, penile curvature, penile shortening, or change in genital sensitivity. Postoperative sexual dysfunction rates can vary greatly in the literature depending on the evaluation tool used.[28] One of the first reports on ED after urethroplasty was by Mundy and colleagues in 1993. He reported 5% of ED after anastomotic urethroplasty and 0.9% after graft augmented urethroplasty.[29] Multiple studies

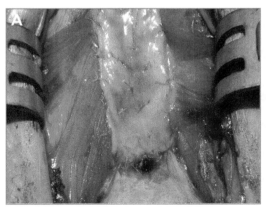
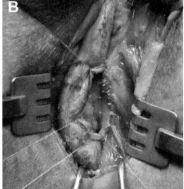

Fig. 1. Urethroplasty using buccal mucosal graft as a dorsal onlay. Once the bulbar urethra is mobilized and hemostasis is achieved, dorsal urethrotomy into normal (>28Fr) urethra is performed. (*A*) Subsequently the buccal mucosal graft is spread-fixed and quilted to underlying corporal bodies and a proximal anastomosis is performed. (*B*) The urethral mucosa and edge of corpus spongiosum is then sewn unilaterally to the buccal mucosal graft. Once the distal anastomosis is complete, the remaining contralateral side is sewn to complete the reconstruction.

have subsequently examined the rate of ED after anterior urethroplasty with a recent meta-analysis concluding there is a 1% to 2% incidence of persisting de novo ED after urethroplasty with a reported range between 0% and 40%.[30] Different etiologies could explain the development of de novo ED after anterior urethroplasty. First, neurologic trauma is possible during surgery. Dissection of the urethra during urethroplasty could potentially lead to cavernosal nerve branch injury, either by direct blunt trauma or with electrocautery. Second, possible vascular injury to the bulbar, bulbospongiosum and perforating arteries during the dissection may result in impaired arterial flow during erection. Finally, it has been hypothesized that there can also be a psychological component to post-operative ED.[31] On balance, sexual dysfunction may arise after urethroplasty, is likely multifactorial in origin and not all cases may be captured with standard measures of erectile function.

Reducing the Risk of Sexual Dysfunction after Anterior Urethroplasty

After examining discrepancies in the literature, it becomes interesting to ask if there is a surgical technique that would prevent or at least reduce the incidence of de novo sexual dysfunction after urethroplasty. Because postoperative sexual dysfunction is strongly associated with patient dissatisfaction, every attempt should be made to reduce its incidence.[32–35]

In the setting of short (<2 cm) bulbar urethral strictures, EPA has historically been the primary urethroplasty for most reconstructive urologists (Video 1) but there has been more recent concern that circumferential transection of the urethra and corpus spongiosum could contribute to ED.[34] This potential concern has prompted some urologists to abandon anastomotic urethroplasty in favor of onlay with oral mucosa, whereas others have innovated and developed nontransecting anastomotic urethroplasty techniques (**Fig. 2**). Multiple studies have compared nontransecting to transecting techniques in heterogeneous urethroplasty cohorts with a suggested association between de novo ED and urethral transection while confirming the often transient nature of posturethroplasty ED.[31,36,37] Although there is no completed randomized study on the subject, a prospective multicentered study of anastomotic urethroplasty demonstrated a significantly lower rate of sexual dysfunction with nontransecting techniques (4.3% vs 14.3%) with no difference in success (97.9% vs 93.8%) or 90-day complications (8.1% vs 4.3%).[38]

With respect to other techniques, studies have compared EPA to substitution urethroplasties with respect to sexual dysfunction. Most of these studies found no difference in rates of sexual dysfunction between these techniques. However, other studies including a 2013 meta-analysis identified a lower rate of ED with graft urethroplasty compared with transecting EPA (16% vs 36%).[39,40] This brings forward the distinct possibility that either less dissection with preservation of perforating arteries between corpora cavernosum and corpus spongiosum or avoiding urethral transection may lead to a reduction in postoperative sexual dysfunction. Thus, whenever possible nontransecting urethroplasty technique should be used at least when considering the perspective of reducing postoperative complications.

Evolving Use of Single Stage Penile Urethroplasty

Penile urethral strictures involving the meatus and fossa navicularis are a reconstructive challenge. Outside of hypospadias, these strictures are most commonly either iatrogenic (from prior urethral instrumentation or catheterization) or caused by LS.[41] Endoscopic treatments such as dilation of urethrotomy with or without intermittent self-catheterization, typically offer only temporary relief, require lifelong instrumentation and may ultimately increase stricture complexity. Although, extended meatotomy offers acceptable urethral patency rates, it is associated with significant cosmetic and functional drawbacks. Reconstruction is often challenging because it requires establishment of a functional and unobstructed urethra while simultaneously creating a cosmetically appealing glans and preserving sexual function. From a reconstructive perspective, the primary dilemma is when a single-stage reconstruction should be used over a multistage repair. Traditionally, a multistage approach with buccal mucosal graft (BMG) has been used. However, this exposes patients to the morbidity of 2 procedures.[42] Recently, there has been an expansion of indications for single-stage repairs for more complex strictures in an attempt to minimize the discomfort and risks associated with multiple procedures. From a patient perspective, single-stage urethroplasty is often preferred over a staged approach in order to reduce the total number of surgeries while avoiding temporary disfigurement of the penis, potential sexual dysfunction and lesser adverse impact on the patient's quality of life.

This preference is exemplified by Andrich and colleagues who identified an approximate 50% revision rate for staged penile urethroplasty,

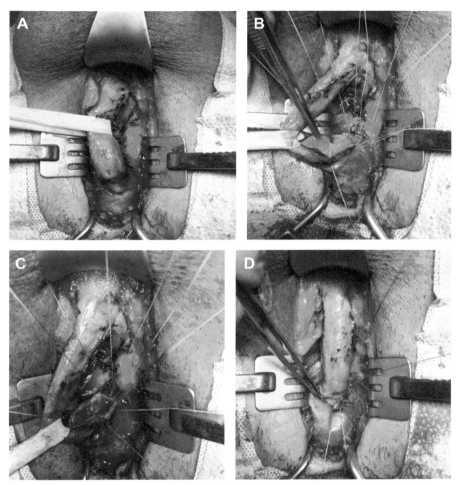

Fig. 2. The technique of nontransecting anastomotic bulbar urethroplasty. (*A*) With this technique, the bulbar urethra is mobilized proximally in the dorsal plane to the bulbomembranous junction. (*B*) Subsequently, the corpus spongiosum is opened in a dorsal manner through the area of stricture until normal caliber urethra is encountered both distal and proximally. Once anastomotic sutures are placed in the proximal spatulation, the area of stricture is localized. (*C*) The mucosal portion of the stricture is then excised while sparing the corpus spongiosum. The urethral mucosa is reapproximated ventrally as a floor strip. The proximal anastomotic sutures are placed at the corresponding opposing distal location. (*D*) Once a catheter is placed the dorsal anastomosis is tied down advancing the distal spatulation and the reconstruction is completed.

meaning that these patients would typically undergo not 2 but 3 surgeries to treat their sricture.[42] Recent evidence suggests that single-stage urethroplasty with BMG offers similar success compared with multistaged urethroplasty (83% vs 87%) with a trend toward more complications with a staged approach.[41] For panurethral strictures, Kulkarni and colleagues described their experience using an inverting perineal single-stage urethroplasty with multiple oral mucosal grafts with an impressive intervention free success rate of 85.9%.[43] Thus, in well-selected patients without complete urethral obliteration and an otherwise healthy glans, single-stage BMG

urethroplasty offers comparable outcomes to a staged approach.[44–46] Single-stage urethroplasty in this context is evolving quickly using various dorsal inlay (Video 2) and transurethral ventral inlay techniques with buccal mucosa.[47] However, patients with multiple prior penile urethral surgeries or complicated prior hypospadias repairs may have higher success rates with multistaged surgeries.[48]

Reduction in Donor Site Morbidity

In cases of substitution urethroplasty, harvest of BMG can be a source of morbidity for the patient with possible complications of bleeding, infection, pain, swelling, wound contraction, and most commonly increased salivation or perioral numbness.[49–53] Although most patients (98.2%) undergoing BMG harvest are satisfied with their surgery with relatively minimal complications, the use of synthetic tissue would be ideal to reduce the morbidity from graft donor site associated with substitution urethroplasty.[51] This would also be beneficial in cases where extensive length of graft is needed or in the setting of revision urethroplasty requiring repeat graft harvest.[54] The first in man study was performed by Bhargava and colleagues[55] This group developed an autologous tissue-engineered buccal mucosa from a buccal mucosa biopsy in 5 men with LS-related urethral strictures. At a mean follow-of 33.6 months, all patients required some form of intervention for either graft contraction of stricture recurrence. El-Kassaby and colleagues performed a randomized study comparing an acellular bladder matrix graft to BMG.[56] The authors concluded that the use of bladder matrix graft may be a viable option but in the instance of an unhealthy urethral bed (defined as 2 or more previous interventions) BMG is the preferred tissue source. More recently in pilot study, 6 patients underwent urethrotomy with subsequent injection of an engineered polymer made from autologous buccal epithelial cells. Of the 6 patients, stricture recurrence occurred in 2 patients within 24 months. The remaining patient did not require any further treatments at 3-year follow-up.[57] A meta-analysis on the subject of tissue-engineered grafts for urethral reconstruction failed to determine the efficacy primarily due to the lack of randomized studies.[58] Overall, BMG remains the first choice for most substitution urethroplasty but future advancements in tissue-engineered graft may soon change the way we treat urethral stricture.

Urethroplasty as a Day Surgery

It is generally well accepted that the treatment with urethroplasty is more cost-effective than repeat urethral dilations. Urethroplasty could be even more cost-effective if these procedures we performed as day-surgery.

In a recent survey of reconstructive urologists, the majority (70.4%) of surgeons have transitioned urethroplasty to either a day surgery or extended day surgery model.[59] This recent and evolving shift likely reflects a need for health-care cost containment, inpatient hospital bed pressures globally, and COVID-19 pandemic restrictions. Theisen and colleagues retrospectively reviewed results of same day discharged anterior urethroplasties.[60]

These patients did not have an increase in 30-day postoperative complications, emergency room visits, unplanned clinic visits, or phone calls. They also had a similar success rate compared with admitted patients.[60] Another study also concluded that with appropriate preoperative education and perioperative analgesia, same-day discharge was possible with comparable complication rates and high patient satisfaction.[60]

Although day surgery urethroplasty certainly seems feasible from a hospital readmission and patient satisfaction perspective, it remains to be seen if complications and outcomes are equivalent to routine inpatient admission.[60–63] The application of an ambulatory model seems most successful in those patients of younger age, shorter strictures, decreased operative times and with minimal medical comorbidities.[60]

STRATIFYING AND OPTIMIZING URETHROPLASTY SUCCESS

Although urethroplasty is likely the most effective treatment of urethral stricture, it is not a perfect procedure. The success rate of bulbar urethroplasties ranges between 80% and 95%, and stricture recurrence occurs even in the most experienced and capable hands.[64] Hampered by the lack of standardized definition of success, comparison between studies is challenging. Previous systematic review identified a lack of repeat intervention as the most common definition of success while stricture recurrence is diagnosed with a mean of 3 different diagnostic tests, most commonly uroflowmetry and retrograde urethrogram (RUG).[65] Despite no consensus regarding the definition of stricture recurrence, evidence suggests that a cystoscopically identified stricture of less than 16Fr caliber is the most sensitive test to detect recurrence.[66]

Factors Associated with Urethroplasty Failure

Further confounding the definition of stricture recurrence is the inconsistency regarding which factors are associated with urethroplasty failure. The factors most often cited in studies are stricture length, prior failed endoscopic treatment, prior urethroplasty, obesity, smoking, diabetes, and LS.[67–72] When performing multivariable analysis, Breyer and colleagues identified that smoking, previous DVIU, and previous urethroplasty were predictive of urethroplasty failure.[68] Although Barbagli and colleagues specifically examined single-stage anterior urethroplasty and found that only substitute tissue type (oral mucosa vs skin) was the only predictor of stricture recurrence.[70] These inconsistencies could be related to heterogeneity in patient populations, surgeon technique, stricture cause, and the type of prior treatment. When analyzing stricture recurrence in a homogenous population of 596 patients undergoing bulbar urethroplasty, Chapman and colleagues found that multiple comorbidities, obesity, longer strictures, and infectious causes were independently associated with stricture recurrence.[71] Although comorbidities are somewhat consistently found to be associated with stricture recurrence, patient age represents an area of disagreement. Levy and colleagues in a multivariable analysis of patients aged older than 60 years undergoing, concluded that comorbidities, but not age, influenced surgery results.[73] In a philosophic sense, it seems that most risk factors for stricture recurrence can be classified as either fibrotic (repeat endoscopic treatments, and so forth) or ischemic (vascular comorbidities, and so forth). This in turn relates to the finding that most stricture causes can also be classified in this manner. For example, traumatic strictures may be primarily a fibrotic process, whereas hypospadias or postprostatectomy strictures may have an ischemic component. When performing urethroplasty, it is therefore important to consider these risk factors in the context of stricture cause when choosing the surgical technique. For example, if a stricture is primarily of fibrotic risk factors and cause (ie, trauma), then the aggressive dissection with resection would seem the most prudent to ensure long-term success. Conversely, when the stricture has potentially significant ischemic components (ie, postprostatectomy), then the preservation of urethral vascularity with avoidance of urethral transection may be the best course of action. Nonetheless, regardless of the circumstance, patients at increased risk for stricture recurrence after surgery should be counseled about risk of failure and their follow-up should be planned accordingly.

Defining Urethroplasty Success

In most studies, urethroplasty success is based on a variable but nonetheless surgeon-derived definition focused primarily on the clinical absence of stricture recurrence. For most patients, postoperative success is more than simply the absence of anatomic stricture. Thus, it has been widely agreed that some form of patient reported outcome measure (PROM) function should be used periodically for follow-up because they are critical when considering the patients' perspective and serve as a baseline evaluation. Most commonly with patient reported outcomes,

the definition of success has been based on uroflowmetry rates, voiding symptom assessment, sexual function, quality of life, or other primarily nonvalidated symptom questionnaires.[66,74] Although further development of PROMs will be of utmost importance, if only patient reported outcomes are considered, then significant anatomic recurrences will likely be missed. In this context, asymptomatic patients with stricture recurrence may be at increased risk for stricture-related complications.[20] On balance, the clinical outcome of urethroplasty is probably more important than a true stricture free postoperative status. For example, a stricture recurrence of 15Fr caliber is unlikely to be overtly symptomatic or morbid for the patient but may serve to portend future stricture recurrence.[75,76] The best way to follow a patient after surgery is yet to be determined. The AUA guideline on urethral strictures states that the surgeons should monitor urethroplasty success after surgery but does not mention with certainty at what frequency or with what modality should be used.[9] According to the SIU/ICUD consultation on urethral strictures, a combination of validated patient-reported outcome measure with an objective measure, such as uroflowmetry or urethroscopy would potentially provide the most accurate results.[66] In a recent survey of perioperative practice patterns for anterior urethroplasty, a total of 142 urologist members of the genitourinary reconstructive surgeons registered their current practice.[59] Seventy-eight percent of these urologists used an objective method to evaluate for stricture recurrence. Uroflowmetry and postvoid-residual were the 2 most prevalent modalities used, closely followed by cystourethroscopy. These were generally performed at 2 to 3 months or 4 to 6 months, postoperatively. Overall, a definitive consensus has not yet reached on the best way to follow-up patients but a combination of patient-reported outcome and anatomic evaluation seems likely to give the best results. Our recommendation is to perform cystourethroscopy in conjunction with a PROM at least once within the first 6 months after intervention as a means to screen for and predict the risk of stricture recurrence. If cystourethroscopy is normal, further follow-up may be performed based on PROMs and other preoperative stricture characteristics. When a failure is detected, RUG should be performed for further staging and decision-making. This is consistent with both the SIU-ICUD, AUA and CUA Guidelines on Male Urethral Strictures.[9,11,66] Although a comprehensive definition of success after treatment is still to be determined, it should incorporate anatomic (urethral) success as well as functional success such as voiding function and other elements of patient satisfaction. **Fig. 3** outlines in flow chart form our preferred approach to patient follow-up after urethroplasty.

Future Considerations for Optimization of Urethroplasty Success

Although there has been emphasis placed on refining urethroplasty technique and the future potential for engineered tissue in urethral reconstruction, focusing on optimizing graft performance after tissue transfer has been somewhat neglected. Most often urethroplasty choice is not limited by a lack of donor tissue except in the infrequent case of treating stricture recurrence after panurethral reconstruction. Additionally, most risk factors for stricture recurrence relate to impaired graft function not availability such as stricture length, prior treatment, and patient comorbidities. Thus, with graft quality not quantity bottlenecking future improvements in urethroplasty success, it would seem beneficial to focus on methods to improve the performance of grafted tissue. Some attention has been paid to the use of amniotic or amnion-chorionic tissue in urethral reconstruction given the potential benefits of inflammation modulation, incorporation of essential growth factors, reduction in postoperative scarring, and overall enhancement of wound healing.[77,78] Potentially, the immunologic status and availability of amniotic tissue could affect its

broad surgical application. Focusing on improved graft take through the application of inflammation modulating and neo-vascularization agents such as exogenous vascular endothelial growth factor (VEGF), epigallocatechin gallate (EGCG), or autologous adipose-derived stem cells remains a largely uninvestigated area of urethral reconstruction.[79–81] In the case of VEGF, it has been shown to promote nutrient flow, angiogenesis, and vascular remodeling necessary for improved graft survival underwent adverse circumstances and can be readily applied in microcapsule form.[79] Similarly, EGCG, the major polyphenol found in green tea, has been found to enhance neovascularization and perfusion of grafts through the endothelial-derived nitric oxide-mediated vasodilator activity.[80] Similarly, the autologous ASC transplantation has demonstrated increased microvessel density with improvement in graft survival in an animal model.[81] Surgically, these agents could be applied to patients at risk for stricture recurrence or urethroplasty complications such as patients with increased comorbidities, panurethral stricture, LS, hypospadias, radiation complications, or those requiring revision surgery. For urethroplasty techniques and success to further improve particularly in these at-risk groups, the synergistic potential of combining wound healing enhancing agents with evolving surgical technologies represents an exciting future opportunity to pursue in the quest to optimize urethroplasty outcomes.

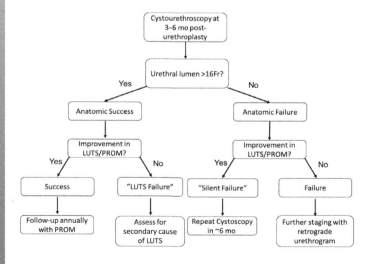

Fig. 3. Flow chart depicting a stratified approach to patient follow-up after urethroplasty. Our recommendation is to perform cystourethroscopy in conjunction with a patient reported outcome measure (PROM) at least once within the first 6 months after intervention. If cystourethroscopy is normal and the patient is functionally improved, further follow-up may be performed annually with a PROM such as IPSS or USS-PROM. When there is no anatomic evidence of stricture identified but the patient fails to report functional improvement (LUTS failure) further evaluation for a secondary cause of voiding dysfunction should be performed. When anatomic recurrence is detected with minimal patient symptoms, further cystoscopic assessment at approximately 6 to 12 months is prudent given the increased risk of stricture progression despite an initial lack of symptoms. Finally, when both anatomic and functional failure occurs, retrograde urethrogram should be performed in order to further stage stricture recurrence and facilitate informed decision-making.

CLINICS CARE POINTS

- Although patient preference often helps guide treatment decisions, poor long-term success, cumulative risk of repeat endoscopic treatments, and the complications innately associated with urethral stricture emphasize that urethroplasty is most often the best choice for successful treatment in the long-term.

- However, widespread urologic society recommendation has placed further emphasis on the need to better refine urethroplasty techniques and optimize patient outcomes.

- Urethroplasty has now largely transitioned to a day-surgery procedure in most centers.

- Although sexual dysfunction after urethroplasty is uncommon, some evidence suggests that avoiding urethral transection and/or avoiding overzealous urethral mobilization may lead to a reduction in postoperative sexual dysfunction.

- The trend toward single-stage penile urethroplasty with buccal mucosal grafts likely minimizes patient morbidity without compromising urethroplasty success.

- Follow-up after urethroplasty should include both a patient-reported outcome combined with an objective measure of success, such as uroflowmetry or urethroscopy.

- For urethroplasty success to further improve particularly in patients at high risk for stricture recurrence, the synergistic potential of combining wound healing enhancing agents with evolving tissue engineering represents an exciting future opportunity in the quest to perfect urethroplasty outcomes.

CONFLICT OF INTEREST

None.

ACKNOWLEDGMENTS

None.

SUPPLEMENTARY DATA

Supplementary data related to this article can be found online at https://doi.org/10.1016/j.ucl.2022.04.002.

REFERENCES

1. Das S. Shusruta of India, the pioneer in the treatment of urethral stricture. Surg Gynecol Obstet 1983; 157(6):581–2.

2. Latini JM, McAninch JW, Brandes SB, et al. SIU/ICUD consultation on urethral strictures: epidemiology, etiology, anatomy, and nomenclature of urethral stenoses, strictures, and pelvic fracture urethral disruption injuries. Urology 2014;83(3 Suppl):S1–7.

3. Rourke K, Hickle J. The clinical spectrum of the presenting signs and symptoms of anterior urethral stricture: detailed analysis of a single institutional cohort. Urology 2012;79(5):1163–7.

4. Stein DM, Thum DJ, Barbagli G, et al. A geographic analysis of male urethral stricture aetiology and location. BJU Int 2013;112(6):830–4.

5. Fenton AS, Morey AF, Aviles R, et al. Anterior urethral strictures: etiology and characteristics. Urology 2005;65(6):1055–8.

6. Lumen N, Hoebeke P, Willemsen P, et al. Etiology of urethral stricture disease in the 21st century. J Urol 2009;182(3):983–7.

7. Breyer BN, Edwards TC, Patrick DL, et al. Comprehensive qualitative assessment of urethral stricture disease: toward the development of a patient centered outcome measure. J Urol 2017;198(5):1113–8.

8. Moynihan MJ, Voelzke B, Myers J, et al. Endoscopic treatments prior to urethroplasty: trends in management of urethral stricture disease. BMC Urol 2020;20(1):68.

9. Wessells H, Angermeier KW, Elliott S, et al. Male Urethral Stricture: American Urological Association Guideline. J Urol 2017;197(1):182–90.

10. Lumen N, Campos-Juanatey F, Greenwell T, et al. European Association of Urology Guidelines on Urethral Stricture Disease (Part 1): Management of Male Urethral Stricture Disease. Eur Urol 2021;80(2):190–200.

11. Rourke KF, Welk B, Kodama R, et al. Canadian Urological Association guideline on male urethral stricture. Can Urol Assoc J 2020;14(10):305–16.

12. Nuss GR, Granieri MA, Zhao LC, et al. Presenting symptoms of anterior urethral stricture disease: a disease specific, patient reported questionnaire to measure outcomes. J Urol 2012;187(2):559–62.

13. Santucci RA, Joyce GF, Wise M. Male urethral stricture disease. J Urol 2003;7177:1667–74.

14. Romero Perez P, Mira Llinares A. Male urethral stenosis: review of complications. Arch Esp Urol 2004;57:485–511.

15. Lazzeri M, Salvatore S, Guazzoni G, et al. Incidence, causes, and complications of urethral stricture disease. Eur Urol Suppl 2016;15(1):2–6.

16. Santucci RA, Joyce GF, Wise M. Male urethral stricture disease in Litwin MS. US Department of Health and Human Services, Public Health Service, National Institutes of Health, National Institute of Diabetes and Digestive and Kidney Diseases.. In: Saigal CS, editor. Urologic diseases in

America5512. Washington (DC): US Government Printing Office; 2007. p. 533–51

17. Anger JT, Santucci R, Grossberg AL, et al. The morbidity of urethral stricture disease among male medicare beneficiaries. BMC Urol 2010;10:3–4.

18. Cinman AC, de Matos RA, van Blerk PJ. Urethral strictures at Baragwanath Hospital. Br J Urol 1980; 52(5):386–9.

19. Van der Merwe J, Basson J, Van der Merwe A, et al. Management of male urethral strictures: evidence-based medicine versus health care economics: Can we afford to practise what we preach? Urology 2009;74(Suppl 4A):S40.

20. King C, Rourke KF. Urethral stricture is frequently a morbid condition: incidence and factors associated with complications related to urethral stricture. Urology 2019;132:189–94.

21. Buckley JC, Heyns C, Gilling P, et al. SIU/ICUD Consultation on Urethral Strictures: Dilation, internal urethrotomy, and stenting of male anterior urethral strictures. Urology 2014;83(3 Suppl):S18–22.

22. Morey AF, Watkin N, Shenfeld O, et al. SIU/ICUD consultation on urethral strictures: anterior urethra–primary anastomosis. Urology 2014;83(3 Suppl):S23–6.

23. Chapple C, Andrich D, Atala A, et al. SIU/ICUD Consultation on Urethral Strictures: The management of anterior urethral stricture disease using substitution urethroplasty. Urology 2014;83(3 Suppl):S31–47.

24. Harris CR, Osterberg EC, Sanford T, et al. National variation in urethroplasty cost and predictors of extreme cost: a cost analysis with policy implications. Urology 2016;94:246–54.

25. Lacy JM, Madden-Fuentes RJ, Dugan A, et al. Short-term complication rates following anterior urethroplasty: an analysis of national surgical quality improvement program data. Urology 2018;111:197–202.

26. Al-Qudah HS, Santucci RA. Extended complications of urethroplasty. Int Braz J Urol Off J Braz Soc Urol 2005;31(4):315–23 [discussion: 324-325].

27. Kim S, Cheng KC, Patell S, et al. Antibiotic stewardship and postoperative infections in urethroplasties. Urology 2021;152:142–7.

28. Calleja Hermosa P, Campos-Juanatey F, Varea Malo R, et al. Trauma and Reconstructive Urology Working Party of the European Association of Urology Young Academic Urologists. Sexual function after anterior urethroplasty: a systematic review. Transl Androl Urol 2021;10(6):2554–73.

29. Mundy AR. Results and complications of urethroplasty and its future. Br J Urol 1993;71(3):322–5.

30. Blaschko SD, Sanford MT, Cinman NM, et al. De novo erectile dysfunction after anterior urethroplasty: a systematic review and meta-analysis. BJU Int 2013;112(5):655–63.

31. Heinsimer K, Wiegand L. Erectile and ejaculatory dysfunction after urethroplasty. Curr Urol Rep 2021;22(4):19.

32. Bertrand LA, Voelzke BB, Elliott SP, et al. Measuring and predicting patient dissatisfaction after anterior urethroplasty using patient reported outcomes measures. J Urol 2016;196(2):453–61.

33. Kessler TM, Fisch M, Heitz M, et al. Patient satisfaction with the outcome of surgery for urethral stricture. J Urol 2002;167(6):2507–11.

34. Maciejewski CC, Haines T, Rourke KF. Chordee and penile shortening rather than voiding function are associated with patient dissatisfaction after urethroplasty. Urology 2017;103:234–9.

35. Barbagli G, De Angelis M, Romano G, et al. Long-term followup of bulbar end-to-end anastomosis: a retrospective analysis of 153 patients in a single center experience. J Urol 2007;178(6):2470–3.

36. Bugeja S, Andrich DE, Mundy AR. Non-transecting bulbar urethroplasty. Transl Androl Urol 2015;4(1): 41–50.

37. Erickson BA, Wysock JS, McVary KT, et al. Erectile function, sexual drive, and ejaculatory function after reconstructive surgery for anterior urethral stricture disease. BJU Int 2007;99(3):607–11.

38. Chapman DW, Cotter K, Johnsen NV, et al. Nontransecting Techniques Reduce Sexual Dysfunction after Anastomotic Bulbar Urethroplasty: Results of a Multi-Institutional Comparative Analysis. J Urol 2019;201(2):364–70.

39. Feng C, Xu YM, Barbagli G, et al. The relationship between erectile dysfunction and open urethroplasty: a systematic review and meta-analysis. J Sex Med 2013;10(8):2060–8.

40. Palminteri E, Berdondini E, De Nunzio C, et al. The impact of ventral oral graft bulbar urethroplasty on sexual life. Urology 2013;81(4):891–8.

41. Hoy NY, Chapman DW, Rourke KF. Better defining the optimal management of penile urethral strictures: A retrospective comparison of single-stage vs. two-stage urethroplasty. Can Urol Assoc J 2019;414–8.

42. Andrich DE, Greenwell TJ, Mundy AR. The problems of penile urethroplasty with particular reference to 2-stage reconstructions. J Urol 2003;170(1):87–9.

43. Kulkarni S, Kulkarni J, Surana S, et al. Management of Panurethral Stricture. Urol Clin North Am 2017; 44(1):67–75.

44. Angulo JC, Arance I, Esquinas C, et al. Treatment of long anterior urethral stricture associated to lichen sclerosus. Actas Urol Esp 2017;41(2):123–31.

45. Xu YM, Feng C, Sa YL, et al. Outcome of 1-stage urethroplasty using oral mucosal grafts for the treatment of urethral strictures associated with genital lichen sclerosus. Urology 2014;83(1):232–6.

46. Chung ASJ, Suarez OA. Current treatment of lichen sclerosus and stricture. World J Urol 2020;38(12): 3061–7.

47. Daneshvar M, Simhan J, Blakely S, et al. Transurethral ventral buccal mucosa graft inlay for treatment of distal

urethral strictures: international multi-institutional experience. World J Urol 2020;38(10):2601–7.

48. Barbagli G, Perovic S, Djinovic R, et al. Retrospective descriptive analysis of 1,176 patients with failed hypospadias repair. J Urol 2010;183(1):207–11.

49. Akpayak IC, Shuaibu SI, Ofoha CG, et al. Dorsal onlay buccal mucosa graft urethroplasty for bulbar urethral stricture: a single centre experience. Pan Afr Med J 2020;36:305.

50. Horiguchi A. Substitution urethroplasty using oral mucosa graft for male anterior urethral stricture disease: Current topics and reviews. Int J Urol 2017; 24(7):493–503.

51. Barbagli G, Fossati N, Sansalone S, et al. Prediction of early and late complications after oral mucosal graft harvesting: multivariable analysis from a cohort of 553 consecutive patients. J Urol 2014;191(3):688–93.

52. Dubey D, Vijjan V, Kapoor R, et al. Dorsal onlay buccal mucosa versus penile skin flap urethroplasty for anterior urethral strictures: results from a randomized prospective trial. J Urol 2007;178(6):2466–9.

53. Soliman MG, Abo Farha M, El Abd AS, et al. Dorsal onlay urethroplasty using buccal mucosa graft versus penile skin flap for management of long anterior urethral strictures: a prospective randomized study. Scand J Urol 2014;48(5):466–73.

54. Mangir N, Wilson KJ, Osman NI, et al. Current state of urethral tissue engineering. Curr Opin Urol 2019; 29(4):385–93.

55. Bhargava S, Patterson JM, Inman RD, et al. Tissue-engineered buccal mucosa urethroplasty-clinical outcomes. Eur Urol 2008;53(6):1263–9.

56. el-Kassaby A, AbouShwareb T, Atala A. Randomized comparative study between buccal mucosal and acellular bladder matrix grafts in complex anterior urethral strictures. J Urol 2008;179(4):1432–6.

57. Vaddi SP, Reddy VB, Abraham SJ. Buccal epithelium Expanded and Encapsulated in Scaffold-Hybrid Approach to Urethral Stricture (BEES-HAUS) procedure: A novel cell therapy-based pilot study. Int J Urol Off J Jpn Urol Assoc 2019;26(2):253–7.

58. Versteegden LRM, de Jonge PKJD, IntHout J, et al. Tissue engineering of the urethra: a systematic review and meta-analysis of preclinical and clinical studies. Eur Urol 2017;72(4):594–606.

59. Hoare DT, Doiron RC, Rourke KF. Determining perioperative practice patterns in urethroplasty: a survey of genitourinary reconstructive surgeons. Urology 2021;156:263–70.

60. Theisen K, Fuller TW, Bansal U, et al. Safety and Surgical Outcomes of Same-day Anterior Urethroplasty. Urology 2017;102:229–33.

61. Hebert KJ, Joseph J, Boswell T, et al. Enhanced ambulatory male urethral surgery: a pathway to successful outpatient urethroplasty. Transl Androl Urol 2020;9(1):23–30.

62. Lewis J, Wolgast K, Ward J, et al. Outpatient anterior urethroplasty: outcome analysis and patient selection criteria. J Urol 2002;168:1024.

63. MacDonald S, Haddad D, Choi A, et al. Anterior urethroplasty has transitioned to an outpatient procedure without serious rise in complications: data from the national surgical quality improvement program. Urology 2017;102:225.

64. Mundy AR, Andrich DE. Urethral strictures. BJU Int 2011;107(1):6–26.

65. Meeks JJ, Erickson BA, Granieri MA, et al. Stricture recurrence after urethroplasty: a systematic review. J Urol 2009;182(4):1266–70.

66. Angermeier KW, Rourke KF, Dubey D, et al. SIU/ICUD Consultation on Urethral Strictures: Evaluation and follow-up. Urology 2014;83(3 Suppl):S8–17.

67. Wood DN, Andrich DE, Greenwell TJ, et al. Standing the test of time: the long-term results of urethroplasty. World J Urol 2006;24(3):250–4.

68. Breyer BN, McAninch JW, Whitson JM, et al. Multivariate analysis of risk factors for long-term urethroplasty outcome. J Urol 2010;183(2):613–7.

69. Gimbernat H, Arance I, Redondo C, et al. Analysis of the factors involved in the failure of urethroplasty in men. Actas Urol Esp 2014;38(2):96–102.

70. Barbagli G, Kulkarni SB, Fossati N, et al. Long-term followup and deterioration rate of anterior substitution urethroplasty. J Urol 2014;192(3):808–13.

71. Chapman D, Kinnaird A, Rourke K. Independent Predictors of Stricture Recurrence Following Urethroplasty for Isolated Bulbar Urethral Strictures. J Urol 2017;198(5):1107–12.

72. Shalkamy O, Abdelazim H, Elshazly A, et al. Factors Predicting Urethral Stricture Recurrence after Dorsal Onlay Augmented, Buccal Mucosal Graft Urethroplasty. Urol Int 2021;105(3–4):269–77.

73. Levy M, Gor RA, Vanni AJ, et al. The Impact of Age on Urethroplasty Success. Urology 2017;107:232–8.

74. Barbagli G, De Angelis M, Romano G, et al. Clinical outcome and quality of life assessment in patients treated with perineal urethrostomy for anterior urethral stricture disease. J Urol 2009;182(2):548–57.

75. Baradaran N, Fergus KB, Moses RA, et al. Clinical significance of cystoscopic urethral stricture recurrence after anterior urethroplasty: a multi-institution analysis from Trauma and Urologic Reconstructive Network of Surgeons (TURNS). World J Urol 2019; 37(12):2763–8.

76. Amend GM, Nabavizadeh B, Hakam N, et al. Urethroscopic Findings Following Urethroplasty Predict the Need for Secondary Intervention in Long-Term: A Multi-Institutional Study from Trauma and Urologic Reconstructive Network of Surgeons. J Urol 2021. https://doi.org/10.1097/JU.0000000000002353. Epub ahead of print. PMID: 34854754.

77. Oottamasathien S, Hotaling JM, Craig JR, et al. Amniotic therapeutic biomaterials in urology: current

and future applications. Transl Androl Urol 2017; 6(5):943–50.

78. DiDomenico LA, Orgill DP, Galiano RD, et al. Aseptically Processed Placental Membrane Improves Healing of Diabetic Foot Ulcerations: Prospective, Randomized Clinical Trial. Plast Reconstr Surg Glob Open 2016 Oct;12(4(10)):e1095. https://doi.org/10.1097/GOX.0000000000001095.

79. Richter GT, Fan CY, Ozgursoy O, et al. Effect of vascular endothelial growth factor on skin graft survival in Sprague-Dawley rats. Arch Otolaryngol Head Neck Surg 2006;132(6):637–41.

80. Cheon YW, Tark KC, Kim YW. Better survival of random pattern skin flaps through the use of epigallocatechin gallate. Dermatol Surg 2012;38(11): 1835–42.

81. Zografou A, Tsigris C, Papadopoulos O, et al. Improvement of skin-graft survival after autologous transplantation of adipose-derived stem cells in rats. J Plast Reconstr Aesthet Surg 2011;64(12): 1647–56.

Pelvic Fracture Urethral Distraction Defect

Kevin Krughoff, MD[a],*, Joshua Shapiro, MD[b,1], Andrew C. Peterson, MD, MPH[a]

KEYWORDS

- PFUDD • Posterior urethroplasty • Pelvic fracture • Urotrauma

KEY POINTS

- The combination of RUG-VCUG is usually all that is needed in the acute setting.
- Coordination of care with an orthopedic surgeon is recommended when considering SPT placement and patient positioning requirements for definitive repair.
- Urinary incontinence is incompletely understood and difficult to predict, likely relying on more than direct injury to the distal urethral sphincter alone.
- A delayed repair using the elaborated perineal approach allows successful tension-free anastomosis in nearly all cases of PFUDD.
- The length of the distraction defect, or urethral gap length, does not predict the number of steps needed in the elaborated perineal approach.

BACKGROUND

In the arena of genitourinary trauma, posterior pelvic fracture urethral distraction defects (PFUDD) can present formidable reconstructive challenges. PFUDD most often occurs in the context of motor vehicle accidents (MVA) and workplace injuries which impart other severe or life-threatening conditions. Expert management of PFUDD requires a comprehensive diagnostic approach, astute clinical judgment, and technical mastery of many reconstructive techniques. While the incidence of PFUDD is fortunately on the decline, the ubiquitous presence of automobiles and the unpredictability of trauma makes the principles of diagnosis and stabilization universally valuable.

NATURE OF THE PROBLEM
Incidence

PFUDD is now, fortunately, a rare occurrence in most developed nations. In countries that experience more traumatic accidents, a single high-volume center may see up to 14 cases per year;

however, the domestic experience is vastly different.[1] Contemporary data from institutional trauma registries and the National Trauma Data Bank report PFUDD in only 2% to 3% of cases of pelvic fracture.[2,3]

Clinical Presentation

Classically described signs and symptoms of PFUDD include the inability to urinate, blood at the meatus, perineal hematoma, or a high riding prostate on DRE. Blood at the meatus is perhaps the most frequent clinical finding along with the inability to urinate; however, voiding assessment may not be testable based on patient condition and in many situations, an unsuccessful attempt at Foley placement may have preceded this part of the assessment.[4–6] Perineal hematoma, while common, may not be seen for several hours after the injury.[4,7] A high-riding prostate is an unreliable finding given the notoriously low sensitivity of DRE for PFUDD and DRE may be best for ruling out other injuries.[8–10]

Pelvic fractures from lateral compression forces are the most common followed by anterior–

---

[a] Division of Urology, Genitourinary Cancer Survivorship Program, Duke University Medical Center, DUMC 3146, Durham, NC 27710, USA; [b] Department of Orthopaedics, University of North Carolina, Chapel Hill, NC, USA
[1] Present address: DUMC 3146, Durham, NC 27710.
* Corresponding author.
E-mail address: kevin.krughoff@duke.edu
Twitter: @kkroogs (K.K.); @APeterson_Duke (A.C.P.)

Urol Clin N Am 49 (2022) 383–391
https://doi.org/10.1016/j.ucl.2022.04.003

posterior compression fractures. The likelihood of a proximal urethral injury increases when there exist multiple fractures of the anterior rami or combined anterior and posterior fractures; however, the fracture pattern itself is a poor predictor of urethral injury or the need for intervention.[11,12]

Evaluation

Nothing beyond a retrograde urethrogram (RUG) (per AUA guidelines) and antegrade cystourethrography (per EUA guidelines) must be conducted before establishing urinary drainage and allowing the stabilization of nonurologic injuries to proceed.[13,14] The AUA guidelines suggest that surgeons proceed directly to suprapubic tube (SPT) placement for most cases of PFUDD. It is not unreasonable for a brief attempt at Foley catheter placement based on the physical examination alone and the needs of the trauma team, but extended efforts at primary realignment (PR) should be abandoned in favor of SPT placement. It is our opinion that a RUG should be performed whenever possible if urethral trauma is suspected before any urethral manipulation. A reasonable exception to this may be when an angiogram is anticipated, such as to avoid imaging interference from superimposed contrast.

After the stabilization of the patient, delayed repair should take place after several months of rehabilitation and recovery. A comprehensive workup should be undertaken before repair, and an array of diagnostic options are at the disposal of the Urologist. Different approaches are advocated by different experts, but the most common starting approach is the combination of a RUG and voiding cystourethrogram (VCUG) to measure the distraction length, rule out the presence of fistulae and assess the location of important landmarks and bony anatomy. A bladder neck that remains open at rest may signify damage to the sphincter mechanism or possibly the sacral plexus, with implications for future urinary incontinence given the pattern of internal sphincter dependency following PFUDD.[15,16]

The potential for ED after PFUDD is well-established; however, the etiology is multifactorial and often thought to be from the primary injury rather than the means of repair. Both the timing and workup for this vary from center to center. Pharmacodynamic penile duplex US, for instance, may uncover penile deformity and curvature that affect management options. When considering urethroplasty, it is the opinion of some experts that data from this investigation provide additional safeguards against necrosis and failed reconstructive efforts.[17]

MRI has been advocated in certain scenarios to provide additional diagnostic and prognostic information which may not be obtained through traditional RUG-VCUG or CT.[18–20] MRI allows the assessment of retropubic fibrosis and in some situations can better define the urethral disruption gap by delineating the displacement and lateralization of the defect.[12] Lateralization of the prostate apex may have implications for sexual dysfunction and incontinence due to the close apposition of the neurovascular bundles, for instance.[19] Blunt trauma to the penis may result in cavernosal hematoma, disruption of the tunica albuginea, or less commonly high flow priapism. MRI studies suggest these injuries may present more frequently than commonly suspected.[21] A useful protocol is available detailing the use of viscous intraurethral lidocaine at the time of MRI to opacify the urethra on T2 weighted images.[22]

ANATOMY

The bony pelvis is a ring formed by the sacrum and 2 innominate bones including the ilium, ischium, and pubis and is stabilized by the interdigitation of the sacral ala and articulating ilium, by the sacroiliac, sacrotuberous, sacrospinous, iliolumbar, and lumbosacral ligaments, by the symphysis pubis, and by the pelvic floor musculature.

The fracture pattern observed can be correlated with the mechanism of injury and is classified by Young and Burgess, Tile, and AO/OTA.[23–25] A lateral compression (LC) force results in an internally rotated hemipelvis with severe injuries causing a windswept deformity of ipsilateral internal rotation and contralateral external rotation. An anterior–posterior compression (APC) injury pattern results in an externally rotated hemipelvis, and an axial directed load results in a vertical shear (VS) injury pattern. Complex injury patterns exist most commonly as a combination of LC and either APC or VS.

Early descriptions of the mechanism of PFUDD entailed a traumatic upward displacement of the bladder and prostate, stretching the urethra and disrupting it at the more fragile membranous component. In milder versions, the separation of the apical prostate from the pelvic floor results in hematoma that elevates the bladder base and imparts a stretching force on the membranous urethra, but we will restrict our discussion to PFUDD and not pelvic fracture urethral injury as a whole.

Urethral Injury

The posterior urethra is directly supported by a periurethral ligamentous support system which fastens to the pubis on either side of the pubic symphysis. The distracting forces exerted on the urethra from the pubourethral ligaments are directly responsible for the type of urethral injury seen in PFUDD cases and an understanding of these structures is central to the understanding of the PFUDD mechanism.

In an extensively cited anatomic study, Steiner found that the band-like condensation of the pubourethral ligament commonly referred to as the puboprostatic ligament was just the cephalad condensation of a more distal ligamentous support system. The pubourethral ligament extends around the posteroinferior surface of the pubic bone to a point midway underneath the pubic arch, terminating at a confluence of subpubic muscle and fascia continuous with the proximal boundary of the suspensory ligament of the penis. The pubourethral ligament system similarly extends down the length of the membranous urethra and in Steiner's report moved in unison when any single component of the ligament was tensioned.[26]

When a deceleration or crush injury generates enough force to fracture the pelvis, the upward displacement of the bladder and prostate is classically said to avulse the puboprostatic ligament, stretching and eventually disrupting the urethra at the bulbomembranous junction. However, the precise location of the defect along the membranous urethra has been a matter of debate, with one group demonstrating injuries at the bulbomembranous junction[27] and another around the same time period finding injuries closer to the apex of the prostate.[28] Given a modern understanding of the broader pubourethral support system along with individual anatomic variation in the arrangement of pubourethral ligaments, prostate shape and size, pelvic arch and angle, and retropubic eminence, a more likely explanation is that several locations are susceptible to injury and exist as variations on the same mechanism.[29,30]

Continence

The muscles of the external urethral sphincter (EUS) are intimately associated with the membranous urethra, separated only by a thin connective tissue sheath.[31] Because distraction defects occur at the level of the membranous urethra, damage tends to extend to the EUS. The proximal urethral sphincter is rarely damaged but can be seen when injury results in the separation of one pubourethral ligament from the other, essentially tearing apart the prostatic urethra and, by extension, the bladder neck.[32]

Early descriptions of PFUDD assumed that the EUS was completely ablated in the course of injury, with continence relying completely on the function of the internal urethral sphincter. More recent urodynamic studies found that the EUS still contributes to continence in the least some portion of these patients, which challenges this notion and suggests that there may be more heterogeneity to which the EUS is affected.[33]

The neurologic arrangement required for proper EUS function is a matter of debate but is most likely a combination of autonomic and somatic nerves, all of which can be injured during a pelvic fracture. Somatic branches can travel to the EUS from the pelvic plexus itself, or can extend from the pudendal nerve either before or after the pudendal nerve emerges from the pudendal canal (as the dorsal nerve of the penis).[34]

PREOPERATIVE

From an orthopedic perspective, the primary management objective in patients with unstable pelvic fractures is to reduce further hemorrhage by reapproximating fractures and dislocations with a pelvic binder. These act to mitigate hemorrhage by compressing bleeding from fractures and decreasing volume within the pelvis via a tamponade effect. Pelvic binders have a time-dependent complication profile and should not be used for more than 24 hours due to the risk of skin necrosis and pressure ulceration.[35] If a patient is not deemed suitable for definitive internal fixation, then a temporizing external fixator may be used to reduce the risk of pressure injury related to a binder.

SPT management is controversial when internal fixation is being considered. One study found that most of the urologists argue that SPTs do not increase the risk of infection while an identical majority of orthopedic surgeons argue that they do, although both positions are largely based on anecdotal evidence.[36] From an orthopedic standpoint, avoidance of SPT in the setting of anterior pelvis fixation is based on the presumption that potential leakage from the SPT tract can increase risks of hardware infection; however, no objective evidence has corroborated this. Accordingly, the 2020 AUA Urotrauma guidelines state that SPTs can be safely placed in patients undergoing anterior pelvic fixation, although this was based on expert opinion.[13] Until these data are widely known and available, open lines of communication are mandatory in the management of complex injuries to the pelvis. Our preference, when confronted with PFUDD, is for SPT drainage with delayed repair.

The decision on when to proceed with definitive repair is a matter of debate. Historic accounts suggested waiting up to a year for fibrosis to resolve[37] while today some experts wait 6 weeks.[38] It remains to be determined if MRI can help dictate the timing of intervention, given the ability of MRI to identify scarring and thickening of pelvic floor muscles, pertinent ligaments, and their relations to nerves, fascia and blood vessels.[39,40] We have found a 3-month period of urethral rest to be sufficient for the multitude of tissue insults from hematoma, extravasation of urine, infection and generalized local inflammation to subside.

PREP AND PATIENT POSITIONING

In the absence of a bladder neck injury, complex fistula, or other complicating injury warranting an abdominoperineal approach, a perineal approach allows reapproximating of even large urethral gaps using a progression of maneuvers originally described by Webster.[41] The patient is placed in the lithotomy position. A perineal Jordan retractor is used along with headlamps and surgical loupes. Ratcheting pediatric malleable retractors often help with deep exposure. Once stabilized, isolated pelvic fractures typically do not impart any positioning limitations if weight-bearing restrictions strictly adhere. Communication with the treating orthopedic team and testing for the safe range of motion is imperative nonetheless to ensure the patient will tolerate the high lithotomy position for several hours.

PROCEDURAL APPROACH

The current approach to PFUDD evolved in a stepwise process from the first operative descriptions in the 1950s. In broad strokes, urethral pull-through techniques and variations on the scrotal-inlay procedure were the first well-known descriptions for the surgical correction of PFUDD. Citing concerns around the associated morbidity related to erectile dysfunction and incontinence associated with immediate repair, delayed urethroplasty after SPT placement was championed by Johanson. Waterhouse and Turner-Warwick then popularized abdominal pubectomy for use in complex cases involving various fistulae. Waterhouse described the removal of a wedge of anterior pubis using a Gigli saw in virtually all cases of PFUDD, whereas Turner-Warwick described a stepwise approach that was guided by the complexity of injury. He excised the pubic bone only when the anastomosis could not be obtained using a perineal approach or if the gap length was over 3 cm.[37]

Webster first described his perineal approach in 1983, which used neither abdominal exposure nor total pubectomy.[42] The key was using a limited wedge excision of the inferior portion of the pubis after carrying out 3–5 cm of corporal splitting. Before 1990, a 1-stage procedure was not thought feasible when the gap was more than 2 cm.[41] The stepwise use of these maneuvers (**Fig. 1**): urethral mobilization, corporal splitting, inferior wedge pubectomy, and supracrural rerouting, was termed the *elaborated perineal approach*, capable of bridging gaps as long as 9 cm and remains today a time-tested approach to PFUDD.

Step 1: Urethral Mobilization

Circumferential mobilization of the distal urethra to the suspensory ligament of the penis is generally sufficient for small gaps. A midline perineal incision is made which may be bifurcated posteriorly. The proximal bulbar urethra is mobilized proximally to the point of traumatic obliteration before transecting it. If the integrity of the vascular supply to the urethra is in question, a bulbar artery-sparing, non-transecting posterior urethroplasty may be considered, with the use of intraoperative ultrasound to select and preserve the stronger artery.[43–45] Mobilization continues distally toward the boundary of the suspensory ligament of the penis. The transected urethra at this point exists as a flap, dependent on retrograde blood flow from the dorsal penile artery and perforating vessels of the corpora.

A urethral sound or flexible cystoscope is passed antegrade through the suprapubic tube tract and down the proximal lumen of the urethra. The proximal stump is identified amidst the scarred pelvic floor by palpating the tip of the instrument and excising the surrounding scar tissue. The proximal stump is generally more posterior than expected given the characteristic upward displacement of the prostate. If the sound cannot be palpated, judicious incision and excavation of the scar along the midline generally assist in locating it. On occasion, the aspiration of urine from the careful placement of a spinal needle has helped identify the proximal stump. There is now also available a hollow sound that accommodates a flexible scope, allowing for easier navigation and avoidance of false passages.[46]

The proximal stump is spatulated on its ventral surface as far back as the boundary of the verumontanum. The proximal urethra is calibrated with bougie a boule to 30F. The distal urethra is spatulated on its dorsal surface. If a tension-free anastomosis can be accomplished, this is carried out using radially placed 4-O polyglycolic acid sutures. A long-bladed nasal speculum and J-shaped needles, either directly supplied or

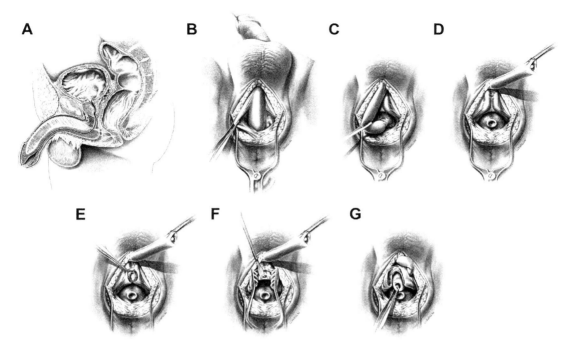

Fig. 1. Procedural approach to PFUDD. (*A*) Saggital section portraying proximity of pubic symphysis to pubourethral ligament complex and dorsal median raphe. (*B-D*) Urethral mobilization. (*E*) Corporal splitting. (*F*) Inferior Wedge Pubectomy. (G)Urethral Rerouting.

simply bent to shape from other needles, are often useful when suturing the proximal urethra by way of a push in–pull out technique. The anastomosis is stented with a 14F silicone catheter.

Pitfalls of this step relate to conditions such as hypospadias or previous interventions which place undue tension on the urethra or compromise retrograde blood flow to the urethral flap. Preoperative vascular evaluation should be considered and a bulbar artery-sparing approach may be warranted for these individuals. Failure to remove sufficient scar tissue adjacent to the proximal stump will not allow for a tension-free anastomosis.

Step 2: Corporal Splitting

If additional length is required after urethral mobilization, a channel for the urethra can be created between the posteriorly separated corporal bodies, straightening the path of the urethra between the tip of the penis and the proximal defect. Corporal splitting can be performed in a bloodless plane for up to 5 cm from the crus before the corporal union becomes too strong. This maneuver provides an extra 1 to 2 cm in length. Corporal splitting has not prohibited future penile prosthesis placement in our experience.

Pitfalls of this step include injury to the dorsal vein which may arise from overly aggressive splitting and dorsal dissection.

Step 3: Inferior Wedge Pubectomy

A partial pubectomy is performed at the inferior pubic arch if further gap length is to be traversed. Lateral retraction of the separated corporal bodies allows the mobilization and ligation of the dorsal vein, thereby exposing the midline symphysis pubis. Our preference is to remove a channel of bone wide enough for the urethra to lie within it using an osteotome and bone rongeurs as opposed to the large anterior wedge historically removed.[37],[47] The bulbospongiosus can be mobilized on its pedicle and interposed around the urethra along this channel to avoid scar encasement. The dorsal penile nerves are naturally lateralized at this location along the corpora, posing minimal risk for injury.[48]

Step 4: Urethral Rerouting

Supracrural rerouting was a maneuver originally performed to facilitate anastomosis during the abdominoperineal approach but can be performed just as well during a perineal approach if tension-free anastomosis is still not possible after the first 3 maneuvers. This serves as the final maneuver in creating the most direct route from the proximal defect. Rerouting takes the urethra dorsally, around the lateral side of the left corporal body and through the inferior pubectomy defect. To accommodate the path of the urethra, an additional small furrow of bone is removed just lateral to the midline partial pubectomy to avoid compression between the corporal body and the bone.

As above, this maneuver does not eliminate the possibility of future placement of a penile prosthesis, nor does it preclude urethral catheterization; however, penile torsion up to 45° can be noted on erection.

Procedural Summary

The degree of tension on the urethra dictates the need to advance to the next maneuver. Achieving an altered geometric path requires a healthy elastic bulbar urethra, and any prior injury or surgery may reduce tensionless gains from each step along the process. In addition, die back of the bulb in the posttraumatic healing process often makes this process more cumbersome than initial imaging might suggest. It is exceedingly difficult to predict the extent of maneuvers that will be ultimately required for successful repair in the preoperative setting. We maintain that the Urologist must be prepared to employ the full breadth of these maneuvers as necessitated during the intraoperative experience.

Equipment advances including flexible scopes, support for high lithotomy and self-retaining retractors likely helped reduce the requirement for more aggressive dissection, and supracrural rerouting is less commonly used today.[49] Regardless, rerouting maintains a role in the experience of many high volume centers.[50–53] Some experts prefer instead to convert to an abdominoperineal approach and perform complete pubectomy if anastomosis cannot be obtained after inferior wedge resection.[12] Due to the associated morbidity and risk for long-term complications, we feel the abdominoperineal approach is best reserved for the most complex of cases such as those with other complicating genitourinary injuries.

RADIATION-INDUCED POSTERIOR URETHROPLASTY STENOSIS

While a complete discussion of all posterior stricture etiologies and considerations for repair are outside of the scope of this article, there exist similarities particularly between PFUDD and radiation-induced posterior urethral stenosis (PUS). Cancer survivors are living longer after their life-saving treatments, which often include radiation, and there exists today a burgeoning conversation around the management of radiation-induced PUS.[54] For this reason we feel that the similarities and discrepancies between these conditions deserve mention. Radiation side effects often take up to 8 to 10 years to present and in this situation typically causes PUS at the bulbomembranous junction, similar to the location of injury in PFUDD. Reconstruction in the setting of radiation-induced PUS presents notable challenges all the same because of the dense fibrosis encountered, and excisional approaches may or may not incorporate some aspects of PFUDD repair such as corporal splitting and urethral rerouting. Success rates of around 70% are reported by individual centers of excellence and by multi-institutional experiences.[55–57] In a radiated field, however, the tissue surrounding the injury is generally further compromised and rarely can a distinction between normal and abnormal tissue be made on gross dissection. Furthermore, complete obliteration of the lumen is more often the exception than the rule. But perhaps the most notable difference in the management discussion for radiation-induced PUS concerns the potential for grafting and substitution urethroplasty.

The tissue bed in radiation-induced PUS is traditionally felt to be compromised and poorly suitable for grafting purposes. Investigating this further, a histologic study compared urethral specimens from radiated and nonradiated patients undergoing dorsal onlay urethroplasty for posterior urethral stenosis. On one hand, the presence of increased fibrosis, higher collagen density and decreased vascularity was, indeed, confirmed in radiated specimens, yet counterintuitively, the presence of these factors was not reflected by surgical outcomes which instead slightly favored patients with a history of radiation.[58] To this end, multi-institutional experiences with graft-based repairs for PUS report recurrence rates of 33% and 17.7% when using ventral and dorsal approaches, respectively, with do novo incontinence rates of 53% reported for the ventral approach and 8% for the dorsal approach.[59,60] The most recent effort from one center of excellence noted an overall 71% success rate; however, a trend of declining success with longer follow-up was noted, decreasing from 90% after 1 year to 39% after 4 years.[61] The most recent consensus panel recommendation is for a graded approach starting with endourologic procedures owing to the high rate of complications associated with reconstructive efforts, with advancement to more invasive options as needed.[62] An updated consensus report incorporating more recent results with graft-based repairs may better illuminate the pros and cons of this potentially promising approach. The inclusion of gracilis muscle transposition with ventral grafting should be considered and will be the focus of discussion in other articles.

Recovery and Rehabilitation

A drain is placed in the superficial perineal pouch and brought out through the lateral scrotum. The suprapubic tube is replaced and capped. A Foley catheter is left in place for 3 to 4 weeks and removed in the clinic after confirming the integrity of the repair on cystourethrography. The suprapubic tube is capped at this time and removed 7 to 10 days later if the patient is urinating without difficulty. No additional antibiotics are given over standard procedural prophylaxis. Erectile dysfunction has long been held to relate more closely to the trauma than the method of management, and delayed recovery may be seen many months after the initial injury.[63]

OUTCOMES

Common complications are usually self-limited such as perineal hematoma or neuropathic complaints, while more serious complications relate to prolonged high lithotomy positioning such as compartment syndrome or decubitus ulcer.[12] Contemporary multi-institutional data report a success rate of 91%, defined as the need for repeat intervention. A third of cases required one or more ancillary maneuvers to gain urethral length. Of these, 36% received corporal splitting, 13% partial or complete pubectomy, 2% supracrural rerouting. An abdominoperineal approach was needed in less than 5%. Younger patients, those with longer distraction defects, and those with a history of angioembolization were more likely to require ancillary maneuvers.[52] Failures are most often detected within the first year; however, late recurrences do occur which warrant long-term follow-up.[12] A qualitative review found that 13% of men reported some degree of incontinence; however, data in this domain are less robust.[12]

SUMMARY

PFUDD entails a distinct mechanism but a wide spectrum of injury to the urethra and organs of the pelvis. As was stated by Turner-Warwick, it is often the Urologist who will help navigate the most devastating and chronic consequences of injury after the acuity of trauma are over.[37]

Trauma is unpredictable and infinitely variable by nature, and for this reason, expert opinion is likely to

continue to dictate several components of management. By the same token, it is unlikely that one approach to PFUDD will prove superior in all cases. Despite this, surgical intervention for PFUDD has evolved significantly over the last 60 years and the elaborated perineal approach proves to be an excellent platform in the vast majority of cases.

CLINICS CARE POINTS

- The combination of RUG-VCUG is usually all that is needed in the acute setting.
- Coordination of care with an orthopedic surgeon is recommended when considering SPT placement and patient positioning requirements for definitive repair.
- Urinary incontinence is incompletely understood and difficult to predict, likely relying on more than direct injury to the distal urethral sphincter alone.
- A delayed repair using the elaborated perineal approach allows successful tension-free anastomosis in nearly all cases of PFUDD.
- The length of the distraction defect, or urethral gap length, does not predict the number of steps needed in the elaborated perineal approach.

DISCLOSURE

The authors have nothing to disclose.

REFERENCES

1. Saini DK, Sinha RJ, Sokhal AK, et al. Analysis of anastomotic urethroplasty for pelvic fracture urethral distraction defect: Decadal experience from a high-volume tertiary care center. Urol Ann 2019;11:77–82.
2. Velazquez N, Fantus RJ, Fantus RJ, et al. Blunt trauma pelvic fracture-associated genitourinary and concomitant lower gastrointestinal injury: incidence, morbidity, and mortality. World J Urol 2020; 38:231–8.
3. Johnsen NV, Dmochowski RR, Young JB, et al. Epidemiology of Blunt Lower Urinary Tract Trauma With and Without Pelvic Fracture. Urology 2017; 102:234–9.
4. Lowe MA, Mason JT, Luna GK, et al. Risk Factors for Urethral Injuries in Men with Traumatic Pelvic Fractures. Journal of Urology 1988;140:506–7.
5. Lückhoff C, Mitra B, Cameron PA, et al. The diagnosis of acute urethral trauma. Injury 2011;42:913–6.
6. Ziran BH, Chamberlin E, Shuler FD, et al. Delays and difficulties in the diagnosis of lower urologic injuries

in the context of pelvic fractures. J Trauma 2005;58: 533–7.

7. Mundy AR, Andrich DE. Urethral trauma. Part I: introduction, history, anatomy, pathology, assessment and emergency management. BJU Int 2011;108: 310–27.

8. Ball CG, Jafri SM, Kirkpatrick AW, et al. Traumatic urethral injuries: Does the digital rectal examination really help us? Injury 2009;40:984–6.

9. Shlamovitz GZ, Mower WR, Bergman J, et al. Poor test characteristics for the digital rectal examination in trauma patients. Ann Emerg Med 2007;50:25–33, 33.e21.

10. Figler BD, Hoffler CE, Reisman W, et al. Multi-disciplinary update on pelvic fracture associated bladder and urethral injuries. Injury 2012;43: 1242–9.

11. Koraitim MM. Predictors of erectile dysfunction post pelvic fracture urethral injuries: a multivariate analysis. Urology 2013;81:1081–5.

12. Cooperberg MR, McAninch JW, Alsikafi NF, et al. Urethral reconstruction for traumatic posterior urethral disruption: outcomes of a 25-year experience. J Urol 2007;178:2006–10 [discussion 2010].

13. Morey AF, Broghammer JA, Hollowell CMP, et al. Urotrauma Guideline 2020: AUA Guideline. J Urol 2021;205:30–5.

14. Martínez-Piñeiro L, Djakovic N, Plas E, et al. EAU Guidelines on Urethral Trauma. Eur Urol 2010;57: 791–803.

15. Iselin CE, Webster GD. The significance of the open bladder neck associated with pelvic fracture urethral distraction defects. J Urol 1999;162:347–51.

16. MacDiarmid S, Rosario D, Chapple CR. The importance of accurate assessment and conservative management of the open bladder neck in patients with post-pelvic fracture membranous urethral distraction defects. Br J Urol 1995;75:65–7.

17. Gomez RG, Scarberry K. Anatomy and techniques in posterior urethroplasty. Translational Andrology and Urology 2018;7:567–79.

18. Sung DJ, Kim YH, Cho SB, et al. Obliterative urethral stricture: MR urethrography versus conventional retrograde urethrography with voiding cystourethrography. Radiology 2006;240:842–8.

19. Koraitim MM, Reda IS. Role of magnetic resonance imaging in assessment of posterior urethral distraction defects. Urology 2007;70:403–6.

20. Horiguchi A, Edo H, Soga S, et al. Pubourethral Stump Angle Measured on Preoperative Magnetic Resonance Imaging Predicts Urethroplasty Type for Pelvic Fracture Urethral Injury Repair. Urology 2018;112:198–204.

21. Armenakas NA, McAninch JW, Lue TF, et al. Post-traumatic impotence: magnetic resonance imaging and duplex ultrasound in diagnosis and management. J Urol 1993;149:1272–5.

22. Joshi PM, Desai DJ, Shah D, et al. Injury in Pelvic Fracture Urethral Injury Is Membranobulbar: Fact or Myth. Urology 2017;102:e9–10.

23. Young JW, Burgess AR, Brumback RJ, et al. Pelvic fractures: value of plain radiography in early assessment and management. Radiology 1986;160: 445–51.

24. Burgess AR, Eastridge BJ, Young JW, et al. Pelvic ring disruptions: effective classification system and treatment protocols. J Trauma 1990;30:848–56.

25. Tile M. Pelvic ring fractures: should they be fixed? J Bone Joint Surg Br 1988;70:1–12.

26. Steiner MS. The puboprostatic ligament and the male urethral suspensory mechanism: an anatomic study. Urology 1994;44:530–4.

27. Mouraviev VB, Santucci RA. Cadaveric anatomy of pelvic fracture urethral distraction injury: most injuries are distal to the external urinary sphincter. J Urol 2005;173:869–72.

28. Myers JB, McAninch JW. Management of posterior urethral disruption injuries. Nat Clin Pract Urol 2009;6:154–63.

29. Becker I, Woodley SJ, Stringer MD. The adult human pubic symphysis: a systematic review. J Anat 2010; 217:475–87.

30. Kim M, Boyle SL, Fernandez A, et al. Development of a novel classification system for anatomical variants of the puboprostatic ligaments with expert validation. Can Urol Assoc J 2014;8:432–6.

31. Dalpiaz O, Mitterberger M, Kerschbaumer A, et al. Anatomical approach for surgery of the male posterior urethra. BJU Int 2008;102:1448–51.

32. Mundy AR, Andrich DE. Pelvic fracture-related injuries of the bladder neck and prostate: their nature, cause and management. BJU Int 2010;105:1302–8.

33. Whitson JM, McAninch JW, Tanagho EA, et al. Mechanism of continence after repair of posterior urethral disruption: evidence of rhabdosphincter activity. J Urol 2008;179:1035–9.

34. Narayan P, Konety B, Aslam K, et al. Neuroanatomy of the external urethral sphincter: implications for urinary continence preservation during radical prostate surgery. J Urol 1995;153:337–41.

35. Jowett AJL, Bowyer GW. Pressure characteristics of pelvic binders. Injury 2007;38:118–21.

36. Johnsen NV, Firoozabadi R, Voelzke BB. Treatment Discrepancy for Pelvic Fracture Patients With Urethral Injuries: A Survey of Orthopaedic and Urologic Surgeons. J Orthop Trauma 2019;33:e280–4.

37. Turner-Warwick R. Prevention of complications resulting from pelvic fracture urethral injuries–and from their surgical management. Urol Clin North Am 1989;16:335–58.

38. Scarberry K, Bonomo J, Gómez RG. Delayed Posterior Urethroplasty Following Pelvic Fracture Urethral Injury: Do We Have to Wait 3 Months? Urology 2018;116:193–7.

39. Hoznek A, Rahmouni A, Abbou C, et al. The suspensory ligament of the penis: an anatomic and radiologic description. Surg Radiol Anat 1998;20:413–7.

40. Lakhoo J, Khatri G, Elsayed RF, et al. MRI of the Male Pelvic Floor. Radiographics 2019;39:2003–22.

41. Webster GD, Ramon J. Repair of pelvic fracture posterior urethral defects using an elaborated perineal approach: experience with 74 cases. J Urol 1991; 145:744–8.

42. Webster GD, Selli C. Management of traumatic posterior urethral stricture by one stage perineal repair. Surg Gynecol Obstet 1983;156:620–4.

43. Jordan GH, Eltahawy EA, Virasoro R. The technique of vessel sparing excision and primary anastomosis for proximal bulbous urethral reconstruction. J Urol 2007;177:1799–802.

44. Kishore TA, Bhat S, John RP. Colour Doppler ultrasonographic location of the bulbourethral artery, and its impact on surgical outcome. BJU Int 2005;96: 624–8.

45. Gomez RG, Campos RA, Velarde LG. Reconstruction of Pelvic Fracture Urethral Injuries With Sparing of the Bulbar Arteries. Urology 2016;88:207–12.

46. Gelman J, Wisenbaugh ES. Posterior Urethral Strictures. Adv Urol 2015;2015:628107.

47. Waterhouse K, Abrahams JI, Gruber H, et al. The transpubic approach to the lower urinary tract. J Urol 1973;109:486–90.

48. Yucel S, Baskin LS. Neuroanatomy of the male urethra and perineum. BJU Int 2003;92:624–30.

49. Kizer WS, Armenakas NA, Brandes SB, et al. Simplified reconstruction of posterior urethral disruption defects: limited role of supracrural rerouting. J Urol 2007;177:1378–81 [discussion: 1381-1372].

50. Singh SK, Pawar DS, Khandelwal AK, et al. Transperineal bulboprostatic anastomotic repair of pelvic fracture urethral distraction defect and role of ancillary maneuver: A retrospective study in 172 patients. Urol Ann 2010;2:53–7.

51. Koraitim MM. Transpubic Urethroplasty Revisited: Total, Superior, or Inferior Pubectomy? Urology 2010;75:691–4.

52. Johnsen NV, Moses RA, Elliott SP, et al. Multicenter analysis of posterior urethroplasty complexity and outcomes following pelvic fracture urethral injury. World J Urol 2020;38:1073–9.

53. Fu Q, Zhang YM, Barbagli G, et al. Factors that influence the outcome of open urethroplasty for pelvis fracture urethral defect (PFUD): an observational study from a single high-volume tertiary care center. World J Urol 2015;33:2169–75.

54. Selph JP, Peterson AC. Review Article: Past, Present and Future of Cancer Survivorship and the Importance of the Urologist. Urology Practice 2017;4: 60–70.

55. Elliott SP, McAninch JW, Chi T, et al. Management of severe urethral complications of prostate cancer therapy. J Urol 2006;176:2508–13.

56. Hofer MD, Zhao LC, Morey AF, et al. Outcomes after urethroplasty for radiotherapy induced bulbomembranous urethral stricture disease. J Urol 2014;191: 1307–12.

57. Meeks JJ, Brandes SB, Morey AF, et al. Urethroplasty for radiotherapy induced bulbomembranous strictures: a multi-institutional experience. J Urol 2011;185:1761–5.

58. Hughes M, Caza T, Li G, et al. Histologic characterization of the post-radiation urethral stenosis in men treated for prostate cancer. World J Urol 2020;38: 2269–77.

59. Vetterlein MW, Kluth LA, Zumstein V, et al. Buccal mucosal graft urethroplasty for radiation-induced urethral strictures: an evaluation using the extended Urethral Stricture Surgery Patient-Reported Outcome Measure (USS PROM). World Journal of Urology 2020;38:2863–72.

60. Policastro CG, Simhan J, Martins FE, et al. A multi-institutional critical assessment of dorsal onlay urethroplasty for post-radiation urethral stenosis. World J Urol 2021;39:2669–75.

61. Ahyai SA, Schmid M, Kuhl M, et al. Outcomes of Ventral Onlay Buccal Mucosa Graft Urethroplasty in Patients after Radiotherapy. Journal of Urology 2015;194:441–6.

62. Herschorn S, Elliott S, Coburn M, et al. SIU/ICUD Consultation on Urethral Strictures: Posterior urethral stenosis after treatment of prostate cancer. Urology 2014;83:S59–70.

63. Golimbu M, al-Askari S, Morales P. Transpubic approach for lower urinary tract surgery: a 15-year experience. J Urol 1990;143:72–6.

Female Urethral Reconstruction
Urethral Diverticulectomy, Urethral Strictures, Vesicovaginal Fistula

Ignacio Alvarez de Toledo, MD, Jessica DeLong, MD, FACS*

KEYWORDS

- Female urethral stricture • Female urethral diverticulum • Vesicovaginal fistula • Urethroplasty
- Urethral diverticulectomy • Buccal mucosa graft • Vaginal flap

KEY POINTS

- Women with urethral pathologic conditions are usually underdiagnosed, with the correct diagnosis often being made years after the onset of symptoms. A high index of suspicion is required.
- Female urethral strictures can be managed with either conservative treatments, such as urethral dilation, or definitive surgeries, such as augmented urethroplasty, using either flaps or grafts.
- Female urethral diverticulum is a challenging diagnostic and reconstructive problem, and its definitive treatment is a urethral diverticulectomy.
- The outcome of a urethral diverticulectomy will depend on the complexity of the diverticulum itself.
- Vesicovaginal fistula is a socially devastating entity, and the treatment is determined by an adequate management of the patient's global health and the following of basic surgical principles such as exposure, mobilization, tension-free closure, and correct bladder drainage.

 Video content accompanies this article at http://www.urologic.theclinics.com.

INTRODUCTION

Much has been written regarding pelvic reconstruction in women. Moreover, many of the early advances that were made in pelvic dysfunction and reconstruction in women were later extrapolated to male patients and to urologic diseases in general. The opposite situation can be found when describing urethral diseases. It took some time for the urologic scientific community to remind us that *women have urethras too*.

For many years, urethral diseases in women have been overlooked and, oftentimes, underdiagnosed. Although most lower urinary tract symptoms (LUTS) in women can be attributed to multiple causes, bladder outlet obstruction (BOO) accounts for 8.3% to 29% of patients.[1,2] Within these patients, it is important to differentiate between functional versus anatomic causes of BOO. Anatomic causes of BOO include a wide variety of pathologic entities such as female urethral stricture (FUS), female urethral diverticulum (FUD), vesicovaginal fistula (VVF), pelvic organ prolapse, post anti-incontinence procedure, and malignancy, among others. FUS disease accounts for a considerable proportion ranging from 4% to 18% of women with BOO[3]. The prevalence of FUD ranges between 0.6% and 4.7% according to the literature,[4] and the real incidence of VVF is unknown, although it has been reported to be between 0.3% and 2.0%.[5]

Department of Urology, Eastern Virginia Medical School, Urology of Virginia, 225 Clearfield Avenue, Virginia Beach, VA 2346, USA
* Corresponding author.
E-mail address: jessicadelong@gmail.com

Urol Clin N Am 49 (2022) 393–402
https://doi.org/10.1016/j.ucl.2022.04.004

Finding a suitable definition for FUS remains controversial. It has been proposed that a urethral lumen too narrow to admit a 17Fr flexible cystoscope or that has the feel of scar tissue by cystoscopic haptic feedback is diagnostic for stricture,[3] whereas others define FUS as a fixed anatomic narrowing of the urethra such that the lumen will not accommodate instrumentation without disruption of the urethral mucosal lining.[6] On the contrary, FUD is well defined as a variably sized urine-filled periurethral cystic structure adjacent to the urethra within the confines of the pelvic fascia, connected to the urethra via an ostium.[7] Finally, VVF is defined as a pathologic connection between the bladder and the vagina.

Most urethral disease in women can be attributed to 4 causes: idiopathic, iatrogenic, inflammatory, or traumatic. There is a small proportion of rare causes that include urethral tuberculosis, urethral carcinoma, locally advanced cervical carcinoma, fibroepithelial polyps, and infection.[8–10] Most patients with FUS disease will have an unknown cause (51.3%). Another large proportion (32.8%) will have a history of past surgical interventions in the form of urethral dilations, anti-incontinence surgery, transurethral bladder surgery, or other types of urethral surgery. A smaller percentage will occur due to inflammation (9.2%) or trauma (6.6%).[11] Regarding FUD, the most accepted etiopathogenic theory relies on a history of chronic inflammation of periurethral ducts, which ultimately result in sacculation and diverticulum formation.[12] Finally, it is important to discriminate between VVF diagnosed in developing versus developed countries. Most VVFs in developing countries occur as a result of obstructed labor during childbirth,[13] whereas in developed countries VVFs are rare and often encountered after hysterectomies or as a consequence of complex pelvic surgery, malignancies, and/or radiation.[14]

The purpose of this article is to describe complex urethral diseases in women such as FUS, FUD, and VVF as well as to review the available reconstructive surgical techniques for these entities. Step-by-step videos of urethral stricture reconstruction and urethral diverticulectomy are included. For instructive videos of VVF repair, we strongly recommend the Lee and colleagues[5] (vaginal approach) and McKay and colleagues[15] (abdominal approach) articles from prior issues of this journal.

DIAGNOSIS

Diagnosing urethral pathologic condition in women can be challenging. Frequently, these patients will see several specialists before a definitive diagnosis is made. Some authors reported that it can take up to 5 years between the onset of symptoms and the definitive diagnosis of FUD.[16] Clinicians should have a high index of suspicion in order to avoid a delay in treatment. Thorough investigation regarding past medical history, surgical history, voiding and sexual habits, and history of malignancies or radiation is crucial to differentiate urethral anatomic pathologic conditions from functional ones.

Physical examination (PE) is mandatory. It is very important to perform a complete PE because it may provide the clinician with key information not only to arrive at a definitive diagnosis but also for surgical planning. Observation of poor tissue quality, meatal stenosis, or lichen sclerosus may guide our diagnosis toward an FUS, whereas a paraurethral bulging mass will be diagnostic of FUD in more than 80% of cases.[17] Continuous vaginal leakage after a pelvic surgical procedure is suspicious for VVF. In every case, PE should be performed thoroughly, including bimanual pelvic, vaginal, and speculum examinations.

Regarding LUTS, there are vague and generally nonpathognomonic signs. Classically, a 3-D Triad (Dysuria, Dyspareunia, and postvoid Dribbling) has been described associated with FUD but studies have shown that only 5% of patients have all 3, and even more, 27% of the patients did not present with any of those symptoms.[18,19] Patients with FUS might have a variety of symptoms ranging from minor discomfort to a wide spectrum of voiding and storage symptoms. Inconsistently, the classic obstructive picture with a weak urinary stream, sensation of incomplete voiding, and straining will suggest FUS. However, as Kuo demonstrated, the differential diagnosis of lower urinary tract dysfunction in women cannot be based on LUTS alone.[20]

Patients with voiding dysfunction and suspicion for obstruction should have a uroflow and a postvoid residual (PVR) checked because it contributes important initial information. Although there are no specific cutoffs for uroflowmetry or PVR volumes, a curve that reaches a plateau, flow less than 12 to 15 mL/s, or PVRs greater than 100, may suggest obstruction.[21] Cystourethroscopy (CU) is very useful in assessing tissue quality, an area of maximal stricture, and/or finding anomalous communication between the urinary tract and the genitalia. When available, we encourage the use of pediatric cystoscopes in cases with a narrow lumen. We generally do not perform an office CU in suspected FUD cases because it will not change our management and can be uncomfortable for patients. Simple urethral calibration with bougie-à-boule can also

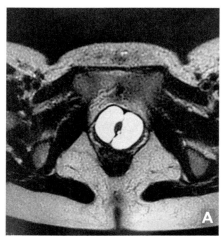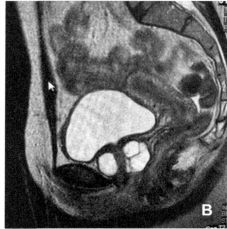

Fig. 1. Complex urethral diverticulum on MRI ((*A*): axial; (*B*): sagittal).

provide important information regarding urethral diameter and stricture location as well as tissue quality although we should not rely on urethral diameter itself to completely rule out FUS.[22] In cases where we want to assess bladder function, a urodynamic study (UDS) might be indicated. In obstructed patients, it will show a classic high-pressure low-flow pattern. To maximize the information provided by UDS, we recommend adding fluoroscopy and performing a video-UDS because it will provide critical anatomic information regarding bladder neck function as well as the location of any obstruction. It has been proposed that a detrusor contraction at a maximum of greater than 25 cm H_2O, with a flow less than 12 cc/s could be diagnostic of BOO, although there is no consensus regarding cutoff values.[23] Other fluoroscopic studies such as retrograde urethrogram or voiding cystourethrogram may be helpful in diagnosing an outpouching diverticulum or an anomalous communication in patients with suspected VVF. These studies may not be as helpful as in male patients because it can often be challenging to distinguish between a primary bladder neck obstruction, a urethral sphincter obstruction, a pelvic floor obstruction, or a urethral stricture itself. Cystoscopy with bilateral retrograde pyelography is often recommended to rule out ureteral involvement in the case of VVF.

Finally, pelvic magnetic resonance imaging (MRI) plays a central role in the diagnosis and management of patients with urethral dysfunction, particularly FUD and VVF. In recent years, there has been an increasing interest in using this diagnostic tool not only for diagnosis but also to rule out other pathologic conditions such as malignancy, concomitant calculus, abscesses, or other findings. MRI's superiority relies on its multiplanar

scanning capability, superior soft tissue differentiation, noninvasive nature, and overall excellent contrast resolution.[24] Additional features such as the ability to provide functional imaging make the MRI the gold standard diagnostic test for diagnosing periurethral pathology[25] (**Fig. 1**).

ANATOMY

Urethral surgery in women requires a great understanding of anatomy and surgical planes. The goal in performing urethral reconstructive surgery is to alleviate symptoms while preserving and hopefully improving voiding and sexual function.

The normal urethra in women is a musculofascial tube approximately 3 to 4 cm in length, extending from the bladder neck to the external urethral meatus. The urethra is suspended by the urethropelvic ligament, which is a bilayered connective tissue. It is between these 2 layers that FUD usually develops.[7]

The urethral lumen is lined proximally by urothelial tissue and distally by nonkeratinized stratified squamous epithelium. The urethra in women is lined by a longitudinal inner smooth muscle layer and outer circular smooth muscle layer. Its striated skeletal muscle component is omega-shaped and is thinner in the dorsal aspect. This sphincteric mechanism is not completely described, and it has been hypothesized that the inner longitudinal layer not only helps with micturition but also acts as a plug while contracted to help with the overall continence mechanism.[26]

Beyond the lamina propria, there are a series of periurethral glands. These are located posterolaterally and have a central role in the pathophysiologic development of FUD. It has been proposed that chronic inflammation and obliteration of these glands may ultimately result in FUD formation. Most of these glands are located in the distal one-third of the urethra. The Skene glands (SGs) are the largest and most distal of these glands. These glands drain outside the urethral lumen, and this is why when they obliterate, they have a similar presentation to FUD but represent a different entity as SG are more distal, almost sub-meatal, and do not communicate with the urethra.[7] Finally, the neurovascular clitoral structures are located cephalad and lateral to the dorsal aspect of the external urethral meatus so the risk of injury is low.

MANAGEMENT
Urethral Diverticulum

FUD has been described as one of the most challenging diagnostic and reconstructive problems in female urology, and we agree with that statement.[7] Its wide variety of clinical presentations and its surgical approach make it a unique challenge. In their series, Pincus and colleagues[27] found that 21% of patients with a UD were asymptomatic, and only 51% of them needed a surgical excision. In patients who do not undergo treatment, it is advisable to monitor the diverticulum. Alternatives to surgical reconstruction can be minimally invasive approaches such as endoscopic coagulation, marsupialization, fulguration or endoscopic or open incision and drainage, although these might have high-recurrence rates.[28] Bodner-Adler and colleagues[4] reported their surgical management as follows: transvaginal resection of the UD $\pm$ reconstruction (84%), marsupialization (3.8%), transurethral endoscopic unroofing (2.0%), and various other techniques (9.7%). Furthermore, some authors propose a robotic approach for proximal dorsal FUD, reporting satisfactory results, and feasibility with this technique.[29] Finally, there is a current debate on whether a concomitant stress urinary incontinence procedure should be done along with the urethral diverticulectomy. Juang and colleagues[30] suggest that meticulous suture of the urethral defect left by the diverticulectomy with reconstruction of the periurethral fascia might enhance urethral resistance and thus overcome the problem of stress urinary incontinence; therefore, a combined antiincontinence procedure should not be mandatory. If done, a bladder neck suspension or autologous fascial pubovaginal sling has proven to be safe and successful.[31]

Urethral Stricture

We separate treatment options into conservative versus definitive management. Conservative management includes urethral dilation, which is the most used treatment modality by urologists.[32] The other minimally invasive option is a direct vision internal urethrotomy, although it is not as popular as urethral dilation, and is only anecdotally reported. Urethral dilation is easy to do and has relatively low morbidity and complication rates.

Within definitive management, options include augmented urethroplasty using either flaps or grafts, and, very rarely, excision and primary anastomosis. Once considered as a second-line treatment, recently it has become more popular due to improved knowledge and training, and has made primary reconstruction a first-line treatment option, as suggested by Önol and colleagues.[33]

Urethral reconstruction using flaps remains a valid option when considering approaches for urethroplasty in women. Flaps can be obtained from vaginal (U-shaped or C-shaped), labial, or vestibular tissue. They are relatively easy to obtain, with low donor site morbidity. One should consider the health of local tissue before deciding to use a flap. In patients with lichen sclerosus or a history of radiation, the use of local flaps is discouraged, and in this case, we strongly recommend the use of non-local grafts.

Within urethral reconstruction using grafts, local grafts or oral mucosa grafts may be used. Local grafts can be obtained from the vagina as well as from the labia minora. As with local flaps, these grafts are contraindicated in patients with unhealthy tissues. Another aspect to consider is treatment with local estrogens when considering local flaps or grafts. This type of adjuvant local treatment has proven to be safe and efficacious by Romero-Maroto and colleagues.[34] As mentioned above, our preferred surgical technique is a urethral reconstruction using a buccal mucosa graft (BMG). As with male patients, BMG is popular because of its versatility and relatively low morbidity. Some authors presented their study using lingual mucosa grafts with acceptable results compared with the available literature.[35] In our experience, we only use lingual mucosa grafts when there is no available healthy buccal mucosa to harvest.

Vesico-Vaginal Fistula

VVF diagnosis includes a heterogeneous group of patients that range from minorly symptomatic to devastating cases, and because of this, it can be difficult to determine management options and treatment algorithms. Principles of VVF repair should include treatment of infection, anemia, and malnutrition and ensure no foreign nondissolving material or malignancy, tension-free watertight repair, and uninterrupted bladder drainage.[5]

These repairs can be classified into simple or complex. Simple fistulas are small (<0.5 cm) and single in nonradiated patients with no associated malignancy. Complex fistulas are large (≥2.5 cm), those that failed previous fistula repair, or are associated with chronic disease or postradiation. A fistula sized between 0.5 and 2.5 cm is considered intermediate.[36]

Conservative management can be attempted when we encounter a simple fistula. The first and simplest option is to insert a Foley catheter, drain the bladder, and prescribe an anticholinergic. This strategy alone has proven to be effective up to 39% of the time.[37] Many other minimally invasive treatments have also been reported, such as injection of fibrin sealant/cyanoacrylic glue and/ or electrocautery with laser or coagulation diathermy, all showing acceptable results although practiced in a small number of patients and with short follow-up.

Finally, if conservative measures do not resolve the VVF or if the fistula is not suitable for conservative management, a formal surgical repair is indicated. In these cases, the surgeon will have to sort through a series of options: mmediate repair versus delayed repair, vaginal approach versus abdominal approach, open procedure or laparoscopic/robotic, interposition of tissue versus no interposition, removal of fistulous tract versus no removal. All of these are still open controversies, and there is a lack of sufficient data to recommend one over the other. In summary, we agree with Malik and colleagues[38] who opined that VVF can be best managed following basic surgical principles, such as adequate exposure, identification of structures, wide mobilization, tension-free closure, good hemostasis, and uninterrupted bladder drainage. Additional discussion can be found in the next headings.

PREOPERATIVE PLANNING

After diagnosis, the reconstructive surgeon must consider additional imaging or studies, if necessary, to adequately plan intervention. Some authors suggest that performing UDS in patients with FUD is helpful as it may diagnose BOO in up to 50% of the cases.[39] Reeves and colleagues[31] propose that in cases where MRI is needed, it should be done sagittal and postvoid, in order to allow the UD to fill with urine and provide better imaging. In patients where a CU might be needed, it may be beneficial to perform under sedation to avoid patient discomfort. Cystoscopy with bilateral retrograde pyelography may be indicated for patients with VVF to rule out ureteral involvement.

There is no consensus on whether or not to perform a preoperative urine culture. If the patient has a history of recurrent UTIs, it is beneficial to obtain one in order to adjust therapy according to the antibiogram. Some authors advocate the idea that a urine culture should be done for every patient before surgery.[40] In cases with VVF where urinoma or urosepsis is present, it is advised to delay the definitive repair for at least 6 weeks after drainage, if possible. This is also the case in a postpartum event because the uterus takes some time to return to its involute state.[5] In postmenopausal women, intravaginal estrogens may be administered preoperatively to treat vaginal mucosal atrophy.[34]

In patients with suspected malignancy, a biopsy should be done before undergoing a reconstructive procedure because this would likely change management. It is in these cases where an MRI is potentially useful as well. Malignancies can present as part of a stricture, diverticulum, or fistula, so in every case, the surgeon should be aware of this possibility and patients properly counseled.

As with male patients, the reconstructive surgeon must be ready to change the plan if intraoperative findings differ from the preoperative plan. It is highly recommended to be precise and clear with the patient before consenting to avoid misunderstandings. It is also of the utmost importance to manage patients' expectations appropriately before performing these procedures as, sometimes, resolving one urethral problem (FUS, FUD, VVF) may bring on an additional urethral problem and more than one procedure may be needed.

PREP AND PATIENT POSITIONING

Patients with urethral pathologic conditions are widely variable and ultimately each treatment option should be adjusted to each particular need. In general, we use the low lithotomy position because it provides us with access to the urethral meatus, vaginal introitus, and the vestibule as well as the abdomen. Interestingly, Reeves and colleagues[31] propose a novel prone position stating it can provide better access in these patients, especially in complex high VVF. We prep and drape our patients in the usual sterile fashion, using 2% chlorhexidine gluconate or povidone-iodine solution according to the surgeon's preference. It is very important to carefully pad all pressure points to avoid nerve injury.

To help with retraction, we use the Lonestar-Scott retractor with 4 to 6 blue (sharp) hooks, although labia minora could also be retracted with sutures. Oftentimes, the FUD ostium is difficult to encounter, so in these cases, we find it very useful to instill diluted methylene blue to help find the ostium and dye the diverticulum, which is helpful during dissection. The same retractor is used in cases where a Martius flap is harvested.

Finally, in cases where we will need to harvest a BMG, the patient's mouth is also prepped and draped. Typically, we harvest our own grafts; however, it is acceptable to have a separate team harvest if desired. There is no need for nasotracheal intubation as this procedure can be done with an orotracheal tube in place carefully secured to one side, harvesting from the opposite inner cheek.

PROCEDURAL APPROACH (OUR TECHNIQUES)
Urethral Diverticulum

We start with 17 Fr rigid cystoscopy to assess the urethra and bladder. We look for the FUD ostium, which is not always found. If found, it is usually in the postero-lateral position. As mentioned prior, we use a Scott retractor and blue hooks for better visualization and instill dilute methylene blue. A 14 or 16 Fr catheter is then placed with 10 cc in the balloon. The bladder neck is marked for reference. A vaginal incision is made in an inverted-U fashion with a wide-based flap and into the lateral sulci to permit the later use of a Martius flap, if needed. Further dissection is done sharply with Metzenbaum scissors. It is critical for the dissection to leave enough tissue to avoid thinning the flap and cause devascularization as well as to avoid entering the diverticulum. Bipolar cautery can be judiciously used to control small bleeders. Dissection continues until the level of the bladder neck. Once the diverticulum is identified, a transverse incision is made overlying it just through the endopelvic and endocervical fascia, and flaps are created in both cranial and caudal directions. The diverticulum is visible with a light blue hue and dissected circumferentially until it is defined in all planes. At this point, the diverticulum is opened in order to better appreciate its borders and avoid entry into the urethra. A lacrimal duct probe can be used to identify the os. Manipulating the Foley catheter can bring fluid into the diverticulum to assist in locating the position of the os. If the os is noted to be in a challenging position, consideration can be made to placing a stay suture to better identify the location for later closure. Once the diverticulum is traced back to the os, it is truncated at that point. We always send the diverticulum as a specimen for pathologic analysis. Interrupted 4/0 absorbable sutures are placed to close the os. The flaps created previously can be closed with 4/0 absorbable sutures with a vest over pants, or pants over vest technique. Care needs to be taken when placing these sutures

to avoid devascularization of the flaps. Over this flap, a Martius flap can be rotated in from either labia majora if the patient has a history of radiation or notably poor tissue quality. The vaginal closure is performed with 2/0 interrupted absorbable sutures and a vaginal packing is left in place overnight. The catheter is left in for 2 to 3 weeks (Video 1).

Urethral Stricture

We prefer the dorsal onlay buccal mucosal graft although some might argue it is a more difficult approach. The risk of sexual dysfunction with this dissection is low, as the plane of dissection is well away from neurovascular clitoral structures. Leaving the ventral plane untouched is useful for a possible continence procedure in the future if indicated. In addition, a dorsal fixation helps prevent sacculation of the graft. We harvest, clean, and fenestrate a 4 × 2cm buccal mucosal graft in the standard fashion. Urethral length is relatively constant, so these graft dimensions are generally sufficient even if the stricture is panurethral. A semilunar, suprameatal incision is made. Careful dissection is carried outside the corpus spongiosum until healthy urethra is encountered. We typically open the meatus; however, an alternate meatus-sparing technique is also acceptable. The dissection may be carried out to the bladder neck when necessary without fear of de novo stress urinary incontinence. The graft is sewn in with delayed absorbable suture; we favor 4-0 PDS. Several quilting sutures of 5-0 Vicryl are placed. We ensure patency to 30 Fr with intraoperative bougie-à-boule. A 14 french silicone catheter is left in place for 3 weeks (Video 2).

Vesico-Vaginal Fistula

For most fistula, we prefer the vaginal approach. When possible the fistula is cannulated with either a 5 Fr ureteral catheter, a wire, or ideally a Fogarty balloon or small foley to aid in identification and manipulation. We start with a U-shaped incision the apex of which is at the fistula and develop a vaginal flap, taking care to preserve the periurethral fascia. Once we encounter the fistula, we dissect and widely mobilize it. Typically, we will excise the tract and send it for pathology. The bladder is then closed in 2 layers and inner running and outer interrupted layer with 4-0 absorbable suture. Based on the quality of the surrounding tissues and fistula cause, a Martius flap may or may not be used. Typically, in radiated patients or redo cases, we recommend the interposition of a Martius flap, which is usually available. The Martius flap is raised based on the upper or lower vascular pedicle depending on the position of the fistula and the patient's anatomy. If the Martius flap is insufficient or not available, other flaps such as peritoneal, omental, or a gracilis interposition flap may be used. The repair is leak tested. The vaginal incision is then closed interrupted 2-0 Vicryl. A 14 Fr silicone catheter is left in place for 2 to 4 weeks. If a suprapubic catheter was present, this is also left in situ for maximal bladder drainage.

For complex, high, or recurrent fistula, an abdominal approach may be used. We prefer a minimally invasive robotic-assisted transvesical approach in these cases. Similar to the vaginal approach, the fistula is cannulated whenever possible. Temporary external ureteral catheters may be placed if the fistula is near the ureteral orifices. The bladder is opened at the posterior dome and the fistula is identified. It is widely mobilized, and the tract is sent for pathology. The vagina is closed with 3-0 or 4-0 absorbable suture, and the bladder is similarly closed, in 1 or 2 layers avoiding overlapping suture lines. The cystotomy is finally closed with running 3-0 or 4-0 suture. The repair is leak tested. A 14 Fr silicone catheter is left in place for 2 to 4 weeks.

Excellent videos of both the vaginal[5] and abdominal approach to VVF[15] are available in a prior volume of Urologic Clinics of North America (Volume 46, Issue 1).

RECOVERY AND REHABILITATION

Recovery from urethroplasty for FUS is generally brief. Minor stress incontinence may be encountered initially, however this generally resolves. In our institution, this is an outpatient surgery. We do leave a small labial drain for 1 to 2 days if a Martius flap was harvested. We usually leave a vaginal packing in place, which will be removed within the first 24 hours postop. We discharge patients with pain medication as needed and also anticholinergic medication to help with bladder spasms. Unless the patient had recurrent urinary tract infection (UTI), we do not provide antibiotics during the catheterization period.

Most patients are seen in the office for a wound check within 1 week, and the catheter is removed between 2 and 4 weeks depending on the procedure performed. Voiding cysto urethrogram (VCUG) or cystogram, as appropriate, is performed in most cases prior to catheter removal. Any relevant pathology results are reviewed.

OUTCOMES
Urethral Diverticulum

Interestingly, some authors propose classification of urethral diverticulum into simple or complex in order to predict their postoperative outcomes. Complex FUD are those extending partially or circumferentially around the urethra. In their series, Nickles and colleagues[41] showed that patients with complex FUD were most likely to present postoperatively with urinary tract symptoms (27% vs 3%) compared with patients following reconstruction for simple FUD. In a different study, Ko and colleagues[42] published an overall cure rate with surgery of 77.9% but when the different FUD were broken down into simple, U-shaped, and circumferential, their cure rates were 100%, 75.0%, and 64.0%, respectively. This demonstrates that successful surgical outcomes in these patients have a direct correlation with anatomic complexity, a very important point for patient counseling.

Regarding complications, the most commonly reported are urethrovaginal fistula, de novo stress urinary incontinence, urethral strictures, recurrent UTIs, and recurrence of the diverticulum.[4] One study showed that the most common pathologic finding was squamous metaplasia (31%) and also reported a 2.5% malignancy rate (adenocarcinoma) within their FUD specimens,[27] which is consistent with other malignancy reports (2%) found in the literature.[31]

Finally, there is currently no data showing a well-documented comparison regarding different surgical approaches for FUD. In the future, a proper randomized controlled trial comparing success and complication rates with each treatment would be useful to help guide practice.

Urethral Stricture

The goals for urethral reconstruction in women are to restore function, urinate without obstruction, maintain continence, prevent vaginal voiding, and maintain sexual function. Although these goals are considered an ideal scenario, there is a dearth of literature considering all 5 variables when analyzing outcomes. Much of the available literature regarding FUS has been published within the last 5 years. The most common management is urethral dilation (UD) although its success rate ranges up to 49%,[11,43] with success defined as the lack of need for further intervention. The mean time to failure was 12 months in one study.[44] In our practice, we follow the same principle as in male patients with no more than one attempt at UD given the poor outcomes of repeated dilations (30%), unless the patient is not a surgical candidate.[45]

There is no statistical difference in terms of success rate among reconstructive options. Both reconstructive surgeries using flaps and grafts have proven to be equally safe and efficacious.[46,47] Success rates using flap urethroplasty were 92% with a mean follow-up of 42 months, whereas success rates with BMG graft urethroplasty were 89% with a mean follow-up of 19 months and 87% with vaginal graft urethroplasty with a mean follow-up of 15 months according to a recent systematic review.[11]

Acceptable complication rates were reported with flap procedures, with only 3.7% de novo SUI noted.[11] Furthermore, in patients with concomitant SUI, a pubovaginal sling could be placed without major morbidity. Where to place the graft still remains a controversy, with some authors advocating to place it dorsally, whereas others opine it should be placed ventrally. There is no data available supporting one over the other so, ultimately, it remains at the surgeon's discretion. Finally, de novo SUI was found to be similar in both approaches (3.6% with a dorsal approach vs 5.8% with a ventral approach).[11]

Vesico-Vaginal Fistula

Traditionally, the classic strategy has always been to repair within 1 week of injury or after a delay of 3 to 6 months to allow for healing of the traumatized tissue. Studies have shown that early repairs have similar rates of success as delayed ones.[48] When a delayed approach is selected, the surgeon must optimize preoperative patient factors such as nutrition, urinary drainage, and skincare. If there is a recurrence, data suggest that a revision VVF repair is less successful, highlighting that generally, the best chance of fistula closure is at the time of the first operation.[13]

VVF can be repaired via a vaginal approach or an abdominal approach. To date, there are no randomized controlled trials comparing the route of repair, so the decision is up to the surgeon's preference. Typically, simple VVF will be approached vaginally first, as the vaginal approach has demonstrated significantly shorter operative times, decreased blood loss, and a shorter duration of hospitalization.[15] Another advantage to the vaginal approach is that it can be done as an outpatient. However, in complex VVF or redo cases, an abdominal approach may be preferred. The estimated success rate of transvaginal repair ranges from 83% to 100%, whereas the overall success rate of laparoscopic/robotic VVF repairs was 80% to 100%.[5] Tissue interposition is advantageous in some cases. In our practice, we use a Martius flap if approached vaginally when necessary but other tissues such as omentum or a peritoneal flap have been described as well. The utilization of minimally invasive techniques has significantly improved recovery times in these cases.

We agree with Lee and colleagues[5] that heterogeneity of the fistula (size, location) and the occasional use of an interposition graft makes treatment standardization very difficult.

SUMMARY

Urethral reconstruction in women is an evolving art that bases its principles on excellent knowledge of vaginal, urethral, and pelvic anatomy. Reconstructive surgeons eager to manage this type of pathologic condition require the right skillset and armamentarium in order to find an appropriate solution for their patients. Oftentimes, the diagnosis will be delayed and in the context of a suffering patient with truly bothersome symptoms such as urinary leakage, recurrent UTIs, dyspareunia, dysuria, voiding and storage symptoms. Managing patient expectations is crucial. The most important consideration when approaching these patients is to follow basic reconstructive surgical principles such as adequate exposure, broad mobilization, gentle handling of tissue, tension-free closure, and satisfactory hemostasis. Finally, in complex cases, it is always a wise option to refer these patients to an experienced specialized center for definitive management.

CONFLICTS OF INTEREST

Dr J. DeLong is a consultant for Urotronic, Inc. and for Urovant. Dr I. Alvarez de Toledo has no conflicts to report.

SUPPLEMENTARY DATA

Supplementary data related to this article can be found online at https://doi.org/10.1016/j.ucl.2022.04.004.

REFERENCES

1. Nitti VW, Tu LM, Gitlin J. Diagnosing bladder outlet obstruction in women. J Urol 1999;161:1535.
2. Blaivas JG, Groutz A. Bladder outlet obstruction nomogram for women with lower urinary tract symptomatology. Neurourol Urodyn 2000;19:553.
3. Blaivas JG, Santos JA, Tsui JF, et al. Management of urethral stricture in women. J Urol 2012;188(5):1778–82.
4. Bodner-Adler B, Halpern K, Hanzal E. Surgical management of urethral diverticula in women: a systematic review. Int Urogynecol J 2016;27:993–1001.
5. Lee D, Zimmern P. Vaginal approach to vesicovaginal fistula. Urol Clin North Am 2019;46:123–33.
6. Smith AL, Ferlise VJ, Rovner ES. Female urethral strictures: successful management with long-term

clean intermittent catheterization after urethral dilatation. BJU Int 2006;98(1):96–9.

7. Rovner ES. Bladder and female urethral diverticula, . Campbell-Walsh Urology. 11th edition. Philadelphia, PA: Elsevier; 2016. p. 2140–68.

8. Keegan KA, Nanigian DK, Stone AR. Female urethral stricture disease. Curr Urol Rep 2008;9(5):419–23.

9. Desai S, Libertino JA, Zinman L. Primary carcinoma of the female urethra. J Urol 1973;110(6):693–5.

10. Indudhara R, Vaidyanathan S, Radotra BD. Urethral tuberculosis. Urol Int 1992;48(4):436–8.

11. Sarin I, Narain TA, Panwar VK, et al. Deciphering the enigma of female urethral strictures: a systematic review and meta-analysis of management modalities. Neurourol Urodyn 2021;40:65–79.

12. Huffman JW. The detailed anatomy of the paraurethral ducts in the adult human female. Am J Obstet Gynecol 1948;55:86–101.

13. Wall LL. Obstetric vesicovaginal fistula as an international public-health problem. Lancet 2006;368: 1201–9.

14. Goodwin WE, Scardino PT. Vesicovaginal and ureterovaginal fistulas: A Summary of 25 years of experience. J Urol 1980;123:370–4.

15. McKay E, Watts K, Abraham N. Abdominal approach to vesicovaginal fistula. Urol Clin N Am 2019;46:135–46.

16. Romanzi LJ, Groutz A, Blaivas JG. Urethral diverticulum in women: diverse presentations resulting in diagnostic delay and mismanagement. J Urol 2000;164(2):428–33.

17. Blaivas JG, Flisser AJ, Bleustein CB, et al. Periurethral masses: etiology and diagnosis in a large series of women. Obstet Gynecol 2004;103(5 Pt 1): 842–7.

18. Ockrim JL, Allen DJ, Shah PJ, et al. A tertiary experience of urethral diverticulectomy: diagnosis, imaging and surgical outcomes. BJU Int 2009;103(11): 1550–4.

19. Baradaran N, Chiles LR, Freilich DA, et al. Female Urethral Diverticula in the Contemporary Era: Is the Classic Triad of the "3Ds" Still Relevant? Urology 2016;94:53–6.

20. Kuo HC. Clinical symptoms are not reliable in the diagnosis of lower urinary tract dysfunction in women. J Formos Med Assoc 2012;111:386–91.

21. Agochukwu-Mmonu N, Srirangapatnam S, Cohen A, et al. Female urethral strictures: review of diagnosis, etiology, and management. Curr Urol Rep 2019; 20(11):74.

22. Kalra S, Gupta P, Dorairajan L, et al. Does successful urethral calibration rule out significant female urethral stenosis? confronting the confounder- an outcome analysis of successfully treated female urethral strictures. Int Braz J Urol 2021;47:829–40.

23. West C, Lawrence A. Female urethroplasty: contemporary thinking. World J Urol 2019;37:619–29.

24. Itani M, Kielar A, Menias CO, et al. MRI of female urethra and periurethral pathologies. Int Urogynecol J 2016;27(2):195–204.

25. Crescenze IM, Goldman HB. Female Urethral Diverticulum: Current Diagnosis and Management. Curr Urol Rep 2015;16(10):71.

26. Mistry MA, Klarskov N, DeLancey JO, et al. A structured review on the female urethral anatomy and innervation with an emphasis on the role of the urethral longitudinal smooth muscle. Int Urogynecol J 2020;31(1):63–71.

27. Pincus JB, Laudano M, Leegant A, et al. Female Urethral Diverticula: Diagnosis, Pathology, and Surgical Outcomes at an Academic, Urban Medical Center. Urology 2019;128:42–6.

28. Aldamanhori R, Inman R. The treatment of complex female urethral pathology. Asian J Urol 2018;5(3): 160–3.

29. Mozafarpour S, Nwaoha N, Pucheril D, et al. Robotic assisted proximal dorsal urethral diverticulectomy. Int Urogynecol J 2021;32(10):2863–6.

30. Juang CM, Horng HC, Yu HC, et al. Combined diverticulectomy and anti-incontinence surgery for patients with urethral diverticulum and stress urinary incontinence: is anti-incontinence surgery really necessary? Taiwan J Obstet Gynecol 2006;45(1):67–9.

31. Reeves FA, Inman RD, Chapple CR. Management of symptomatic urethral diverticula in women: a single-center experience. Eur Urol 2014;66(1):164–72.

32. Heidari F, Abbaszadeh S, Ghadian A, et al. On demand urethral dilatation versus intermittent urethral dilatation: results and complications in women with urethral stricture. Nephrourol Mon 2014;6(2): e15212.

33. Önol FF, Antar B, Köse O, et al. Techniques and results of urethroplasty for female urethral strictures: our experience with 17 patients. Urology 2011; 77(6):1318–24.

34. Romero-Maroto J, Verdú-Verdú L, Gómez-Pérez L, et al. Lateral-based anterior vaginal wall flap in the treatment of female urethral stricture: efficacy and safety. Eur Urol 2018;73(1):123–8.

35. Sharma GK, Pandey A, Bansal H, et al. Dorsal onlay lingual mucosal graft urethroplasty for urethral strictures in women. BJU Int 2010;105(9):1309–12.

36. Stamatakos M, Sargedi C, Stasinou T, et al. Vesicovaginal fistula: diagnosis and management. Indian J Surg 2014;76:131–6.

37. Fouad LS, Chen AH, Santoni CJ, et al. Revisiting Conservative Management of Vesicovaginal Fistula. J Minim Invasive Gynecol 2017;24(4):514–5.

38. Malik MA, Sohail M, Malik MT, et al. Changing trends in the etiology and management of vesicovaginal fistula. Int J Urol 2018;25(1):25–9.

39. Lin KJ, Fan YH, Lin AT. Role of urodynamics in management of urethral diverticulum in females. J Chin Med Assoc 2017;80(11):712–6.

40. Waterloos M, Verla W. Female Urethroplasty: A Practical Guide Emphasizing Diagnosis and Surgical Treatment of Female Urethral Stricture Disease. Biomed Res Int 2019;2019:6715257.

41. Nickles SW, Ikwuezunma G, MacLachlan L, et al. Simple vs complex urethral diverticulum: presentation and outcomes. Urology 2014;84(6):1516–9.

42. Ko KJ, Suh YS, Kim TH, et al. Surgical Outcomes of Primary and Recurrent Female Urethral Diverticula. Urology 2017;105:181–5.

43. Osman NI, Mangera A, Chapple CR. A systematic review of surgical techniques used in the treatment of female urethral stricture. Eur Urol 2013;64(6):965–73.

44. Romman AN, Alhalabi F, Zimmern PE. Distal intramural urethral pathology in women. J Urol 2012; 188:1218–23.

45. Popat S, Zimmern PE. Long-term management of luminal urethral stricture in women. Int Urogynecol J 2016;27(11):1735–41.

46. Kowalik C, Stoffel JT, Zinman L, et al. Intermediate outcomes after female urethral reconstruction: graft vs flap. Urology 2014;83(5):1181–5.

47. Lane GI, Smith AL, Stambakio H, et al. Treatment of urethral stricture disease in women: a multi-institutional collaborative project from the SUFU research network. Neurourol Urodyn 2020;39(8): 2433–41.

48. Blandy JP, Badenoch DF, Fowler CG, et al. Early repair of iatrogenic injury to the ureter or bladder after gynecological surgery. J Urol 1991;146(3):761–5.

Male Stress Urinary Incontinence

George E. Koch, MD*, Melissa R. Kaufman, MD, PhD

KEYWORDS

- Stress incontinence ● Incontinence after prostate treatment ● Artificial urinary sphincter ● Male sling
- Adjustable balloon

KEY POINTS

- The artificial urinary sphincter remains the gold standard for male stress urinary incontinence for its efficacy and durability in both nonirradiated and irradiated patients.
- Male slings and adjustable balloon devices offer a passive mechanism of action that may be desirable for select, nonirradiated patients.
- Persistent and recurrent incontinence following artificial urinary sphincter placement poses a potentially complex conundrum and should be evaluated thoroughly and thoughtfully.
- Evaluation and treatment of men with stress urinary incontinence is becoming more nuanced with the growing landscape of prostate treatment modalities and may require more sophisticated strategies in the future.

INTRODUCTION

Stress urinary incontinence (SUI) is the involuntary loss of urine on effort or physical exertion.[1] In men, SUI is primarily due to inadequate outlet resistance, often as a result of iatrogenic interventions that impair the innervation or structural components of the internal and external urethral sphincters. The goal of surgical intervention for male SUI is to regain social continence by increasing the patient's outlet resistance.

SUI following treatment of benign prostatic hyperplasia (BPH) and prostate cancer (PCa) represent the most common scenarios for male SUI; however, SUI secondary to trauma, iatrogenic injuries, and neurologic disorders are also frequently encountered. Selecting the appropriate treatment for each patient should consider their level of continence, the mechanism of their lower urinary tract dysfunction, and shared decision-making to define personal goals of care.[2]

NATURE OF THE PROBLEM AND ITS DIAGNOSIS

Diagnosis and management of male SUI continue to evolve in complexity with the expansion of treatment modalities for BPH and indications for radiation in PCa. Therefore, clinicians need to be meticulous in the characterization of the severity and symptoms of a patient's incontinence. Severity can be explored by focusing on objective measures of incontinence, such as the number and type of pads used per day (PPD), and the specific maneuvers that lead to leakage. The type of pad being used and its level of saturation when changed are key parameters but vary widely and should be considered in the context of the bother level and treatment desires of the individual.

Signs of primary urgency incontinence should be ruled out. Determining the contribution and association of storage dysfunction manifesting as urgency, frequency, and urgency incontinence,

Department of Urology, Vanderbilt University Medical Center, 1211 Medical Center Drive, Nashville, TN 37215, USA

* Corresponding author. Vanderbilt University Medical Center, 1161 21st Ave., South A-1302 Medical Center North Nashville, TN 37232-2765.

E-mail address: George.e.koch@vumc.org

urologic.theclinics.com

particularly in irradiated patients, is critical to selecting the appropriate therapy. Inquiring about supine leakage may uncover storage dysfunction not described during daily activities. Pad weights, voiding diaries, and urodynamics can all be used to supplement a complex history and should be used when there is doubt about the character of a patient's incontinence.[3,4] A detailed medical history should include evaluation of health literacy, neurologic dysfunction, infectious conditions, and diabetes. A surgical history should inform the surgeon of past abdominal, inguinal, and perineal surgeries, especially previous hernia repairs with mesh and urologic prosthetics.

A focused physical exam is mandated to assess the patient's incontinence during stress maneuvers and manual dexterity, as well as to evaluate the groin, perineal and genital skin for surgical scarring, and signs of cutaneous infection, inflammation, or chemical irritation. Cystoscopy both rules out a variety of pathologies that should be managed before embarking on surgical therapies for incontinence and also allows for the evaluation of sphincteric tone and control. **Fig. 1** shows an example algorithm for SUI diagnosis and management.

NONOPERATIVE MANAGEMENT

Counseling the patient with SUI should always include a discussion about nonoperative interventions. Pelvic floor muscle exercises (PFME) and pelvic floor muscle training (PFMT) are the mainstays of nonoperative treatment. These exercises consist of training patients to strengthen and coordinate the fast-twitch skeletal muscles of the levator ani to volitionally increase outlet resistance. Exercises can be done alone (PFME), or in one-on-one training sessions with a physical therapist (PFMT). Patients are encouraged to complete at least four sets of 10 to 20 repetitions of each exercise daily.[5] PFME/PFMT is recommended to decrease the time to continence within 1 year of radical prostatectomy, although the studies of PFME/PFPT are limited by protocol and outcome heterogeneity.[2] For patients who continue to have bothersome incontinence outside of this window, PFME/PFMT have not demonstrated durable benefit. Following a transurethral resection of the prostate, PFME/PFMT has not been shown to improve continence rates or time to continence.[5]

Incontinence clamps, external devices that increase outlet resistance by compressing the penile urethra, may be offered to patients who cannot, or prefer not to, undergo a surgical procedure. Patient counseling regarding external clamp usage is key. Evaluation of penile perfusion

demonstrated that devices can be safely worn for up to an hour, followed by an hour of recovery time. However, the effects of longer application have not been studied.[6] Patients therefore must possess the understanding and dexterity to apply and remove these devices appropriately. Both quantitative and qualitative studies have shown incontinence clamps to be effective for stopping urine leakage, but patient comfort varies by device design.[7]

ADJUSTABLE BALLOON DEVICES

Adjustable balloon devices (ABDs) mark the newest surgical technology available for male SUI. The ProACT system, currently approved for use in the United States, consists of two paired silicone balloons placed percutaneously through the perineum along either side of the bladder neck with tubing that extends into the subcutaneous tissues of the scrotum for in-office adjustments.[8] ABDs passively apply coapting pressure on the bladder neck and represent a minimally invasive surgical option for SUI. The passive mechanism offers improvement of continence without the need for device manipulation by the patient, and the ability to adjust the balloon volume in the office allows the urologist to tailor the device to patient continence.

ABDs have demonstrated up to 81.9% success in nonirradiated patients with mild incontinence following prostate treatment, defined as at least 50% improvement in leakage.[2,9] However, given this narrow indication, they are not commonly offered. When extended to patients with prior radiation, ABDs display treatment failure rates as high as 83% coupled with an increased rate of urethral erosion.[10] Subsequent studies have also demonstrated diminished success: 48.8% with at least 50% improvement in leakage, for patients with neurogenic SUI, coupled with a 58.3% complication rate.[11]

Procedural Approach

The key to the successful placement of ABDs is limiting overdissection around the bladder neck and ensuring easy access to the adjustment port under the scrotal skin.

On the day of surgery, patients should undergo one final screen for cutaneous, urinary, and systemic infection. If there is concern for infection, implant surgery should be postponed. This principle should be implemented for all male stress incontinence procedures. Preoperative antibiosis is achieved with weight-based cefazolin, culture-directed antibiotics for prior positive cultures, or dependent on the local antibiogram.

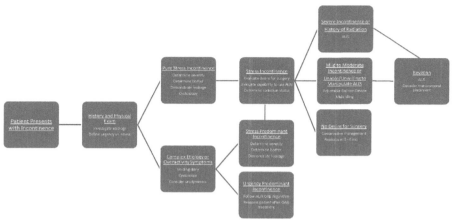

Fig. 1. Sample male stress incontinence algorithm.

For placement of ABDs, male slings, and artificial urinary sphincters (AUS), positioning remains the same, with the patient in high-lithotomy. Care should be taken to ensure that the bony prominences of the spine and lower extremities are well padded to avoid injury and neuropraxia. The hips and knees are flexed to a less than 90°angle to safeguard against nerve or vessel impingement and the bed is moved to a slight Trendelenburg position, 30°above the horizon. A rolled blanket under the sacrum can improve the sightline into the pelvis further. The patient is then prepped with a chlorhexidine gluconate scrub followed by an alcohol-based chlorhexidine prep.

Balloon implantation begins with rigid cystoscopy to confirm urethral patency and ensure no pathology has emerged since diagnostic screening. The bladder is then emptied and refilled with contrast to ensure good visualization of the bladder neck fluoroscopically. The cystoscope with a blind obturator remains in the urethra and bladder.

Through a stab incision, 3 cm below the scrotum and 2 cm laterally, the blunt insertion trocar and sheath are advanced fluoroscopically to the bladder neck. Meticulous placement ensures the trocar is parallel to the cystoscope. If the blunt trocar cannot pierce the pelvic floor, a sharp trocar may be used. The obturator is replaced by a grasper, which is opened to bluntly dissect a pocket for the adjustable balloon just lateral to the bladder neck. The adjustable balloon and preloaded guidewire are advanced to the pocket through the sheath fluoroscopically. The balloon is filled with 0.5 to 1.5 cc of isotonic contrast solution, and the sheath is removed. The procedure is repeated contralaterally.

A retrograde urethrogram ensures that the ABDs are compressing the bladder neck and rules out urethral injury before the guidewires are removed. Finally, two subcutaneous tracts are tunneled from the perineal incisions to the inferolateral scrotum and the adjustment port is placed into this space. Incisions are closed in two layers and a 12 Fr urethral catheter is placed, typically to be removed on postoperative day 1.

Follow-Up Adjustments

Patients may require up to 5 in-office adjustments before reaching social continence. Adjustments are performed by inserting a 23-gauge noncoring needle into the adjustment port to add or remove 1 cc of normal saline. The adjustment port is rated for up to 45 needle punctures and each balloon for up to 8 cc.

Adjustable Balloon Device Outcomes

A 2019 meta-analysis demonstrated good functional outcomes for ABDs although paired with relatively high complication rates compared with male slings and AUS.[9] Pooled efficacy data demonstrated improvements in mean pad usage from 4.0 to 1.1 PPD. Sixty percent of patients reported complete continence with another 21.7% reporting at least 50% improvement in leakage. Patients also displayed 66.2% improvement in quality-of-life scores.

These positive outcomes should be weighed against high complication rates and limited long-term experience. Intraoperative urethral and bladder perforations occurred in 5.3% of procedures whereas subsequent device erosions were seen in 3.8% of patients and balloon migration in another 6.5%. The pooled overall revision rate was 22.2%. Device durability also remains debatable. A 2019 study of 240 patients who underwent adjustable balloon implantation demonstrated that the rate of at least 50% improvement in continence dropped to 67.1% at 24 months.

MALE SLINGS

Male slings are indicated for mild-to-moderate SUI, preferentially in the nonradiated patient. There are two current male sling designs on the US market. The Advance XP sling utilizes a double-armed transobturator mesh that repositions the bulbar urethra proximally, lengthening the functional membranous urethra and optimizing the patient's native sphincteric tone while theoretically avoiding significant urethral compression.[12] This is contrasted to the four-armed Virtue sling that repositions the bulbar urethra with transobturator arms while also compressing the distal urethra with arms affixed to the inferior pubic rami.[13] Given the less-established evidence base for the Virtue sling, the technical descriptions of implantation below apply only to the Advance XP sling.

Patient selection remains an essential component to male sling success. Although most reports of male sling implantation exclude previously radiated patients, smaller series that included irradiated patients demonstrated far inferior outcomes.[14,15] However, though outcomes are less impressive compared with the AUS, Kumar and colleagues demonstrated that patients remain more likely to choose a sling due to its passive mechanism of action.[16] The lack of required manipulation makes the sling an option for men with suboptimal neuromuscular coordination as well as for men with cognitive barriers to AUS use. These should be clinical considerations when counseling patients between active and passive continence implants and may justify a male sling for select irradiated patients.

Procedural Approach

The key to successful sling placement includes safe passage of the trocar at the inferomedial border of the obturator foramen and adequate but not excessive bulbar urethral mobilization.

After draping, a 14 to 16 Fr urethral catheter is placed to empty the bladder via suction and then plugged. Before incision, 5 cc of 0.5% bupivacaine may be infiltrated just medial to the ischial tuberosity bilaterally as a pudendal block.

A 5 to 6 cm longitudinal incision in the median raphe of the perineum is made, centered at the turn of the bulbar urethra (**Fig. 2**). A self-retaining retractor with dull hooks is used for exposure as the bulbospongiosus muscle is cleared off and then split sharply down the middle. Hooks should be adjusted dynamically to ensure adequate exposure. Alternatively, for a patient with a particularly

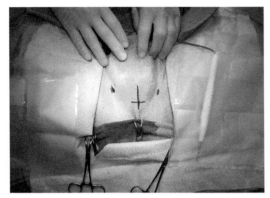

Fig. 2. Perineal incision centered over the bulbar urethra and stab incisions marked inferior to the tendonous insertion of the adductor longus on the pelvis.

deep perineum, a circumferential wound retractor can be used in place of, or in addition to, a self-retaining retractor.

The plane between the muscle and the corpus spongiosum is developed laterally but not circumferentially. The central tendon is identified and a 4 to 0 absorbable suture is placed on the urethral origin to identify the most proximal location for the sling. The needle is left hanging to facilitate later fixation to the sling. Transection of the origin of the central perineal tendon is performed sharply and slowly, with small excursions to allow mobilization of the urethra only 2 cm proximal to its original position. Complete transection may result in urethral hypermobility and worsening incontinence.

The bladder should be emptied before trocar passage to avoid injury. The edge of the obturator foramen can be localized with a spinal needle to determine the optimal entry point for the helical trocars. A stab incision is made 1 to 2 cm below the tendinous insertion of the adductor longus on the pelvis, and the tip of the helical trocar is placed into this incision with the handle 45° lateral to the midline (**Fig. 3**). The tip is advanced cranially, and two distinct "pops" should be felt as the tip pierces the obturator internus and the obturator membrane along the inferomedial border of the obturator foramen. This ensures that the trocar is well away from the neurovascular bundle in the superolateral corner.

On the right side, once the tip is through the obturator foramen, the trocar handle is simultaneously rotated counterclockwise while its angle is dropped medially to the midline to be perpendicular to the floor. As the surgeon's right hand manipulates the trocar, the left hand protects the urethra by keeping it firmly on the dorsal aspect of the fingers while the index finger pad feels for

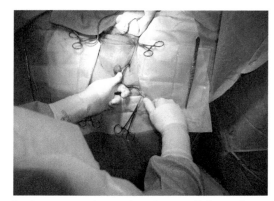

Fig. 3. Trocar with initial angle 45° off the midline.

the trocar tip. The tip of the trocar should appear at the angle created by the urethra and the ipsilateral corporal body. If the trocar tip meets resistance against the inferior pubic ramus, the tip should be withdrawn, and the obturator foramen reentered slightly more inferior and lateral. The mesh sling is then secured to the trocar tip and drawn into the perineal wound as the trocar is withdrawn along the same path it was inserted. Trocar and sling placement are then repeated contralaterally. Notably, on the left side, the trocar is rotated clockwise and the surgeon's hands are switched. Once both sling arms and sheaths are retracted out of the inguinal incisions, the trocars can be removed.

The saddle of the sling is then secured to the corpus spongiosum using three 4 to 0 absorbable sutures, one in each of the superior corners of the saddle and the third in the inferior center, using the suture placed at the origin of the common perineal tendon (**Fig. 4**). By ensuring the sling is secured at the distalmost portion of the common perineal tendon, the surgeon safeguards against securing the sling too proximally on the spongiosum.

The catheter is removed and flexible cystoscopy is undertaken to rule out urethral or bladder injury and assist with appropriate sling tensioning. With the cystoscope observing the external sphincter, the sling is tensioned by gentle traction on the mesh arms at the groin incisions with the vector of effort toward the ceiling. Proper tensioning improves coaptation of the external urethral sphincter with very mild urethral compression. Once the desired tension is achieved, the sling arms are cut at the appropriate location to allow the sheath to be withdrawn, leaving only the mesh sling in situ. The mesh in the groin incisions is then trimmed at the skin. The groin incisions can be closed with surgical adhesive only, the perineal incision should be closed in three layers to reapproximate muscle and close all dead space.

Finally, the 14 to 16 Fr catheter is replaced, to be removed on postoperative day 1.

Male Sling Outcomes

Long-term efficacy of the Advance XP male sling has proven encouraging. In a cohort of 59 patients followed for 5 years, 83% were found to be either cured (57.6%) or improved by at least 50% (25.4%) as seen in **Table 1**.[17] These results may even underestimate the sling's efficacy, as much of the long-term data was produced with a prior version of the sling, the Advance, which did not have the Advance XP's chevron anchors to improve arm fixation. In patients stratified by incontinence severity, patients with mild, moderate, and severe incontinence were found to have success rates of 65%, 62%, and 47% respectively at a median of 5.7 years.[18] These studies demonstrate both the relative long-term durability of slings as well as the decreasing efficacy for more severe incontinence. Radiotherapy prior to male sling implantation has demonstrated inferior outcomes and durability with long-term complete continence rates of 25.0%.[15]

Regarding complications, multiple large series report pain (3%–8%), urinary retention (10%–16.7%), and perioperative infections (0.9%–3%) as the main perioperative and short-term complications.[14,15,18,19] In 426 patients undergoing Advance or Advance XP male sling placement, urinary retention was seen in 48 of 426 (14.1%) patients.[20] Retention resolved following short-term catheterization in 42 of 48 (76.3%) with four of the six remaining patients electing intermittent catheterization and two electing mesh excision. Rates of "de-novo" overactive bladder (OAB) requiring treatment ranged from 1.8% to 11%, with interventions including oral medications, chemical denervation and, rarely, mesh excision.[19] Regarding sling durability, at a follow-up of at least 24 months, 12.4% to 24% of patients had been offered a second anti-incontinence procedure.[18,19]

CLINICS CARE POINTS

- Patients should be counseled that adjustable balloon devices and male slings do not have long-term outcomes data comparable to the artificial urinary sphincter.
- Carefully selected patients who may not be ideal artificial urinary sphincter candidates

due to mental or physical limitations may be offered adjustable balloons or male slings after appropriate counseling on risks and expectations.

ARTIFICIAL URINARY SPHINCTER

The AUS is the gold standard therapy for male SUI and is the only guideline-recommended treatment of both severe incontinence and SUI in irradiated patients.[2] The AMS 800, manufactured by Boston Scientific, is the most commonly implanted AUS and consists of three components: the urethral cuff, the pressure regulating balloon (PRB), and the scrotal pump. At rest, fluid fills the urethral cuff resulting in occlusion via circumferential pressure. When the scrotal pump, which lies in series between the cuff and the PRB, is cycled, it pumps fluid into the PRB against its native pressure gradient, thereby drawing fluid out of the urethral cuff. The PRB then passively empties fluid back into the urethral cuff via the scrotal pump as it returns to its resting pressure.[21]

Patient selection for an AUS is absolutely key to the procedure's success. First, although the AUS is the only guideline endorsed surgical option for irradiated patients, revision is more likely in this setting even though continence rates and patient satisfaction remain high.[22] Further, given both the dexterity required to cycle the device and the patient health literacy needed to appropriately use the device, AUS patient selection must evaluate a number of nonurologic criteria.[23]

Preoperative antibiotics include coverage of both gram-positive and gram-negative pathogens, typically with weight-based vancomycin and gentamicin, ideally with complete infusion 1 hour before incision. A 12 Fr catheter and pudendal block are completed as above. The corpus spongiosum is exposed after opening of the bulbospongiosus muscle in the same manner as for a sling, without incising the common perineal tendon. Sharp dissection is facilitated posteriorly by identifying the groove deep to the spongiosum

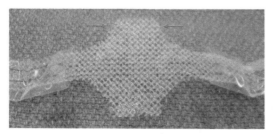

Fig. 4. Arrows denote the location of fixation sutures.

(**Fig. 5**). The space is further widened to 2 cm to accommodate the cuff and should be at or proximal to the confluence of the corporal bodies for optimal bulk of spongiosum (**Fig. 6**).

The circumference of the spongiosum is next measured with the supplied measuring tape. A proper measurement should be snug around the spongiosum without indentation of the tissue below the measuring tape (**Fig. 7**). The appropriate cuff size is rounded up to the nearest half centimeter. While the cuff is being prepped, the measuring tape is left in place and the perineal incision is packed with an antibiotic soaked gauze.

A 4 cm transverse right lower quadrant incision is made along the crease between the abdominal and suprapubic fat pads and carried down to the fascia of the anterior rectus sheath. Before opening the fascia, the bladder is emptied to protect it from injury. The fascia is incised and the underlying rectus muscle split. A pocket is bluntly created under the rectus muscle. Several 0 absorbable interrupted fascial stitches are preplaced, and then the PRB is placed into the pocket. The vast majority of implants use 61 to 70 cm H_2O PRB. The fascial closing stitches are tied down and the balloon is filled with 23 cc of normal saline.

To place the scrotal pump, a ringed forceps is gently inserted into the right lower quadrant incision and passed through fat and areolar tissue to the dependent scrotum, ensuring that the channel is uniformly 1 to 2 cm below the skin. Once in the scrotum, the instrument is tracked so that the final pocket is superficial enough for easy pump manipulation. The pump is then passed into this pocket and secured in place with a babcock clamp on the scrotal skin. If the scrotal skin is violated in this process, resite the pump and close the wound in three layers.

The gauze is removed from the perineal incision, as is the measuring tape, placing a right-angle clamp into the space behind the corpus spongiosum with the pass starting on the side of the PRB. The right angle is then used to bring the tab of the urethral cuff behind the corpus spongiosum. The cuff tubing is then passed through the hole in the tab, using shod hemostats to ensure that no air enters to tubing. The cuff is locked in place by pulling the tab over the tubing adapter (button) at the insertion of the tubing on the cuff, which should then be rotated slightly to orient the button laterally (**Fig. 8**). The tab should not be trimmed, as it can be a convenient handle for future device explant or revision.

Passage of the urethral cuff tubing is accomplished by placing the right index finger in the perineal incision, lateral to the urethra and feeling for the ipsilateral ischial spine, while a tonsil clamp is

Table 1
Long-term outcomes and complications following male sling placement[a]

Male Sling	Virgin Outcomes	Post-Radiation Outcomes	Complications
Bauer et al.,[15] 2011 (N = 24)		Dry: 25.0% ≥50% improvement: 25.0% Refractory SUI: 50.0%	Urethral injury: 4.2% Acute urinary retention: 16.7%
Wright et al.,[14] 2017 (N = 52)	PPD improvement: 2.3 Patient satisfaction: 80.0%	PPD improvement: 1.1 Patient satisfaction: 33.0%	Acute urinary retention: 9.6% Chronic urinary retention: 1.9% Perineal pain: 7.7% No XRT group 1.9% XRT group
Ye et al.,[19] 2018 (N = 113)	Dry: 22.6% ≤1 PPD: 58.0% Refractory SUI: 19.4%		Fluid collection requiring drainage: 2.7% Acute urinary retention: 2.7% De novo OAB: 1.8%
Rizvi et al.,[18] 2021 (N = 91)	≤1 PPD: 58.0% Refractory SUI: 24.0%		SSI infection: 3.0% Acute urinary retention: 10.0% Chronic urinary retention: 1.0% De novo OAB: 11.0%
Mumm et al.,[17] 2021 (N = 59)	Dry: 57.6% ≥50% improvement: 25.4% Refractory SUI: 16.9%		Urinary tract infection: 0.9% De novo OAB requiring medical therapy: 4.3% Sling excision for OAB or retention: 7.8%
Zheng et al.,[20] 2021 (N = 391)			Acute urinary retention: 10.7% Chronic urinary retention: 1.5%

[a] Rates are reported from latest recorded follow-up; OAB: overactive bladder

placed into the abdominal incision with the left hand. The clamp is felt on the index finger of the right hand and can be gently advanced until it is visible in the perineal wound. The cuff tubing is then grasped to ensure no air enters the system and pulled through to the abdominal incision. Alternately, the tubing passer provided with the system can be used to pass the tubing from the perineal incision up to the abdominal incision for connection to the other components. The tubing is trimmed and connected with the quick connect system. Finally, the device should be cycled several times while the cuff is inspected for proper function and then left deactivated.

The abdominal incision is closed in at least two layers, and the perineal incision in at least three, with surgical adhesive for the skin. The catheter can be removed at the end of the case or kept until the first postoperative day based on surgeon discretion. Patients with a history of diabetes, radiation, or undergoing revision may be discharged with five to 7 days of oral antibiotics, but perioperative coverage is generally sufficient for routine cases. Patient follow-up should include a wound check at 2 weeks and device activation at 6 weeks.

Artificial Urinary Sphincter Outcomes

The increased quality of life, continence rates, and durability of the AUS distinguish it as the gold standard therapy for male SUI. Complete continence in 50% of patients and 1 PPD or less in another 40% has been demonstrated out to 4.5 years as

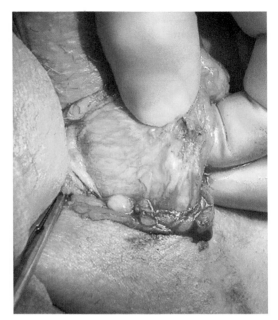

Fig. 5. Identifying the groove deep to the spongiosum facilitates sharp dissection.

reported in **Table 2**.[24] When followed to 7.7 years, patients with an AUS remained dry in 27% of cases and use 1 PPD or less in 32%.[25] Patient satisfaction correlates with these decreases in pad usage and has been reported as high as 92%.[25,26] Although studies show decreased continence rates for previously irradiated patients versus those without a history of radiation, the AUS remains the optimal option for these patients (see **Table 2**).[2,27]

Kretschmer and colleagues identified intraoperative complications, postoperative bleeding, wound healing disorders, postoperative infections, and the penoscrotal surgical approach as independent risk factors for explantation within 6 months.[28] Therefore, current AUA guidelines

recommend perineal implantation. Using a single-cuff perineal approach, Clavien–Dindo scale grade 3 complications occur in 5% to 21% of patients overall leading to an explantation within 6 months in as high as 8.6% of patients.[24,28] Delayed complications at a median follow-up of 4.1 years include device infection and erosion (4.9% total), as well as urethral atrophy (4.9%) and device malfunction (14.7%) with the former mandating explantation and the later requiring revision for continued continence.[29] The overall rate of revision increases by 5% for every year the device has been implanted.[29]

Sphincter efficacy (≤1PPD in 55% vs 56%) and patient satisfaction (90% vs 94%) remained high for revision devices when compared with primary implants in a 2016 study by Viers and colleagues[30] However, subsequent device survival has been shown to decrease from the first AUS to the second (**Table 3**). Hebert and colleagues reported in a large 2021 cohort study that the 5-year device survival for a second implant is 61% compared with 74% for a primary implant ($P < .001$).[31] Further, the same study reported an increased rate of infections and erosion (13.5% vs 8.5%, $P = .02$) for revision devices.

Radiation worsens outcomes for both primary and revision devices. The average revision rate for initial sphincters was increased from 19.8% in nonirradiated patients to 37.3% in irradiated patients in a 2015 meta-analysis (see **Table 2**).[32] This increase was thought to be secondary to

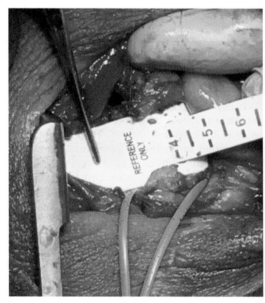

Fig. 7. Measurement of the corpus spongiosum for cuff placement.

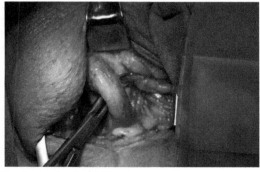

Fig. 6. Urethral mobilization prior to measurement.

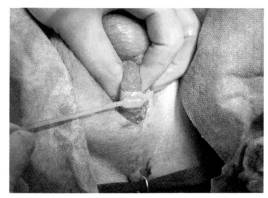

Fig. 8. Appropriately seated urethral cuff with the tab pulled over the tubing adapter (button) prior to rotating the adaptor laterally.

increase in both device infection (52.3%) and urethral atrophy (36.7%). In the revision setting, radiation shortened the time to second AUS explantation (30.1 vs 38.7 months) in a study by Fuller and colleagues[33] In this series when considering only radiated patients, the survival of an initial device was similar to a second device. However, revision device survival has been shown to decrease in irradiated patients in other studies, and patients should therefore be appropriately counseled on their risk of revision in both the primary and revision setting, based on their personal history of radiation.[34]

CLINICS CARE POINTS

- Patients with severe incontinence or previous radiation should be counseled that the artificial urinary sphincter would provide the most robust outcomes.
- Patient counseling regarding goals and expectations should drive the decision to pursue an anti-incontinence implant and be informed by the individualized risk factors for short- and long-term complications.

TRANSCORPORAL CUFF PLACEMENT

This approach can be used when the circumference of the corpus spongiosum does not allow for at least a 4.0 cm cuff, due to urethral atrophy or radiation, and is a helpful tool for revisions. In these cases, patients should be counseled that this approach will likely have a negative impact on erectile function.

For transcorporal cuff placement, bilateral 2 cm longitudinal corporotomies are made 4 mm from the corpus spongiosum. Stay sutures are placed in a longitudinal fashion on either side of each corporotomy with 2 to 0 absorbable sutures (**Fig. 9**). These are analogous to the corporotomy stitches placed during an inflatable penile prosthesis insertion. A right-angle clamp is then placed through the corporotomy incisions, across the septum (**Fig. 10**). Cuff measurement can then proceed normally with the caveat that the corporal holding stitches will be used to close the corporotomies behind the cuff prior to placement (**Fig. 11**).

In smaller series, as outlined in **Table 4**, transcorporal cuff placement has demonstrated increased continence rates and decreased revision rates when used for patients with a "fragile urethra."[35,36] Although the largest comparative study to date reported no difference in social continence or 5-year reoperation rates for transcorporal devices compared with standard bulbar urethral placement, this demonstrates that transcorporal placement can achieve similar AUS outcomes in higher risk patients.[37] Therefore, for patients with a history of urethroplasty, device erosion, infection or radiation, transcorporal cuff placement should be considered.

COMPLICATION MANAGEMENT

All foreign body implants have the potential to become infected. Infections in the early period may be due to device contamination during surgery or iatrogenic urethral or bladder injury and in follow-up are thought to be secondary to hematogenous seeding. Infections present with pain, swelling, and edema and can lead to a systemic response including sepsis. Regardless of the device, infection mandates explant, except in very rare circumstances. Most often, explant is performed in an expedited fashion and augmented by culture-directed antibiotics for 10 to 14 days. Device replacement should not be considered until at least 3 months after catheter removal, and an AUS is preferred in this setting.[38]

For urinary retention following an anti-incontinence device implant, each device has a different strategy for revision. ABDs can be easily titrated in office. Retention after a sling can be temporarily treated with intermittent catheterization and will resolve in most cases. For refractory retention, patient preference plays a role in management as some may be more inclined to self-catheterize over the long term as opposed to leak. For patients who do not wish to catheterize, one arm of the sling can be incised via a perineal approach. Patients with an AUS may self-catheterize, albeit with an increased risk of erosion. Thus, it is paramount that the cuff is appropriately sized in the operating room, and the patient is confirmed to be voiding and leaking before discharge. In cases of refractory retention, a 12 Fr urethral catheter can be placed for up to 48 hours, and options include suprapubic catheter placement or upsizing of the patient's cuff.

PERSISTENT OR RECURRENT INCONTINENCE AFTER ARTIFICIAL URINARY SPHINCTER IMPLANTATION

Incontinence following an AUS should first be categorized as "persistent" (early complication) or "recurrent" (late complication or expected device failure).[39] This distinction is important given varying etiologies and treatment options between the two categories. Persistent incontinence is defined as greater-than-expected leakage soon after device activation. Recurrent incontinence presents following an initially positive outcome. It should be reiterated to patients that the latter is not unexpected and increases in prevalence over time. It is also important in the case of recurrence to ensure the patient's medical condition and goals of care still align with device revision, as they may no longer be good candidates for an AUS.[23]

Cystoscopic Evaluation of an Artificial Urinary Sphincter

Complete evaluation of an AUS includes cystoscopic assessment. Cystourethroscopy can be done with a flexible cystoscope in the office and should be completed in three stages. First, the distal urethra and urethral cuff should be examined with the device activated and in the coapted position. A properly functioning device should show symmetric coaptation with no mucosal changes of the urethral tissue. Next, the device is cycled under direct vision to observe the opening and closing of the cuff. Finally, the entirety of the lower tract should be evaluated with the device deactivated.

Persistent Incontinence: Counseling and Device Usage

For patients with persistent incontinence in the early period following an AUS, a complete history and physical exam should precede any intervention. Eliciting the specific circumstances surrounding the patient's incontinence episodes is essential as many issues can be managed with improved expectation counseling and device education. Does your patient complain of dribbling due to urine-trapping under the foreskin, is the patient giving the device adequate time to cycle before leaving the toilet, and are they experiencing overflow incontinence due to infrequent device cycling, are all questions that may lead to resolution of the patient's issues with counseling alone. Inadvertent device deactivation is not uncommon and should be ruled out. Ensuring the patient is able to reach and manipulate his device is important as well. Finally, the physical examination should include device cycling by the provider to rule out mechanical dysfunction and the patient to evaluate proper handling and usage.

Persistent Incontinence: Storage Dysfunction

Patients with preexisting or de novo urgency, incontinence while lying supine or a history of pre-prostatectomy lower urinary tract symptoms or pelvic radiation should be considered for urodynamic evaluation. Infection should also be ruled out. If symptoms are found to be a manifestation of storage dysfunction, further treatment should proceed along the non-neurogenic overactive bladder pathway.[40]

Persistent Incontinence: Early Mechanical Failure

Early mechanical failure is often a manifestation of complicated device placement. Intraperitoneal PRB placement, improper seating of the cuff tab on the tubing adapter (button), and inadvertent kinking of the tubing or air introduced into the hydraulic circuit can all lead to suboptimal sphincter function. Furthermore, PRB herniation, a postoperative hematoma or infection, or lack of early device manipulation to ensure healing of the scrotal pump in a patient-accessible location can all lead to early mechanical failures. Therefore, a thorough understanding of the intraoperative and early postoperative course for each patient is essential to ensuring correction of an early mechanical failure. This process is aided by a complete history and physical examination, including cuff cycling by the surgeon as well as cross-sectional imaging to evaluate the volume of fluid in, and the location of, the PRB. On imaging, a PRB with a diameter of 3.5 cm is appropriately filled.[41]

Early mechanical failures, while rare, often require surgical intervention for resolution, and single-component revision should be prioritized when a definitive diagnosis is made. However, when a specific component malfunction cannot be definitively identified, the entire device should be removed and replaced.

Table 2
Long-term outcomes and complications following artificial urinary sphincter Placement[a]

Artificial Urinary Sphincter	Virgin Outcomes	Post-Radiation Outcomes	Complications[b]
Gousse et al,[25] 2001 (N = 71)	Dry: 26.8% ≤1 PPD: 32.4% Refractory SUI: 26.8% Revision rate (all-cause): 29.6%		Mechanical failure: 28.2% Erosion: 4.2% Infection: 1.4% De novo OAB requiring medical therapy: 4.2%
Walsh et al.[22] 2022 (N = 98)	Dry: 20.5% ≤1 PPD: 70.0% Refractory SUI: 9.6% Revision rate (all-cause): 23.7%	Dry: 11.1% ≤1 PPD: 72.2% Refractory SUI: 16.6% Revision rate (all-cause): 36.4%	Pump migration: 6.1% Hematoma: 2.0% Urethral atrophy *Non-irradiated: 7.9%* *Irradiated: 13.6%* Infection/Erosion: *Non-irradiated: 1.3%* *Irradiated: 22.7%* Mechanical failure: 1.0%
Trigo Rocha et al.,[24] 2008[c] (N = 40)	Dry: 50.0% ≤1 PPD: 40.0%		Hematoma: 2.5% Infection: 7.5% Mechanical failure: 5.0% Urethral atrophy: 5.0% De Novo OAB: 10.0%
Sacomani et al.,[43] 2018[c] (N = 121)	Dry: 67.8% ≤1 PPD: 19.8% Revision rate (all-cause): 19.8%		Urethral erosion *Non-irradiated: 25.5%* *Irradiated: 4.0%* Skin extrusion: 7.4%
Ravier et al.[44] 2015 (N = 122)	Dry: 53.8% Social Continence: 21.6% Revision rate (all-cause): 32.2%	Dry: 45.6% Social continence: 18.3% Revision rate (all-cause): 29.5%	Erosion: 9.0% Infection: *Non-irradiated: 3.2%* *Irradiated: 16.3%* Urethral atrophy: 15.6%
Bates et al.[32] 2015 (N = 1886)	Refractory SUI: 12.1% Revision rate (all-cause): 19.8%	Refractory SUI: 29.5% Revision rate (all-cause): 37.3%	

Abbreviation: OAB: overactive bladder
[a] Rates are reported from latest recorded follow-up
[b] Complications are broken down by radiation status if there was a significant difference in the rate between groups.
[c] Includes irradiated patients.

Persistent Incontinence: Early Cuff Erosion

Erosion can present with pain and perineal swelling, recurrent urinary tract infections, hematuria, or most commonly, recurrent incontinence. Similar to early mechanical failure, early cuff erosions are often the result of either known patient risk factors or a complex AUS placement and the intraoperative and early postoperative course must be examined in the context of a patient's past medical and surgical history. Patients with a history of urethral surgery, previous urologic prosthetics, and pelvic radiation are all at risk for more difficult device placements and resultant iatrogenic injuries.[41] Blood at the meatus after cuff placement or greater-than-expected bleeding during dissection may indicate an unrecognized urethral injury. Difficulty in seating the cuff may imply inappropriate urethral sizing. The need for prolonged postoperative catheterization also puts the patient at risk for erosion. Cuff erosions should be confirmed cystoscopically before intervention and mandate device explant due to device colonization. Even in the absence of overt infection at the time of diagnosis, urethral erosions will not heal with the device in situ and put the patient at risk for a catastrophic device infection.

If there are no concerns about the other components, a tubing plug can be used to preserve the

Table 3
Outcomes following artificial urinary sphincter revision

Study	Cohort	Control Group	Outcomes/Complications[a]
Hebert et al.,[31] 2021 (N = 1360)	Revision	First-time implant	Revision rate: *Revision: 30.6%* *First-time implant: 18.1%* 5-y device survival: $P < .001$ *Revision: 61%* *First-time implant: 74%* Infection/erosion: $P = .02$ *Revision: 13.5%* *First-time implant: 8.5%*
Viers et al.[30] 2016 (N = 278)	Revision	First-time implant	≤1 PPD post-activation: *Revision: 55%* *First-time implant: 56%* ≥1 episode of leakage per day post-activation: *Revision: 81%* *First-time implant: 71%* Patient would undergo surgery again: *Revision: 90%* *First-time implant: 94%*
Fuller et al.,[33] 2020 (N = 324)	Revision with a history of XRT	Revision without a history of XRT	Months to explant of initial AUS: $P = .043$ *Irradiated: 26.4* *Non-irradiated 35.6* Survival rate of 2nd AUS: $P = .86$ *Irradiated: 56.9%* *Non-irradiated: 57.9%* Months to explanation of 2nd AUS: $P = .034$ *Irradiated: 30.1* *Non-irradiated: 38.7* Indication for explant of 2nd AUS: *Mechanical failure: 25.4% vs. 33.3%, $P = .31$* *Infection/Erosion/Atrophy: 58.5% vs. 50.0%, P = .32*
Manka et al.,[34] 2020 (N = 527)	Revision with a history of XRT	Revision without a history of XRT	5-y survival of 2nd AUS: $P = .07$ *Irradiated: 51%* *Non-irradiated: 64%*

[a] *P*-values reported if available.

closed hydraulic system during cuff explant. The cuff should be removed in the standard fashion, using the cutting current when dissecting around the device. After the cuff is mobilized, the tab should the cut, allowing removal. The tubing should be secured with a rubber shod, 2 cm from the tubing adapter. The tubing can then be cut and the tubing plug applied. The plug should be secured with a 3 to 0 prolene. Although some studies would suggest that outcomes are not linked to urethral repair following cuff removal, we generally advocate primary repair of any type to avoid stricture formation whenever possible.[42] Urethroplasty is sometimes not feasible due to local inflammation and tissue friability and should be omitted in these cases. A new AUS cuff can be reimplanted after at least 3 to 6 months to allow for healing and following cystoscopic confirmation of a widely patent urethra. Transcorporal device placement should be considered in the revision setting.

Recurrent Incontinence: Cuff-Urethra Mismatch

Cuff-urethra mismatch is a condition in which the urethral cuff has loosened around the corpus spongiosum, leading to decreased pressure

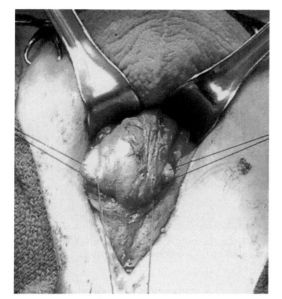

Fig. 9. Exposure of the corpora and placement of stay sutures.

transmission and incomplete urethral coaptation. This may occur secondary to fluid loss from the device or urethral atrophy from the chronic pressure of the cuff. Regardless of the mechanism, both pathologies will present with slowly worsening stress incontinence after an initial positive result. In this setting, the physical examination

may reveal the need for additional pumps of the scrotal pump to completely empty the fluid from the cuff. This signals that the AUS's hydraulic mechanism may be compensating for the increased space between the cuff and the urethral tissue by transferring more fluid to the cuff. Even when this is evident, cystourethroscopy is required to confirm cuff-urethra mismatch and rule out urethral erosion.

Pale urethral tissue at the site of the cuff is suggestive of urethral atrophy whereas visualization of urethral tissue proximal to the coapted cuff is diagnostic of cuff-urethra mismatch. After confirmation of the cuff-urethra mismatch, treatment consists of device replacement. Although some urologists will attempt a capsule release to improve cuff coaptation, most advocate for downsizing the urethral cuff, moving the cuff site to a more robust section of the urethra, transcorporal placement, or a combination of these. Few surgeons routinely use PRBs with pressure regulation higher than 61 to 70 cm of H_2O. It is recommended that for later recurrences, juxtaposed with early device malfunction, the entire device be replaced.

Recurrent Incontinence: Late Urethral Erosion

Although hematuria and recurrent infections are classically thought to herald identification of a urethral erosion, the diagnosis is often more subtle, requiring a higher index of suspicion. Patients with an erosion will most often complain of recurrent incontinence, mandating urethroscopy. Although an erosion may appear as frank exposure of the device, urothelial bullae, bleeding, and pitting may signify a small or pending erosion

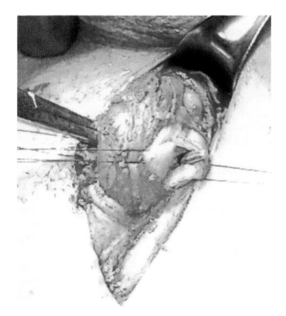

Fig. 10. Right-angle clamp spanning the corporotomies.

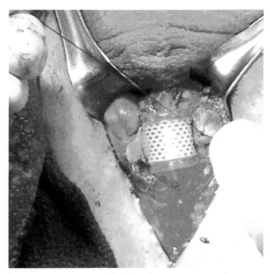

Fig. 11. Stay sutures closing the corporotomies.

Table 4
Outcomes for transcorporal placement for fragile urethra

Study	Outcomes/Complications[a]
Aaronson et al.,[35] 2008 (N = 26)	Social continence: *Transcorporal: 87.5%* *Standard: 61.1%* Explant rate: *Transcorporal: 12.5%* *Standard: 27.7%*
El-Akri et al.,[37] 2021 (N = 464)	Social continence: *P* = .94 *Transcorporal: 60.3%* *Standard: 60.6%* 5-y reoperation-free survival: *P* = .51 *Transcorporal: 42.0%* *Standard: 44.6%*
Redmond et al.,[36] 2020 (N = 67)	Decrease in PPD: *P* = .02 *Transcorporal: 6.5* *Standard: 5.0* Revision rate: *P* = .05 *Transcorporal: 20.8%* *Standard: 36.5%*

Abbreviation: PPD: pads per day
[a] *P*-values reported if available.

and should be treated as such (**Fig. 12**). Late erosions are treated in the same fashion as early erosions, with device explant, urethroplasty, and consideration of reimplantation after 3 to 6 months.

Recurrent Incontinence: Late Mechanical Failure

Similar to the cuff-urethra mismatch, mechanical failures are expected to increase in prevalence as time passes, and patients should be counseled that this is a function of the lifespan of the device. Mechanical failures should be considered the norm in the long-term, as opposed to the exception. Unlike the cuff-urethra mismatch, patients may describe an abrupt change in their symptoms, corresponding to a failure of a specific device component. If the patient is more than 2 years out from their original implantation, the entire device should be exchanged, even if a single component is identified as having failed.

FUTURE DEVELOPMENTS

Implantable devices are the backbone of male SUI treatment, meaning that device development will drive future advances. As of 2022, AUS technologies utilizing magnetic closing mechanisms, electronic control, and dynamic pressure changes

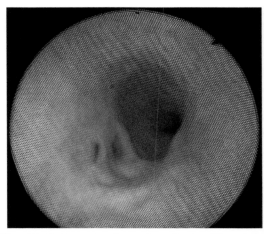

Fig. 12. Cystoscopic view of urethral pitting, later confirmed to be a urethral cuff erosion.

are in various stages of development, but not yet to market. These device innovations are not only aimed at improving continence outcomes while decreasing complications but may also broaden the patient populations eligible for an implant.

As prostate treatment remains the biggest contributor to male SUI, increase in the number of available treatment modalities for both BPH and PCa may drive the development of a more variable approach to SUI management. In addition to a historical increase in the use of radiation for PCa, technologies like holmium and thulium lasers used for enucleation, steam ablation, aquablation, and greenlight laser ablation for BPH may create more heterogeneous complexes of incontinence symptoms necessitating new diagnosis and treatment algorithms.

DISCLOSURE

Dr G.E. Koch has no financial disclosures. Dr M.R. Kaufman has no financial disclosures. Dr Kaufman is the national PI for the Artificial Urinary Sphincter Clinical Outcomes clinical trial (NCT04088331).

REFERENCES

1. Abrams P, Cardozo L, Fall M, et al. The standardisation of terminology in lower urinary tract function: report from the standardisation sub-committee of the International Continence Society. Urology 2003; 61(1):37–49.
2. Sandhu JS, Breyer B, Comiter C, et al. Incontinence after Prostate Treatment: AUA/SUFU Guideline. J Urol 2019. https://doi.org/10.1097/JU.0000000000000314.
3. Malik RD, Cohn JA, Fedunok PA, et al. Assessing variability of the 24-hour pad weight test in men

with post-prostatectomy incontinence. Int Braz J Urol Off J Braz Soc Urol 2016;42(2):327.

4. Huckabay C, Twiss C, Berger A, et al. A urodynamics protocol to optimally assess men with post-prostatectomy incontinence. Neurourol Urodyn 2005;24(7):622–6.

5. Anderson C, Omar M, Campbell S, et al. Cochrane library cochrane database of systematic reviews conservative management for postprostatectomy urinary incontinence (Review). Cochrane Database Syst Rev 2015;1(1). https://doi.org/10.1002/14651858.CD001843.pub5.

6. Lemmens JM, Broadbridge J, Macaulay M, et al. Tissue response to applied loading using different designs of penile compression clamps. Med Devices (Auckl) 2019;12:235.

7. Lee A, Mmonu NA, Thomas H, et al. Qualitative analysis of Amazon customer reviews of penile clamps for male urinary incontinence. Neurourol Urodyn 2021;40(1):384–90.

8. PMA P130018: FDA Summary of Safety and Effectiveness Data SUMMARY OF SAFETY AND EFFECTIVENESS DATA (SSED). Available at: https://www.accessdata.fda.gov/cdrh_docs/pdf13/P130018B.pdf.

9. Larson T, Jhaveri H, Yeung LL. Adjustable continence therapy (ProACT) for the treatment of male stress urinary incontinence: a systematic review and meta-analysis. Neurourol Urodyn 2019;38(8):2051–9.

10. Lebret T, Cour F, Benchetrit J, et al. Treatment of postprostatectomy stress urinary incontinence using a minimally invasive adjustable continence balloon device, ProACT: results of a preliminary, multicenter, pilot study. Urology 2008;71(2):256–60.

11. Ronzi Y, Le Normand L, Chartier-Kastler E, et al. Neurogenic stress urinary incontinence: is there a place for Adjustable Continence Therapy (ACT™ and ProACT™, Uromedica, Plymouth, MN, USA)? A retrospective multicenter study. Spinal Cord 2019;57(5):388–95.

12. AdVance™ XP male sling system instructions for use. Boston Scientific Corporation; 2018. Available at: https://www.bostonscientific.com/content/dam/bostonscientific/uro-mh/resources/male-incontinence/advance-xp/MH-662703-AA-AdVance-XP-Web-Prescriptive-Information-FINAL.pdf.

13. Rubin RS, Xavier KR, Rhee E. Virtue Quadratic Male Sling for stress incontinence—surgical guide for placement and delayed revision. Transl Androl Urol 2017;6(4):666.

14. Wright HC, McGeagh K, Richter LA, et al. Transobturator sling for post-prostatectomy incontinence: radiation's effect on efficacy/satisfaction. Can J Urol 2017;24(5):8998–9002. Available at: https://pubmed-ncbi-nlm-nih-gov.proxy.library.vanderbilt.edu/28971786/. Accessed September 16, 2021.

15. Bauer RM, Soljanik I, Füllhase C, et al. Results of the AdVance transobturator male sling after radical prostatectomy and adjuvant radiotherapy. Urology 2011;77(2):474–9.

16. Kumar A, Litt ER, Ballert KN, et al. Artificial urinary sphincter versus male sling for post-prostatectomy incontinence-what do patients choose? J Urol 2009;181(3):1231–5.

17. Mumm J-N, Klehr B, Rodler S, et al. Five-Year results of a prospective multicenter trial: AdVance XP for Postprostatectomy-Incontinence in Patients with Favorable Prognostic Factors. Urol Int 2021;105(5–6):421–7.

18. Rizvi IG, Ravindra P, Pipe M, et al. The AdVance™ male sling: does it stand the test of time? Scand J Urol 2021;55(2):155–60. https://doi-org.proxy.library.vanderbilt.edu/101080/2168180520211877342.

19. Ye H, Haab F, de Ridder D, et al. Effectiveness and Complications of the AMS AdVance™ Male Sling System for the Treatment of Stress Urinary Incontinence: A Prospective Multicenter Study. Urology 2018;120:197–204.

20. Zheng Y, Major N, Silverii H, et al. Urinary retention after AdVance™ Sling: a multi-institutional retrospective study. Neurourol Urodyn 2021;40(1):515–21.

21. Boston Scientific. AMS 800TM Artificial Urinary Sphincter for Male Patients.; 2019.

22. Walsh IK, Williams SG, Mahendra V, et al. Artificial urinary sphincter implantation in the irradiated patient: safety, efficacy and satisfaction. BJU Int 2002;89(4):364–8.

23. Lavi A, Boone TB, Cohen M, et al. The patient beyond the sphincter–cognitive and functional considerations affecting the natural history of artificial urinary sphincters. Urology 2020. Available at: https://www-sciencedirect-com.proxy.library.vanderbilt.edu/science/article/pii/S0090429519310866?via%3Dihub. Accessed November 28, 2021.

24. Trigo Rocha F, Gomes CM, Mitre AI, et al. A Prospective Study Evaluating the Efficacy of the Artificial Sphincter AMS 800 for the Treatment of Postradical Prostatectomy Urinary Incontinence and the Correlation Between Preoperative Urodynamic and Surgical Outcomes. Urology 2008. https://doi.org/10.1016/j.urology.2007.09.009.

25. Gousse AE, Madjar S, Lambert M-M, et al. Artificial urinary sphincter for post-radical prostatectomy urinary incontinence: long-term subjective results. J Urol 2001;166(5):1755–8.

26. Litwiller SE, Kim KB, Fone PD, et al. Post-Prostatectomy incontinence and the Artificial Urinary Sphincter: a long-term study of patient satisfaction and criteria for success. J Urol 1996;156(6):1975–80.

27. Guillaumier S, Solomon E, Jenks J, et al. Radiotherapy is associated with reduced continence outcomes following implantation of the artificial urinary sphincter in men with post-radical prostatectomy incontinence. Urol Ann 2017;9(3):253.

28. Kretschmer A, Hüsch T, Thomsen F, et al. Complications and short-term explantation rate following artificial urinary sphincter implantation: results from a large middle european multi-institutional case series. Urol Int 2016;97(2):205–11.

29. Linder BJ, Rivera ME, Ziegelmann MJ, et al. Long-term outcomes following artificial urinary sphincter placement: an analysis of 1082 cases at mayo clinic. Urology 2015;86(3):602–7.

30. Viers BR, Linder BJ, Rivera ME, et al. Long-term quality of life and functional outcomes among primary and secondary artificial urinary sphincter implantations in men with stress urinary incontinence. J Urol 2016;196(3):838–43.

31. Hebert KJ, Linder BJ, Morrisson GT, et al. A comparison of artificial urinary sphincter outcomes after primary implantation and first revision surgery. Asian J Urol 2021;8(3):298–302.

32. Bates AS, Martin RM, Terry TR. Complications following artificial urinary sphincter placement after radical prostatectomy and radiotherapy: a meta-analysis. BJU Int 2015;116(4):623–33.

33. Fuller TW, Ballon-Landa E, Gallo K, et al. Outcomes and risk factors of revision and replacement artificial urinary sphincter implantation in radiated and nonradiated cases. J Urol 2020;204(1):110–4.

34. Manka MG, Linder BJ, Rangel LJ, et al. The impact of prior external beam radiation therapy on device outcomes following artificial urinary sphincter revision surgery. Transl Androl Urol 2020;9(1):67–72.

35. Aaronson DS, Elliott SP, McAninch JW. Transcorporal artificial urinary sphincter placement for incontinence in high-risk patients after treatment of prostate cancer. Urology 2008;72(4):825–7.

36. Redmond EJ, Tong S, Zemp L, et al. Improved artificial urinary sphincter outcomes using a transcorporal cuff placement in patients with a "fragile urethra." Can Urol Assoc J 2020;14(12):E621.

37. El-Akri M, Bentellis I, Tricard T, et al. Transcorporal vs. bulbar artificial urinary sphincter implantation in male patients with fragile urethra. World J Urol 2021;39(12):4449–57.

38. Ajay D, Zhang H, Gupta S, et al. The artificial urinary sphincter is superior to a secondary transobturator male sling in cases of a primary sling failure. J Urol 2015;194(4):1038–42.

39. Kaufman MR. Options for persistent incontinence after artificial urinary sphincter placement. AUANews 2021. Available at: https://www.auanet.org/membership/publications-overview/aua-news/all-articles/2021/july-2021/options-for-persistent-incontinence-after-artificial-urinary-sphincter-placement.

40. Lightner DJ, Gomelsky A, Souter L, et al. Diagnosis and treatment of overactive bladder (non-neurogenic) in adults: AUA/SUFU Guideline Amendment 2019. J Urol 2019;202(3):558–63.

41. Khouri RK, Ortiz NM, Dropkin BM, et al. Artificial urinary sphincter complications: risk factors, workup, and clinical approach. Curr Urol Rep 2021;22(5):1–12.

42. Gross MS, Broghammer JA, Kaufman MR, et al. Urethral stricture outcomes after artificial urinary sphincter cuff erosion: results from a multicenter retrospective analysis. Urology 2017;104:198–203.

43. Sacomani CAR, Zequi S de C, da Costa WH, et al. Long-term results of the implantation of the AMS 800 artificial sphincter for post-prostatectomy incontinence: a single-center experience. Int Braz J Urol 2018;44(1):114–20.

44. Ravier E, Fassi-Fehri H, Crouzet S, et al. Complications after artificial urinary sphincter implantation in patients with or without prior radiotherapy. BJU Int 2015;115(2):300–7.

Complex Penile Surgery
Plication, Grafting, and Implants

Ziho Lee, MD[a],*, Jolie Shen, MD[b], Hunter Wessells, MD[b]

KEYWORDS

- Erectile dysfunction • Grafting • Penile implant • Peyronie's disease • Plication

KEY POINTS

- Penile plication may be used in patients with a wide range of curvature, including severe (>60°) or multiplanar deformity, but it is not applicable in patients with hourglass deformity, severe penile shortening, and large ossified plaques.
- Plaque incision (or excision) and grafting of the tunica albuginea may be used in all patients with complex Peyronie's disease, but decision-making should consider the risk-benefit ratio in light of a higher rate of *de novo* erectile dysfunction.
- Penile implant surgery with plication or grafting effectively restores function in patients with concomitant Peyronie's disease and erectile dysfunction.
- In the setting of severe corporal fibrosis, placement of a penile implant may be facilitated via dilation with cavernotomes, use of a counter incision with or without minimal scar tissue extraction, transcorporal scar resection, and wide scar excision with or without tunical grafting.
- When erectile dysfunction or tunica albuginea fibrosis is associated with superficial penile tissue loss from injury, ischemia, infection, or prior surgical complications, flaps should be used preferentially to achieve staged soft tissue coverage to the penile shaft and glans in anticipation of eventual implant surgery.

INTRODUCTION

The pathophysiology of penile defects requiring surgical reconstruction may be classified into injuries of the soft tissue and skin, tunica albuginea (TA), and corpora cavernosa. Although most patients requiring penile reconstruction have a single anatomic defect to the TA or corpora cavernosa, there are a subset of patients with overlapping defects involving multiple anatomic sites (**Fig. 1**). Herein, we focus our discussion on surgical management of patients with Peyronie's disease (PD), which primarily affects the TA and erectile dysfunction (ED) which primarily affects the corpora. Additionally, we discuss complex decision-making and surgical management of patients with PD and ED with overlapping defects involving multiple anatomic sites including defects in skin and soft tissues of the glans and shaft.

Surgical treatments for PD and ED are associated with excellent outcomes. However, certain clinical factors may make reconstruction more challenging. In patients with PD, severe (>60°) and multidirectional curvature, hourglass deformity, and severe penile shortening and an ossified plaque benefit from the application of reconstructive principles including mobilization and resection of scarred and damaged tissue; use of grafts and flaps according to the vascularization of the affected tissue; and a willingness to embark on time-consuming and difficult surgeries. Similarly, severe corporal fibrosis related to prior surgery (ie, infected implant), injury, or priapism may complicate implant surgery in men with ED and

Funding: None.
[a] Department of Urology, Northwestern University, Northwestern University Feinberg School of Medicine, 675 North Saint Clair Street, Galter Pavilion, Suite 20-150, Chicago, IL 60611, USA; [b] Department of Urology, University of Washington School of Medicine, 1959 Northeast Pacific Street, Seattle, WA 98195, USA
* Corresponding author.
E-mail address: Ziho.lee@nm.org

0094-0143/22/© 2022 Elsevier Inc. All rights reserved.

urologic.theclinics.com

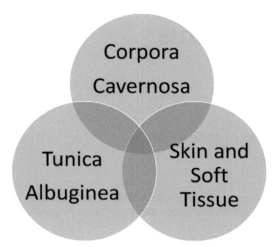

Fig. 1. Venn diagram depicting pathophysiological processes involved in complex penile surgery. Whereas corporal and tunical processes frequently overlap, only rarely will soft tissue defects complicate reconstructive approaches to ED and PD.

cannot be solved solely by implant selection and application of standard techniques. Although there are numerous studies that have reported encouraging surgical outcomes in the setting of complex PD and ED, the current literature highlights the vast variation in surgical techniques and the limitations of retrospective study designs with short-term follow-up and small sample sizes.

The purpose of our report is to review the literature regarding surgical management of complex PD and ED with emphasis on plication, grafting, and implants. Where appropriate, we have illustrated this review of the literature with our own observations and technical solutions to some of the challenging problems in complex penile surgery.

COMPLEX PEYRONIE'S DISEASE

PD is an acquired disorder that is characterized by fibrosis of the TA of the corpora cavernosa. The formation of scar tissue may lead to the development of penile curvature and deformity such as hourglass and hinge defects, which may result in penile pain, ED, and emotional distress.[1] For patients with stable clinically significant PD, in which symptoms have been clinically quiescent or unchanged for at least 3 months, surgical reconstruction provides the most reliable and durable clinical outcomes.[2,3] Intralesional collagenase, approved by the Food and Drug Administration under the trade name Xiaflex (Endo Pharmaceuticals Inc., Malvern, United States), has expanded nonsurgical options for PD.[4] When insufficient correction of curvature is achieved, surgeons

face the additional complexity of post-Xiaflex inflammatory changes, and rarely, rupture in the area of the plaque.[5,6] In patients with complex PD, which we define as severe (>60°) and multidirectional curvature, hourglass deformity, severe penile shortening, and an ossified plaque, surgical reconstruction requires the creative application of multiple techniques to achieve successful outcomes.

The AUA Guideline on PD[1] outlines the complete evaluation of men with PD. A detailed sexual history with documentation of the nature of the penile deformity when erect is essential. Erectile and ejaculatory function must be documented as well. The physical examination should assess plaque size, location, and penile length. Photographs of the erect penis help estimate severity of curvature and narrowing if present.

Straightforward unidirectional curvature in a PD patient with no report of ED can be corrected by penile plication without additional workup. When considering surgical options for patients with complex PD, we cannot overemphasize the importance of performing a detailed assessment of preoperative erectile function including subjective and objective measurement of erectile function. At our institution, we routinely perform color duplex Doppler ultrasound assessment to assist with surgical decision-making (**Fig. 2**). Patients with sufficient preoperative erectile function are counseled toward penile plication or plaque incision or excision and grafting. Those with ED refractory to oral medications, and those found to have arterial insufficiency or evidence of veno-occlusive dysfunction on color Doppler ultrasound, are steered toward reconstructive strategies using a penile implant (**Fig. 3**).[7,8]

Penile Plication

Penile plication, which involves shortening the convex (longer) side of the penis, is the most common surgical technique used to reconstruct patients with PD.[9] Since Nesbit described penile plication technique in 1965,[10] numerous variations of penile plication techniques have been reported. Although penile plication is generally recommended for patients with adequate erectile function, and penile curvature less than 60°,[1,11] there is literature to support its use in the setting of complex PD. In a seminal study, Gholami and Lue described the 16-dot plication technique for the management of patients with PD.[12] This technique involved making a circumcising incision with subsequent degloving dissection or a longitudinal incision over the convex portion of the penis. For patients with multidirectional curvature, or those

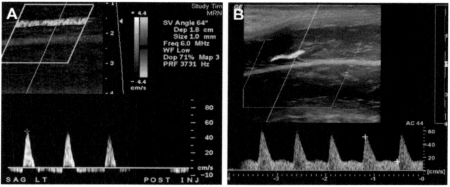

Fig. 2. Duplex Doppler tracings from patients with PD. (*A*) Normal tracing demonstrating peak systolic velocity (PSV) > 40 cm/s and absence of end diastolic flow during full erection (eg, end diastolic velocity (EDV) = 0). Resistive index (RI (PSV – EDV/PSV)) = 1.0. (*B*) Normal PSV with persistent diastolic flow suggestive of veno-occlusive dysfunction (PSV 55 cm/s; EDV 15 cm/s. RI = 0.72).

with significant hourglass narrowing, we generally opt for a degloving incision to allow better visualization of the deformity and maximum flexibility in placement of plication sutures. An erection is induced with intracavernosal papaverine or alprostadil. We supplement the rigidity of the erection with saline injected via a butterfly needle to achieve maximal demonstration of the curvature. After dissecting down to the level of the TA, a marking pen is used to mark the entry and exit points of sutures with 16 (2 pairs) or 24 (3 pairs) dots. Full-thickness bites of the TA are then taken with 2-0 nonabsorbable braided suture to plicate the penis. Tying the suture imbricates and shortens the TA, leading to penile straightening. Although the authors did not specifically set out to evaluate the utility of the 16-dot plication in patients with complex PD, they did perform their technique in patients with curvature greater than 60° and multiplanar curvature. Of 132 total patients, 34% had multidirectional curvature, and the average degree of curvature was 64° (range 30–120). At a mean follow-up of 2.6 years (range 7 months to 6 years), 15% of patients had recurrence of penile curvature. The most common postoperative complaint was penile shortening, which was noted in 41% of patients; loss of penile length ranged from 0.5 to 1.5 cm. Additionally, 12% of patients complained of bother from palpable suture knots, 6% complained of decrease in penile sensation, and 3% had worsening erectile function.

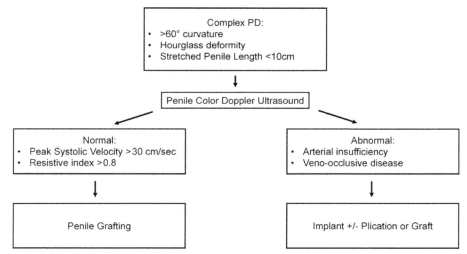

Fig. 3. Flow chart depicting surgical decision-making in patients with complex PD. Patients with normal penile vascular parameters undergo penile grafting. Patients with abnormal penile vascular parameters demonstrating significant arterial insufficiency and/or veno-occlusive dysfunction undergo penile implantation and grafting.

In a report by Adibi and colleagues, 43 patients underwent penile plication for complex PD, which was defined as those with curvature greater than 60° or multiplanar curvature.[13] Penile plication was performed via a penoscrotal incision just lateral to the urethra (for dorsal and lateral curvature) or a dorsal penile incision (for ventral curvature), which was mobilized along the most convex surface of the penile curvature. Penile degloving and dorsal neurovascular mobilization was not performed. A series of parallel sutures was placed in an interrupted vertical mattress fashion along the convex surface of the penis using 2-0 nonabsorbable braided suture until the curvature was completely corrected. There was no predetermined number of plication sutures for reconstruction. With regards to patients with greater than 60° curvature, the mean number of sutures used for plication was 11 (range 7–21) and the mean degree of correction per suture was 6°. With regard to patients with multiplanar curvature, the mean number of sutures used for plication was 7 (range 4–10), and the mean degree of correction per suture was 5°. At a mean follow-up of 15.3 months, 39/43 (92%) men had satisfactory results, defined as curvature less than 30° during erection. Two out of 43 (4%) patients required repeat plication, and 2/43 (4%) developed progressive ED resulting in penile prosthetic implantation. No patients had persistent penile pain with erections, complained of significant penile shortening, or loss of sensation.

Worsening erectile function is a potential complication associated with penile plication. The rate of de novo ED has been reported to occur in 0% to 4% of patients undergoing penile plication.[12–14] Injury to the neurovascular bundle can generally be avoided when placing plication stitches, which minimizes the risk of de novo ED. In patients undergoing dorsal plication for ventral curvature, an intervascular space between the dorsal vein and paired dorsal arteries may be developed. Placing plication sutures in this space reduces the risk of injury to the neurovascular bundle as the dorsal nerve fibers typically run lateral to the dorsal arteries. Although the risk of de novo ED is low, this potential complication should be discussed with all patients undergoing penile plication.

Although penile plication may be an effective option for patients with curvature greater than 60° or multiplanar curvature,[12,13] there are several limitations with its use in patients with complex PD. Penile plication is not well suited for patients with significant hourglass deformities and ossified plaques as these deformities persist after straightening of the penis.[13,15] Patients should be extensively counseled that the goal of penile plication in the setting of severe and multiplanar curvature is not to correct the penis to zero degrees of curvature but to make the penis functional.[13,16] In the aforementioned study by Adibi and colleagues,[13] among patients with greater than 60° curvature, the median degree of preoperative curvature was 70° (range 60–88), and median degree of postoperative curvature was 15° (range 0–30). In patients with multiplanar curvature, the median degree of preoperative curvature in the primary and secondary planes was 45° (range 20–90) and 35° (range 20–75), respectively; and the median degree of postoperative curvature in the primary and secondary planes was 10° (range 0–20) and 5° (range 2–10), respectively. Finally, penile shortening is a relatively common postoperative complaint and has been reported by 36% to 74% of patients after penile plication.[14,17,18] As penile length loss after penile plication is a major concern for many patients, this technique may not be suitable for patients with a shortened penis. Subjective length loss by patients in the postoperative setting has been reported in up to 75% of patients whereas provider-performed objective measures of length loss has been reported in 20% to 40% of patients. Penile length loss has generally been reported to range between 0 to 2.5 cm[13,19] and has been reported to be as much as 5 cm.[17] Although Greenfield and colleagues demonstrated that penile shortening is variable and depends on preoperative penile length (higher preoperative penile length was associated with more length loss) and direction/degree of curvature (ventral or ventrolateral curvature was associated with more length loss),[19] further studies specifically evaluating penile shortening after penile plication in the setting of complex PD are necessary to adequately counsel patients in this subset of patients.

Tunica Albuginea Grafting

Grafting for the management of PD involves incising or excising the TA at the most concave side of the penis and applying a graft to the tunical defect to lengthen the concave side of the penis. This technique is generally indicated in patients with adequate erectile function, and severe (>60°) and multidirectional curvature, hourglass deformity, severe penile shortening, and an ossified plaque. Traditionally, the favored approach to penile grafting has been to excise the entire penile plaque, but there is a direct correlation between the size of the tunical defect and degree of ED.[7,20,21] More recent literature has favored plaque incision or partial excision to minimize the risk of compromising the underlying veno-occlusive mechanism of the TA and causing postoperative ED. Accessing the dorsal TA to repair dorsal curvature requires careful mobilization of the neurovascular bundle whereas accessing the ventral TA to repair ventral curvature requires careful mobilization of the corpus spongiosum. Plaque incision is typically performed using an H-shaped[22] or double-Y[23] incision onto the TA. The primary incision is transverse for a unidirectional dorsal or ventral curvature. In the absence on narrowing, the lateral "darts" of the double-Y incision allow a rectangular graft (**Fig. 4**A). For an hourglass deformity (**Fig. 4**B) in addition to dorsal or ventral curvature, an H-shaped incision allows the correction of curvature and narrowing (**Fig. 4**C). The resulting tunical defect may be filled using an autograft (ie, detubularized saphenous vein[22,24] and buccal mucosa[25]), allograft (ie, human pericardial tissue[26] and human fibrinogen and thrombin coated onto equine collagen sponge[27]), or xenografts (ie, bovine pericardial[28] and bovine intestinal submucosal tissue[29]). Currently, there is no consensus on the most suitable graft material for penile grafting. However, synthetic grafts, such as polyester and polytetrafluoroethylene, have largely fallen out of favor given the risk of formation of a reactive capsule that can alter adaptability of the TA,[30] increased risk of infections,[31] and allergic reactions.[32] Despite heterogeneity in surgical approach (plaque incision vs partial plaque excision) and graft material used, penile grafting has been shown to be an effective option for the management of patients with complex PD.

Penile grafting effectively allows reconstruction in patients with severe (>60°) and multiplanar curvature and adequate erectile function. Sayedahmed and colleagues evaluated 42 patients with a mean degree of curvature of 73° (range 60–90), who underwent plaque incision and grafting using porcine small intestinal submucosa; 74.4% had a completely straight penis at a mean follow-up of 33.0 months (range 10–59).[33] In a report by Hatzichristodoulou and colleagues that evaluated 319 patients who underwent partial plaque excision and grafting with collagen fleece, 249 patients had dorsal curvature and 70 patients had dorsolateral curvature. The median curvature was 73.5° (range 45–110) dorsally and 23.2° (range 15–40) laterally. At a median follow-up of 47.2 months (range 12–100), 91.2% of patents had a completely straight penis.

Hourglass deformity, which refers to bilateral notching or indentation at the same level of the penile shaft, is rare and occurs in approximately 1% of patients with PD.[8] Surgical reconstruction of hourglass deformity is complex not only because of its significant effect on the structural integrity of the penis but also because of its high association with ED. Notching or hourglass deformity is associated with concomitant ED in approximately 61% to 68% of cases.[8,34] Furthermore, Kendirci and colleagues[8] noted that patients with hourglass deformity were more likely to have decreased peak systolic velocities on penile duplex ultrasound. This finding led the authors to hypothesize that hourglass deformity may be a surrogate for more extensive plaque volume that may cause compression of the penile arterial system and subsequent arterial insufficiency. In a report by Yafi and colleagues that evaluated outcomes of surgical management of patients with hourglass deformity, 26 patients underwent partial plaque excision and grafting, and 24 patients underwent inflatable penile prosthetic (IPP) placement.[35] In patients undergoing partial plaque excision and grafting, a 2.0 cm × 0.5 cm spindle-shaped portion of the TA was excised. The tunical defect was then extended laterally in the transverse direction on both sides of the penile shaft to expand the area of the hourglass narrowing. Tachosil (Baxter, Deerfield, IL, USA) graft was used to fill the tunical defect. At a mean follow-up of 20.7 months (SD ± 11.6), 85% of patients reported resolution of hourglass deformity, mean improvement in curvature was 68.1° (SD ± 12.7), and mean postoperative curvature was 2.7° (SD ± 5.3). All patients undergoing partial plaque excision and grafting were able to have intercourse postoperatively. With regard to complications, 2/26 (8%) patients had glans hypoesthesia.

As an alternative to classic H-shaped grafts in patients with severe narrowing and angulation, we combined a modified 16-dot technique with lateral incision and grafting. In 45 consecutive patients (unpublished data, University of Washington, 2022), grafts were placed unilaterally (38%) or bilaterally (62%) to correct narrowing at the same time that plication sutures corrected curvature (median 45°). In a subset evaluable with long-term follow-up (median 8 years), curvature was resolved (67%) or significantly improved (22%), and 61% were able to achieve satisfactory erections without use of aids. This technique avoids extensive neurovascular bundle mobilization and the higher risk of ED associated with "classic" incision and grafting.

Penile shortening is a known sequela of PD. In a nonrandomized prospective trial by Martinez-Salamanca and colleagues comparing penile traction therapy to no therapy in men in the active phase of PD, those in the no therapy group were

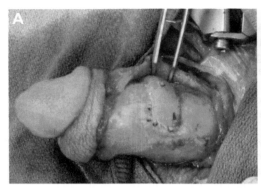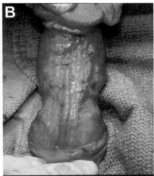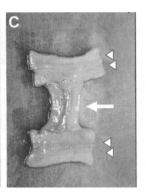

Fig. 4. Considerations in grafting of tunica albuginea. (*A*) Single large saphenous vein graft sutured in place with transverse orientation using "Double Y" incision of plaque. (*B*) Hourglass deformity after degloving and artificial erection (curvature not evident in this photograph). (*C*) H-shaped saphenous vein graft assembled from multiple pieces of vein to correct combination of curvature and narrowing. Arrow denotes middle segment to correct curvature. Arrowheads denote lateral segments to correct severe narrowing.

noted to have an average of 2.4 cm loss of penile length during 6 months of follow-up.[36] As penile shortening secondary to PD is associated with a high degree of distress and dissatisfaction,[36,37] treatment strategies that minimize the risk of penile shortening are paramount. In the setting of penile shortening, penile grafting is well suited for reconstruction because it involves use of a graft to lengthen the concave side of the penis and minimizes the risk of penile shortening. In a report by Egydio and colleagues that evaluated the outcomes of 33 patients who underwent plaque incision and grafting with bovine pericardium graft, the average increase in penile length was 2.2 cm (range 1–4).[38] The authors performed an incomplete circumferential transversal incision with forking at the extremities at an angle of approximately 120°. Sharp dissection along the borders of the incision for 3 to 5 mm was performed between the tunica and spongy tissue of the cavernous body to transform the linear incision in the tunica into a rectangular or trapezoidal tunical defect. This maneuver was critical in lengthening the concave side of the penis to the same length as the convex side. A bovine pericardium graft was then sutured to the tunical defect in a running fashion. In a study by Sansalone and colleagues that evaluated outcomes of 157 patients who underwent plaque incision and grafting, the average increase in penile length after surgery was 2.5 cm (range 1.7–4.1).[28] Although penile grafting is associated with a lower risk of penile shortening compared with penile plication, objective measures of penile length loss have been noted to occur in up to 17% to 22.4% of patients undergoing penile grafting procedures.[39,40] As such, patients should be counseled on the risk of penile shortening after penile grafting.

Ossified plaques present a unique problem because these lesions may cause issues with plaque palpability and persistent penile curvature if they are not excised. Not all calcified plaques warrant the same approach, however. Surgical management of patients with large ossified plaques generally involves plaque excision and grafting despite the risk of postoperative de novo ED. In selected circumstances involving lesser plaque volumes, alternatives have been described (**Fig. 5**). Eisenberg and colleagues described penile plication and tunica-sparing plaque excision in a series of 12 patients with PD and ossified plaques.[41] After performing a penile ultrasound to confirm that the thickness of the TA above the ossified portion of the plaque was more than 1.5 mm thick, a 16-dot plication was performed to straighten the penis. The corporal body was then opened longitudinally, and the ossified plaque was shaved off the undersurface of the tunica. The remnant tunica was then closed primarily. Of 10 patients who had follow-up beyond the period of postoperative sexual abstinence, 7 (70%) had a straight phallus at follow-up. Our own experience with resection of plaque has been disappointing; plaque excision and grafting remains the favored approach at our institution (**Fig. 6**) because the thickness and robustness of the overlying TA is difficult to establish preoperatively.

Although penile grafting may be an effective option for patients with complex PD, there are several limitations with its use. De novo ED is a major risk of penile graft surgery; its etiology is likely multifactorial. Disruption of the veno-occlusive mechanism as a result of incision and excision of the TA and insertion of a graft, and injury to the neurovascular bundle during mobilization while accessing the dorsal TA are the major proposed mechanisms

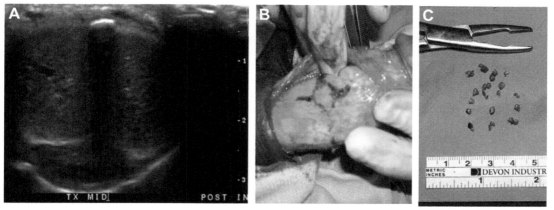

Fig. 5. Examples of minimal plaque ossification. (*A*) Sonographic image showing small midline calcification with acoustical shadowing. (*B*) Marking out a focal plaque for limited excision. (*C*) Use of a rongeur to remove calcified plaque from edge of tunica to facilitate suturing of graft without complete plaque excision.

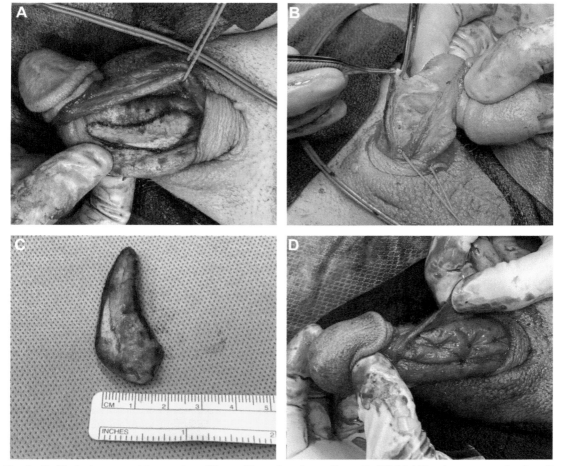

Fig. 6. Ossified plaque excision and grafting with pericardium allograft. (*A*) Mobilized neurovascular bundle marked by vessel loops. Ossified plaque along left dorsolateral aspect marked in pen. (*B*) Excision of ossified plaque preserving underlying cavernosal erectile tissue. (*C*) Excised ossified plaque. (*D*) Completion of grafting of tunical defect with pericardium allograft.

for ED after penile graft surgery.[7] It is generally accepted that graft material is not an important determinant of risk of de novo ED after penile graft surgery, with the caveat that ballooning of the graft may contribute to ED (see Discussion section).[42] Rates of ED after penile graft surgery have been wide ranging and reported to be between 4% to 67%.[7,43,44] Despite this, the specific risk factors that account for the wide-ranging differences in de novo ED after penile graft surgery are poorly understood and future studies are necessary to further elucidate these risk factors.

Glans hypoesthesia secondary to neuropraxia is a well-recognized complication after penile grafting surgery. Fortunately, this complication is generally temporary, and most patients have resolution within 3 to 6 months, although rarely it may require 12 months for recovery.[7] In a report by Terrier and colleagues examining penile sensory changes after penile incision and grafting surgery, 21% of patients developed some degree of penile sensation loss. After 12 and 24 months of follow-up, only 3% and 1.5% of patents had hypoesthesia, respectively.[45] Finally, ballooning of the graft site due to redundancy of the graft material and structural laxity of the graft material has been infrequently reported in the literature. In a report by Kalsi and colleagues that evaluated 113 patients who underwent plaque incision and grafting with saphenous vein, ballooning of the graft site was noted to occur in 2.7% of patents.[46]

Penile Implant Surgery

Insertion of a penile implant with or without adjunctive maneuvers is indicated in patients with PD and concomitant ED.[7] In patients with mild curvature less than 30° and ED, insertion of an implant alone without any adjunctive maneuvers may be sufficient to progressively correct curvature with subsequent device cycling.[7,47] In patients with mild-to-moderate degrees of penile curvature, manual modeling may be performed at the time of implant placement. This technique involves forcefully bending the penis and holding steady pressure for up to 90 seconds, which allows for the stretching and rupturing of the fibrotic bands within the Peyronie's plaque to straighten the penis.[48] Although this technique has been associated with an 80% to 100% rate of satisfactory straightening,[49–51] undue pressures on the distal cylinder tips may cause urethral perforation in up to 3% of patients.[51] As more significant curvature generally requires more pressure to alleviate curvature, modeling may have limited utility in patients with more pronounced curvature. We do not attempt modeling in patients

with ossified plaques out of dual concerns that the device may be injured by the plaque and that the TA may fail at the junction between the calcified and uncalcified tissue.

In patients with ED and complex PD, adjunctive maneuvers in conjunction with insertion of penile implant are indicated. Although penile plication is most useful in patients with mild-to-moderate curvature,[48] there is literature to support its use in the setting of severe curvature, with the caveat that the degree of penile shortening will be greater. Rahman and colleagues evaluated the role of inflatable penile prosthesis (IPP) placement in 5 patients with complex PD.[52] More specifically, the average curvature was 90° and 3/5 (60%) patients had multiplanar curvature. At a mean follow-up of 22 months, none of the patents had recurrence of penile curvature. Further studies evaluating the role of concomitant penile plication and insertion of penile implant in the setting of complex PD are necessary. We generally choose modeling or plaque incision when performing correction of curvature in conjunction with IPP to avoid further penile shortening.

In patients with complex PD and ED, tunical incision with or without grafting may be utilized. Levine and Dimitrou described a step-wise algorithm for management of patients with PD and ED.[53] If a patient had persistent penile curvature after insertion of penile implant and penile modeling, a transverse incision was made into the tunica over the area of maximal curvature. A polytetrafluoroethylene graft was only used if the tunical defect was more than 2 cm in length. Using this algorithm in a cohort of 46 men with PD and ED with a mean preoperative penile curvature of 53°, 12 patients underwent implant with plaque incision and 9 patients underwent implant with plaque incision and graft. The authors noted that almost all deformities less than 60° only required manual modeling alone. At a median follow-up of 39 months, all patients had full erectile capacity with a straight penis. None of the patients experienced herniation of the penile implant and 1/46 (2%) patient developed an infection.

Penile implant placement has also been shown to be useful in the setting of hourglass deformity. In the aforementioned report by Yafi and colleagues, 24 patients with a hourglass deformity and mean pretreatment curvature of 58.3° underwent IPP placement with adjunctive maneuvers for concomitant management of PD and ED.[35] All patients had resolution of hourglass deformity and the mean postoperative curvature was 8.8°. Interestingly, 19/24 (79%) patients required modeling only and 1/24 (4%) patients required modeling and plication. None of the patients required tunical incision or partial excision. Only 2 (8%) of patients had residual curvature greater than 20° and hourglass deformity resolved in all patients over 3 to 6 months. The authors hypothesized that chronically inflating the cylinders alone will induce remodeling of the fibrotic tunical tissues and correct hourglass deformity. There was one postoperative complication wherein the patient developed a cylinder aneurysmal dilation that required surgical revision.

Penile implant placement may compound the naturally occurring penile shortening secondary to PD. In a study by Levine and colleagues IPP placement was associated with penile length loss ranging from 0.25 to 4.0 cm.[47] As such, in patients with a shortened penis, several intraoperative maneuvers for length optimization at time of penile implant placement have been described. Although aggressive corporal dilation with the penis on full stretch has been described, this technique is limited by inherent tunical scarring of the existing corporal body that results in lack of penile elasticity.[48] Techniques involving various tunical incisions with and without grafting to allow for greater tunical stretching have been described. Rolle and colleagues described the sliding technique in which the urethra and neurovascular bundle are dissected off of the TA.[54] After making longitudinal incisions in each corporal body, these incisions are connected by hemicircular incisions along the dorsal aspect proximally and along the ventral aspect distally. A graft is then used to fill in the resulting tunical defect. In a multi-institutional study by Rolle and colleagues that used the sliding technique in 28 patients, the mean length gain was 3.2 cm.[55] Egydio and Kuehhas reported the multiple slice technique, a modification of the sliding technique, in a cohort of 103 patients.[56] The technique involved making multiple paired hemicircumferential tunical incisions in conjunction with two longitudinal incisions, which resulted in a series of smaller tunical defects. Although the authors noted an average length gain of 3.1 cm, one patient developed glans necrosis likely secondary to disruption of the glanular arterial supply from the dorsal penile arteries during neurovascular bundle mobilization and terminal spongiosal arteries during urethral mobilization. Although the risk of glans necrosis is rare, extreme caution should be exercised when performing penile lengthening procedures in this setting. At our institution, we prefer to use the "finger trap" technique described by Santucci and Berger.[57] After mobilizing the neurovascular bundle and corpus spongiosum, hemicircumferential staggered incisions of the TA are made according to a template. These relaxing incisions allow for the expansion of the corporal bodies and accommodate placement

of a penile implant. The defects in the TA are left to heal by secondary intention with the device inflated for 3 to 4 weeks. We generally do not use grafts (**Fig. 7**). We have performed this in 7 patients with length increase of 2 to 3 cm without device herniation; one postoperative infection required temporary placement of a malleable device, and later replacement of an IPP.

PENILE IMPLANT SURGERY FOR CORPORAL FIBROSIS

Penile implant placement is indicated in patients with ED who are refractory to less invasive treatment options or elect definitive surgical correction. In uncomplicated first time cases, penile implant placement is well tolerated with low complication (5%–11%[58,59]) and infection rates (0.8%–8.3%[60,61]), minimal postoperative pain,[58] and high satisfaction rates of 85% to 95%.[62,63]

Corporal fibrosis significantly complicates the insertion of a penile implant, imparting a higher risk of septal and crural perforation, urethral injury, surgical site infection, penile shortening, hypoesthesia, and procedural abandonment.[64–67] Severe corporal fibrosis generally occurs following explantation of an infected implant,[68–71] trauma,[72] chronic intracavernosal injection,[73,74] priapism requiring corporal shunting procedures,[70,75–77] and in patients who have undergone construction of a neophallus. Rarely, PD, poorly-controlled diabetes or end stage renal disease can result in severe corporal fibrosis.[78] Of these etiologies, the most severe fibrosis generally occurs after removal of the infected implant, as the empty and inflamed corporal body space allows for excessive deposition of collagen and extracellular matrix.[79] Although no standards exist to define or quantify "severe" corporal fibrosis, a clinical history of inability to passively dilate the corporal bodies at time of penile implant placement is generally used as inclusion criteria in the literature.[78]

Patients with severe fibrosis may require advanced maneuvers for successful penile implant placement. Although a number of options for placement of penile implants in this setting have been described in the literature, the data are limited by small cohorts and intermediate-term follow-up. Furthermore, there are no comparative studies among techniques and there are no guidelines to direct intraoperative decision-making in this setting. Herein, we will review the literature on surgical techniques and the risks and benefits of the placement of penile prostheses for severe corporal fibrosis. Of note, surgeons may be able to anticipate the location and severity of maximum scarring based on the

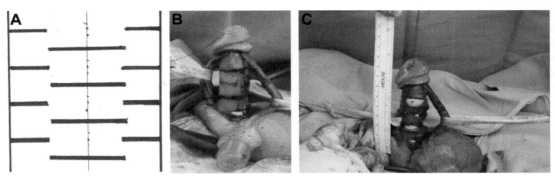

Fig. 7. Finger trap method for penile lengthening. (*A*) Template for tunical incisions on corporal bodies. (*B*) Template for tunical incisions marked on corporal bodies with first incision made at base of penis. Note both the neurovascular bundle and corpus spongiosum have been completely mobilized off the corporal bodies. (*C*) Completed "Finger Trap" method for penile lengthening and placement of penile implant. Defects in the TA are allowed to heal by secondary intention.

original etiology of the fibrosis. For example, a prior penile implant that has eroded likely will pose the greatest degree of scarring at the old corporotomy sites and at sites of distal erosion. Gunshot, stab wounds, and blunt penile injury will create localized fibrosis commensurate with the kinetic energy of the injury. In contrast, priapism with extensive ischemic necrosis of corporal tissue may cause a pan-corporal fibrosis.

Dilation

Dilation techniques in the setting of severe corporal fibrosis generally involve using sharp dilators to facilitate creation of a space to allow for implant placement. Although dilation techniques do not require advanced surgical maneuvers, these techniques generally have the highest risk of corporal body and urethral perforation, and often require implantation of decreased diameter or noninflatable implants. Cavernotomes are dilators with sharp ends that may be used to enhance the effectiveness of dilation into fibrous cavernosa, and there are two major cavernotomes that may be used in the setting of severe corporal fibrosis.

The Carrion–Rossello cavernotome (Coloplast A/s, Humlebæk, Denmark) is an instrument with teeth projecting from either side that can be pronated and supinated to dilate the corporal body. Dilation also is achieved when the device is removed, engaging the teeth in the fibrotic corporal tissue. Importantly, the teeth allow the instrument to be advanced through scar tissue and also protects from perforation from sudden inadvertent forward movement. These cavernotomes range in diameter from 9 to 12 mm. As the smallest Carrion–Rossello cavernotome is 9 mm in diameter, it often requires creation of an initial space within the fibrotic cavernosal tissue via sharp dissection before the cavernotome can be

introduced. Wilson and colleagues first described using the Carrion–Rossello cavernotome to dilate the corporal bodies in 32 patients undergoing complex IPP placement.[80] The authors noted an 87% 1-year success rate and no cases of urethral perforation. Complications included 2 (6%) cases of inadequate proximal dilation and 2 (6%) cases of prosthesis infection.

The Uramix cavernotome (Uramix Inc., Lansdown, United States) is an instrument with a longitudinal blade that rises 1 mm from a beveled surface to incise or sharply drag across the fibrotic layers of tissue. These cavernotomes range in diameter from 6 to 13 cm. In a cohort of 16 patients with severe corporal fibrosis from either explant of infected implant or priapism, Mooreville and colleagues utilized Uramix cavernotomes to dilate the corporal bodies.[71] Similar to the technique described by Wilson and colleagues,[80] Mooreville and colleagues described the creation of an initial space within the fibrotic corporal bodies via sharp dissection using a scalpel and Metzenbaum scissors prior to initiating dilation.[71] Although all patients underwent successful implantation of IPPs, proximal crural perforation occurred in 5 (31%) patients and corporal crossover occurred in 3 (19%) patients. Moreover, 4 (25%) patients required revision surgery for impending cylinder erosion distally. Finally, 14 (88%) patients received a downsized implant as the fibrotic corpora would not allow dilation large enough to place a standard sized cylinder. The performance of downsized implants is especially important in men with longer penile length; the aspect ratio of length to girth makes it harder for these longer narrower implants to resist buckling.

In a multicenter report by Krughoff and colleagues that evaluated penile implant placement in 42 patients with severe corporal fibrosis, the authors described their corporal dilation technique using a combination of Uramix and Carrion–Rossello cavernotomes.[78] Although standard dilators were used in 15/42 (36%) of patients, 25/42 (60%) patients required dilation with cavernotomes and 1/42 (2.4%) required limited sharp corporal excision and dilation with cavernotomes. More specifically, when standard dilation technique was unsuitable for dilation, the authors used a 6-mm Uramix cavernotome to create the initial channel and serially advanced up to 11-mm Uramix cavernotomes. In the setting of very severe fibrosis, the authors instead used Rossello cavernotomes to expand the fibrotic tissue. All patients underwent successful placement of a penile implant, with 10/42 (24%) patients requiring a decreased diameter cylinder and 10/42 (24%) patients requiring a malleable penile prosthetic (MPP). There was one major complication in which 1/42 (2%) patient suffered a distal erosion and required device explant.

Counter Incision

Use of a counter incision may assist with dilation of the distal corporal body in the setting of distal fibrosis, which may complicate surgery for PD as well as ED. In a report by Ghanem and colleagues, 17 patients with severe corporal fibrosis secondary to explantation of an infected penile implant or priapism underwent insertion of MPP.[81] Intraoperatively, the authors accessed the corporal bodies via an infrapubic and subcoronal incisions. Initial dilation was carried sharply using Metzenbaum scissors and small caliber Heggar dilators. During initial dilation, the authors created lateral subtunical tracts to minimize the risk of urethral perforation. The authors did not reconstruct the corporal bodies using grafts and utilized Buck's fascia to cover defects that were all less than 4 cm. There was one case of a crural perforation that was repaired intraoperatively. All patients underwent successful placement of an MPP, and there were no postoperative infections or reoperations. As this technique relies on tissue stretching without creating a wide corporal tunnel by excising the fibrous core, it is best suited for insertion of MPP. The authors preferred not to perform corporal reconstruction with grafts given their concern for postoperative infection with excessive manipulation of the corporal bodies and use of synthetic material.

Minimal Scar Tissue Extraction and Counter Incision

George and colleagues described a technique in which a minimal amount of scar is excised at the location of the initial corporotomy.[82] This is then followed by corporal body dilation using blunt-tipped Metzenbaum scissors and then 7 to 11-gauge Hegar dilators and/or a Dilamezinsert (Cooper Surgical, Trumbull, CT United States). If there was difficultly in dilating the distal corporal body, an additional subcoronal incision was made to facilitate distal dissection. After insertion of the penile implant, if closure of the TA of the corporal bodies was difficult, a polytetrafluoro-ethylene graft was used. In a follow-up to the initial report of this technique by George and colleagues,[82] Rajpurkar and colleagues described their experience with this technique in 34 patients with severe corporal fibrosis.[83] Intraoperatively, 32 (94%) patients were noted to have bilateral severe corporal fibrosis, and 2 (6%) patients were noted to have unilateral severe corporal fibrosis. The subcoronal counter incision was required in 30/34 (88%) patients, and grafting was required in 13/34 (38%) patients. All patients underwent successful placement of a penile prosthesis. Although semirigid implants were required in 4/34 (12%) patients, two patients underwent subsequent surgery for exchange of their semirigid implant to an inflatable implant. There was 1/34 (3%) complication related to the index surgery in which a patient had an unrecognized crural perforation. This patient required revisional surgery with grafting. None of the patients developed any early postoperative complications, including infection. The authors attributed their excellent surgical outcomes to two aspects of their technique. First, by making a small corporal excision rather than a wide excision, there was less compromise to the blood supply to the penis, thus assisting with healing of the surgical wound and delivery of antibiotic to the surgical site. Second, the use of a counter incision allowed for more controlled dilation over smaller distances and under better visualization.

Transcorporal Scar Resection

Shaeer described an endoscopic technique in which fibrotic corporal body is resected transcorporally.[84] An endoscopic urethrotome is used to incise the corporal body and create a channel for endoscopic resectoscope insertion. Although the technique was used successfully in 6 patients without any intraoperative complications or postoperative infections, a subsequent technical modification suggests that the original method has been abandoned. In the later description, a linear 7.5 MHz ultrasound probe was used to monitor and guide trans-corporal excavation.[85] A urethrotome was advanced over the guidewire and used to incise the corporal body in 1 to 2 cm increments.

All 12 patients undergoing this technique had successful placement of a 13 mm diameter IPP.

These approaches may have specific applications for milder degrees of corporal fibrosis; nevertheless, the lack of replication of the results at other centers, and concerns about the potential for perforation and inadequate resection of scar tissue in more severe cases limits our enthusiasm for this technique.

Wide Scar Excision

Wide scar excision involves dissecting the fibrotic scar within the corporal body free from the TA. Early studies describing the technique of wide scare excision in patients with severe corporal fibrosis have noted a significant complication rate, which includes infection (18%–20%),[64,86,87] pain (6%),[87] penile angulation (6%),[88] reoperation (30%–50%),[89] and device malfunction (6%–12%).[90] Early and late complication rates have been reported to be as high as 30% and 50% to 65%, respectively.[91] However, more recent literature has shown that variations of this technique may be performed with excellent outcomes. Montague and Angermeier described complete corporal excavation in 2006.[70] This technique involved a long penoscrotal incision to allow for exposure of the entire corpus cavernosum with subsequent sharp excision of all fibrotic intracorporal tissue. In all 9 patients who underwent this technique, the corporal bodies were able to be closed primarily over the penile prostheses without the use of grafts. However, 7/9 (78%) patients required reduced diameter devices. There were no intraoperative or postoperative complications noted. The authors highlighted that this technique was particularly useful because it allowed for a reduced risk of perforation given that all of the dissection was under direct visualization.

Given the degree of scarring and contracture often encountered in the setting of severe corporal fibrosis, closing the resulting corporal defect over a cylinder of a penile implant may be difficult. Although some authors have suggested leaving the tunical defect open and closing the overlying fascia and skin over the implant, this strategy has been associated with an increased risk for infection, migration and deformity during device use, malfunction, and erosion.[92,93] In this setting, a graft may be used for corporal reconstruction to allow for adequate closure of the corporal body around the penile implant. Although there have been numerous studies using various graft materials, there is no consensus on the ideal graft material for use in corporal reconstruction. There are three major classes of grafts that may be used for corporal reconstruction: (1) synthetic (ie, polytetrafluoroethylene), (2) autologous (ie, saphenous vein, tunica vaginalis, fascia lata, rectus fascia, and buccal mucosa), and (3) extracellular matrix (ie, cadaveric pericardium, porcine submucosal intestinal substance).[32,94,95] Synthetic grafts such as polytetrafluoroethylene have tensile strengths far greater than that of normal tunica, which may help prevent corporal body ruptures and aneurysms. However, synthetic grafts may limit implant expansion given their propensity for fibrosis. Additionally, synthetic grafts are associated with an increased rate of infection, and has been reported to be as high as 30% in some cases.[96] Although autologous grafts have decreased infection and immunogenic risk, they come at the expense of increased donor morbidity/availability, increased operative time, and variable tensile strength, which can limit full expansion of cylinder.[32] Use of cadaveric pericardial tissue for corporoplasty has been associated with lower rates of infection and fibrosis compared to synthetic grafts.[97] Additionally, cadaveric pericardial tissue was associated with improved graft elasticity due to its tensile strength and multidirectional elasticity compared to TA, especially when considering the physiologic dynamics of erection.

Sansalone and colleagues used simultaneous corporal reconstruction and porcine patch grafts to facilitate IPP placement in 18 patients with severe corporal fibrosis.[69] An MPP was inserted in 4/18 (22%) patients and an IPP was inserted in 14/18 (78%) patients. Postoperative complications included superficial scrotal wound dehiscence in 2/18 (11%) patients and small scrotal hematoma in 3/18 (17%) patients, which were all managed with a prolonged course of antibiotics. At an average follow-up of 26 months (range 6–36), revision surgery was required in 4 patients (3 patients for elective exchange to IPP, and 1 patient for upsizing of the implant). All patients were able to achieve penetrative sexual intercourse.

Between 2006 and 2021, we performed 10 cases of IPP placement in severe corporal fibrosis due to infected IPP explant, trauma, and ischemic priapism at our institution.[98] Our approach is to make a midline ventral penoscrotal incision, which can, if necessary, be extended as far distally as necessary. Of 10 patients, 1 (10%) underwent corporal excavation only, 4 (40%) underwent excavation with corporal grafting with polytetrafluoroethylene, and 5 (50%) underwent excavation with corporal grafting with pericardium allograft (**Fig. 8**). Although all patients underwent implantation with an IPP, 5 (50%) patients required insertion of a reduced diameter implant. We use polytetrafluoroethylene if the graft is required at

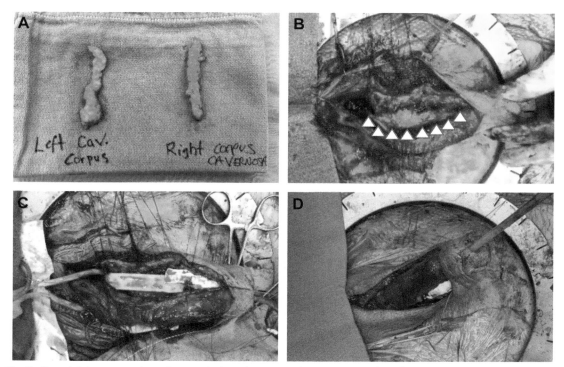

Fig. 8. Pictorial demonstration of our technique for corporal excavation and grafting and placement of an inflatable penile implant. (*A*) Excavated scar tissue from corporal bodies. (*B*) Corporal bodies after scar excavation. Arrowheads denote right corporal body that has been opened and splayed out. (*C*) Corporal body reconstruction with polytetrafluoroethylene graft with inflatable penile implant in place. Note that polytetrafluoroethylene was used because the narrowing extended distally to tip of corporal body, and thus graft strength needed to keep tip of implant within proper glans location was considered (*D*) Completed corporal excavation and grafting with inflatable penile prosthesis fully inflated. Note polytetrafluoroethylene graft incorporated into the left corporal body. Same patient as in **Fig. 9** and 9 months after flap reconstruction.

the distal most portion of the corporal body to ensure proper positioning of the distal tip of the IPP in relation to the glans. If the graft is required more proximally, and does not involve the distal corporal body, we use the pericardium allograft. At a median follow-up of 6.8 months, surgical success was demonstrated in 90% of cases. Postoperative complications included 2 (20%) superficial skin infections requiring an extended course of oral antibiotics and 1 (10%) patient with temporary postoperative neuropathic pain/distal glans numbness. The one surgical failure was in a patient who experienced severe penile shortening and required a penile lengthening procedure and upsizing of the IPP 10 months post-operatively.

Soft Tissue Defects and Penile Implants

Patients with ED and concomitant penile skin and soft tissue loss from injury, ischemia, infection, or prior surgical complications pose unique challenges and require particularly creative reconstructive solutions. In such cases, penile skin and soft tissue must be restored before penile implant surgery to allow adequate coverage of implant components and graft materials. We preferentially use flaps to achieve coverage in these circumstances. Whereas a skin graft will bring only dermis and epidermis, flaps provide a robust subcutaneous tissue that can be remobilized at a subsequent implant surgery. Originally proposed by Jordan[99] in the context of penile reconstruction, we have found radial forearm free flaps to be versatile in this setting. The size of the penile skin or soft tissue defect generally is amply covered by a small RFFF, which allows for a simplified donor site closure compared with flaps harvested for phalloplasty. One example of this technique is shown in **Fig. 9**. A 54-year-old man presented with ED after prolonged ischemic priapism and multiple shunts and complications. Our strategy for IPP was impeded by a substantial defect of the skin and right hemiglans soft tissue after multiple distal shunts for priapism (**Fig. 9**A,B). Thus, we performed a radial forearm free flap to fill in the skin and soft tissue glans defect in a first stage

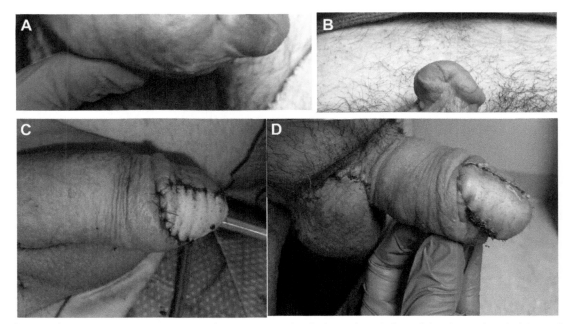

Fig. 9. Soft tissue coverage in patient with severe ED and right hemiglans defect of the skin and underlying soft tissue after multiple distal shunts for priapism and corpora-cutaneous fistula. (*A, B*) Preoperative images showing right hemiglans defect. (*C*) Intraoperative image at the completion of flap interposition into glans defect. (*D*) Postoperative image 4 weeks status post radial forearm free flap reconstruction of the right hemiglans (same patient as in **Fig. 8**)

(see **Fig. 9**C,D). Nine months after glans reconstruction, we were able to perform penile excavation, corporal grafting and distal corporal windsock with polytetrafluoroethylene, and IPP implantation (see **Fig. 8**). Six months after the second stage surgery, the patient's IPP is functional and there have been no complications.

SUMMARY

Surgical management of patients with complex PD and ED may be challenging and necessitate sophisticated techniques for reconstruction. Although patients with severe or multiplanar curvature may be managed with penile plication or grafting, patients with hourglass deformity and severe penile shortening require penile grafting. Patients with complex PD and ED generally require penile plication or grafting in conjunction with penile implant placement. In the setting of severe corporal fibrosis, placement of a penile implant may be facilitated via dilation with cavernotomes, utilization of a counter incision with or without minimal scar tissue extraction, transcorporal scar resection, and wide scar excision with or without grafting. With extensive soft tissue defects, additional tissue transfer techniques should be considered to allow adequate coverage of implants and grafts.

FINANCIAL CONFLICTS OF INTEREST

All authors have no conflicts of interest or financial ties to disclose.

REFERENCES

1. Nehra A, Alterowitz R, Culkin DJ, et al. Peyronie's Disease: AUA Guideline. J Urol 2015;194(3):745–53.
2. Ottaiano N, Pincus J, Tannenbaum J, et al. Penile reconstruction: An up-to-date review of the literature. Arab J Urol 2021;19(3):353–62.
3. Garcia-Gomez B, Gonzalez-Padilla DA, Alonso-Isa M, et al. Plication techniques in Peyronie's disease: new developments. Int J Impot Res 2020; 32(1):30–6.
4. Gelbard M, Goldstein I, Hellstrom WJ, et al. Clinical efficacy, safety and tolerability of collagenase clostridium histolyticum for the treatment of peyronie disease in 2 large double-blind, randomized, placebo controlled phase 3 studies. J Urol 2013;190(1): 199–207.
5. Cocci A, Ralph D, Djinovic R, et al. Surgical outcomes after collagenase Clostridium histolyticum failure in patients with Peyronie's disease in a multicenter clinical study. Sci Rep 2021;11(1):166.
6. Levine LA, Larsen SM. Surgical correction of persistent Peyronie's disease following collagenase

clostridium histolyticum treatment. J Sex Med 2015; 12(1):259–64.

7. Osmonov D, Ragheb A, Ward S, et al. ESSM position statement on surgical treatment of Peyronie's Disease. Sex Med 2021;10(1):100459.

8. Kendirci M, Nowfar S, Gur S, et al. The relationship between the type of penile abnormality and penile vascular status in patients with peyronie's disease. J Urol 2005;174(2):632–5 [discussion 635].

9. Oberlin DT, Liu JS, Hofer MD, et al. An analysis of case logs from american urologists in the treatment of Peyronie's Disease. Urology 2016;87:205–9.

10. Nesbit RM. Congenital curvature of the phallus: report of three cases with description of corrective operation. J Urol 1965;93:230–2.

11. Mandava SH, Trost LW, Hellstrom WJ. A critical analysis of the surgical outcomes for the treatment of Peyronie's disease. Arab J Urol 2013;11(3):284–93.

12. Gholami SS, Lue TF. Correction of penile curvature using the 16-dot plication technique: a review of 132 patients. J Urol 2002;167(5):2066–9.

13. Adibi M, Hudak SJ, Morey AF. Penile plication without degloving enables effective correction of complex Peyronie's deformities. Urology 2012; 79(4):831–5.

14. Van Der Horst C, Martinez Portillo FJ, Seif C, et al. Treatment of penile curvature with Essed-Schroder tunical plication: aspects of quality of life from the patients' perspective. BJU Int 2004;93(1):105–8.

15. Chung E. Penile reconstructive surgery in Peyronie disease: challenges in restoring normal penis size, shape, and function. World J Mens Health 2020; 38(1):1–8.

16. Cordon BH, Osmonov D, Hatzichristodoulou G, et al. Peyronie's penile plication. Transl Androl Urol 2017; 6(4):639–44.

17. Schneider T, Sperling H, Schenck M, et al. Treatment of penile curvature–how to combine the advantages of simple plication and the Nesbit-procedure by superficial excision of the tunica albuginea. World J Urol 2003;20(6):350–5.

18. Syed AH, Abbasi Z, Hargreave TB. Nesbit procedure for disabling Peyronie's curvature: a median follow-up of 84 months. Urology 2003;61(5): 999–1003.

19. Greenfield JM, Lucas S, Levine LA. Factors affecting the loss of length associated with tunica albuginea plication for correction of penile curvature. J Urol 2006;175(1):238–41.

20. Chung E, Ralph D, Kagioglu A, et al. Evidence-based management guidelines on Peyronie's Disease. J Sex Med 2016;13(6):905–23.

21. Hatzichristodoulou G, Osmonov D, Kubler H, et al. Contemporary review of grafting techniques for the surgical treatment of Peyronie's Disease. Sex Med Rev 2017;5(4):544–52.

22. Lue TF, El-Sakka AI. Venous patch graft for Peyronie's disease. Part I: technique. J Urol 1998;160(6 Pt 1):2047–9.

23. Egydio PH, Lucon AM, Arap S. A single relaxing incision to correct different types of penile curvature: surgical technique based on geometrical principles. BJU Int 2004;94(7):1147–57.

24. Yurkanin JP, Dean R, Wessells H. Effect of incision and saphenous vein grafting for Peyronie's disease on penile length and sexual satisfaction. J Urol 2001;166(5):1769–72 [discussion: 1772-1763].

25. Liu B, Zhu XW, Zhong DC, et al. [Replacement of plaque by buccal mucosa in the treatment of Peyronies disease: a report of 27 cases]. Zhonghua Nan Ke Xue 2009;15(1):45–7.

26. Taylor FL, Levine LA. Surgical correction of Peyronie's disease via tunica albuginea plication or partial plaque excision with pericardial graft: long-term follow up. J Sex Med 2008;5(9):2221–8. ; [discussion: 2229-2230].

27. Hatzichristodoulou G. Partial Plaque Excision and Grafting With Collagen Fleece in Peyronie Disease. J Sex Med 2016;13(2):277–81.

28. Sansalone S, Garaffa G, Djinovic R, et al. Long-term results of the surgical treatment of Peyronie's disease with Egydio's technique: a European multi-centre study. Asian J Androl 2011;13(6):842–5.

29. Knoll LD. Use of small intestinal submucosa graft for the surgical management of Peyronie's disease. J Urol 2007;178(6):2474–8. ; [discussion: 2478].

30. Brannigan RE, Kim ED, Oyasu R, et al. Comparison of tunica albuginea substitutes for the treatment of Peyronie's disease. J Urol 1998;159(3):1064–8.

31. Garcia-Gomez B, Ralph D, Levine L, et al. Grafts for Peyronie's disease: a comprehensive review. Andrology 2018;6(1):117–26.

32. Kadioglu A, Sanli O, Akman T, et al. Graft materials in Peyronie's disease surgery: a comprehensive review. J Sex Med 2007;4(3):581–95.

33. Sayedahmed K, Rosenhammer B, Spachmann PJ, et al. Bicentric prospective evaluation of corporoplasty with porcine small intestinal submucosa (SIS) in patients with severe Peyronie's disease. World J Urol 2017;35(7):1119–24.

34. Cakan M, Akman T, Oktar T, et al. The clinical characteristics of Peyronie's patients with notching deformity. J Sex Med 2007;4(4 Pt 2):1174–8.

35. Yafi FA, Hatzichristodoulou G, Wang J, et al. Outcomes of surgical management of men with peyronie's disease with hourglass deformity. Urology 2016;91:119–23.

36. Martinez-Salamanca JI, Egui A, Moncada I, et al. Acute phase Peyronie's disease management with traction device: a nonrandomized prospective controlled trial with ultrasound correlation. J Sex Med 2014;11(2):506–15.

37. Yafi FA, Hatzichristodoulou G, DeLay KJ, et al. Review of management options for patients with atypical Peyronie's Disease. Sex Med Rev 2017;5(2):211–21.

38. Egydio PH, Lucon AM, Arap S. Treatment of Peyronie's disease by incomplete circumferential incision of the tunica albuginea and plaque with bovine pericardium graft. Urology 2002;59(4):570–4.

39. Akkus E, Ozkara H, Alici B, et al. Incision and venous patch graft in the surgical treatment of penile curvature in Peyronie's disease. Eur Urol 2001;40(5):531–6 [discussion: 537].

40. El-Sakka AI, Rashwan HM, Lue TF. Venous patch graft for Peyronie's disease. Part II: outcome analysis. J Urol 1998;160(6 Pt 1):2050–3.

41. Eisenberg ML, Smith JF, Shindel AW, et al. Tunica-sparing ossified Peyronie's plaque excision. BJU Int 2011;107(4):622–5.

42. Kadioglu A, Kucukdurmaz F, Sanli O. Current status of the surgical management of Peyronie's disease. Nat Rev Urol 2011;8(2):95–106.

43. Zucchi A, Silvani M, Pastore AL, et al. Corporoplasty using buccal mucosa graft in Peyronie disease: is it a first choice? Urology 2015;85(3):679–83.

44. Chung E, Clendinning E, Lessard L, et al. Five-year follow-up of Peyronie's graft surgery: outcomes and patient satisfaction. J Sex Med 2011;8(2):594–600.

45. Terrier JE, Tal R, Nelson CJ, et al. Penile sensory changes after plaque incision and grafting surgery for Peyronie's Disease. J Sex Med 2018;15(10):1491–7.

46. Kalsi J, Minhas S, Christopher N, et al. The results of plaque incision and venous grafting (Lue procedure) to correct the penile deformity of Peyronie's disease. BJU Int 2005;95(7):1029–33.

47. Levine LA, Benson J, Hoover C. Inflatable penile prosthesis placement in men with Peyronie's disease and drug-resistant erectile dysfunction: A single-center study. J Sex Med 2010;7(11):3775–83.

48. Ziegelmann MJ, Farrell MR, Levine LA. Modern treatment strategies for penile prosthetics in Peyronie's disease: a contemporary clinical review. Asian J Androl 2020;22(1):51–9.

49. Chung E, Solomon M, DeYoung L, et al. Comparison between AMS 700 CX and Coloplast Titan inflatable penile prosthesis for Peyronie's disease treatment and remodeling: clinical outcomes and patient satisfaction. J Sex Med 2013;10(11):2855–60.

50. Montague DK, Angermeier KW, Lakin MM, et al. AMS 3-piece inflatable penile prosthesis implantation in men with Peyronie's disease: comparison of CX and Ultrex cylinders. J Urol 1996;156(5):1633–5.

51. Wilson SK, Delk JR 2nd. A new treatment for Peyronie's disease: modeling the penis over an inflatable penile prosthesis. J Urol 1994;152(4):1121–3.

52. Rahman NU, Carrion RE, Bochinski D, et al. Combined penile plication surgery and insertion of penile prosthesis for severe penile curvature and erectile dysfunction. J Urol 2004;171(6 Pt 1):2346–9.

53. Levine LA, Dimitriou RJ. A surgical algorithm for penile prosthesis placement in men with erectile failure and Peyronie's disease. Int J Impot Res 2000;12(3):147–51.

54. Rolle L, Ceruti C, Timpano M, et al. A new, innovative, lengthening surgical procedure for Peyronie's disease by penile prosthesis implantation with double dorsal-ventral patch graft: the "sliding technique." J Sex Med 2012;9(9):2389–95.

55. Rolle L, Falcone M, Ceruti C, et al. A prospective multicentric international study on the surgical outcomes and patients' satisfaction rates of the 'sliding' technique for end-stage Peyronie's disease with severe shortening of the penis and erectile dysfunction. BJU Int 2016;117(5):814–20.

56. Egydio PH, Kuehhas FE. The multiple-slit technique (MUST) for penile length and girth restoration. J Sex Med 2018;15(2):261–9.

57. Santucci RA, Berger RE. Finger trap" penile lengthening after partial penectomy by multiple incisions in the tunica albuginea. J Urol 1995;154(2 Pt 1):530–2.

58. Jorissen C, De Bruyna H, Baten E, et al. Clinical outcome: patient and partner satisfaction after penile implant surgery. Curr Urol 2019;13(2):94–100.

59. Scherzer ND, Dick B, Gabrielson AT, et al. Penile prosthesis complications: planning, prevention, and decision making. Sex Med Rev 2019;7(2):349–59.

60. Miller JA, Bennett NE. Comparing risk factors for adverse outcomes in virgin inflatable penile prosthesis implantations and revisions: a retrospective cohort study. Sex Med 2020;8(3):388–95.

61. Ghanem HM, Fahmy I, Fallon B. Infection control in outpatient unicomponent penile prosthesis surgery. Int J Impot Res 1999;11(1):25–7.

62. Akin-Olugbade O, Parker M, Guhring P, et al. Determinants of patient satisfaction following penile prosthesis surgery. J Sex Med 2006;3(4):743–8.

63. Govier FE, Gibbons RP, Correa RJ, et al. Mechanical reliability, surgical complications, and patient and partner satisfaction of the modern three-piece inflatable penile prosthesis. Urology 1998;52(2):282–6.

64. Wilson SK, Delk JR. Inflatable penile implant infection: predisposing factors and treatment suggestions. J Urol 1995;153(3 Pt 1):659–61.

65. Levine LA, Becher EF, Bella AJ, et al. Penile prosthesis surgery: current recommendations from the International Consultation on Sexual Medicine. J Sex Med 2016;13(4):489–518.

66. Hellstrom WJ, Montague DK, Moncada I, et al. Implants, mechanical devices, and vascular surgery for erectile dysfunction. J Sex Med 2010;7(1 Pt 2):501–23.

67. Yafi FA, Sangkum P, McCaslin IR, et al. Strategies for penile prosthesis placement in Peyronie's disease and corporal fibrosis. Curr Urol Rep 2015;16(4):21.

68. Garber BB, Lim C. Inflatable penile prosthesis insertion in men with severe intracorporal fibrosis. Curr Urol 2017;10(2):92–6.

69. Sansalone S, Garaffa G, Djinovic R, et al. Simultaneous total corporal reconstruction and implantation of a penile prosthesis in patients with erectile dysfunction and severe fibrosis of the corpora cavernosa. J Sex Med 2012;9(7):1937–44.

70. Montague DK, Angermeier KW. Corporeal excavation: new technique for penile prosthesis implantation in men with severe corporeal fibrosis. Urology 2006;67(5):1072–5.

71. Mooreville M, Adrian S, Delk JR, et al. Implantation of inflatable penile prosthesis in patients with severe corporeal fibrosis: introduction of a new penile cavernotome. J Urol 1999;162(6):2054–7.

72. Orvis BR, McAninch JW. Penile rupture. Urol Clin North Am 1989;16(2):369–75.

73. Larsen EH, Gasser TC, Bruskewitz RC. Fibrosis of corpus cavernosum after intracavernous injection of phentolamine/papaverine. J Urol 1987;137(2):292–3.

74. Shaeer O. Penile prosthesis implantation in cases of fibrosis: ultrasound-guided cavernotomy and sheathed trochar excavation. J Sex Med 2007;4(3):809–14.

75. Bertram RA, Carson CC, Webster GD. Implantation of penile prostheses in patients impotent after priapism. Urology 1985;26(4):325–7.

76. Stember DS, Mulhall JP. Ischemic priapism and implant surgery with sharp corporal fibrosis excision. J Sex Med 2010;7(6):1987–90.

77. Macaluso JN, Sullivan JW. Priapism: review of 34 cases. Urology 1985;26(3):233–6.

78. Krughoff K, Bearelly P, Apoj M, et al. Multicenter surgical outcomes of penile prosthesis placement in patients with corporal fibrosis and review of the literature. Int J Impot Res 2022 Jan;34(1):86–92. https://doi.org/10.1038/s41443-020-00373-9.

79. Wilson SK. Reimplantation of inflatable penile prosthesis into scarred corporeal bodies. Int J Impot Res 2003;15(Suppl 5):S125–8.

80. Wilson SK, Delk JR, Terry T. Improved implant survival in patients with severe corporal fibrosis: A new technique without necessity of grafting. J Urol 1995;153:359A.

81. Ghanem H, Ghazy S, El-Meliegy A. Corporeal counter incisions: a simplified approach to penile prosthesis implantation in fibrotic cases. Int J Impot Res 2000;12(3):153–6.

82. George VK, Shah GS, Mills R, et al. The management of extensive penile fibrosis: a new technique of 'minimal scar-tissue excision. Br J Urol 1996;77(2):282–4.

83. Rajpurkar A, Li H, Dhabuwala CB. Penile implant success in patients with corporal fibrosis using multiple incisions and minimal scar tissue excision. Urology 1999;54(1):145–7.

84. Shaeer O. Penoscopy: optical corporotomy and resection for prosthesis implantation in cases of penile fibrosis, Shaeer's technique. J Sex Med 2007;4(5):1214–7.

85. Shaeer O. Implantation of penile prosthesis in cases of corporeal fibrosis: modified Shaeer's excavation technique. J Sex Med 2008;5(10):2470–6.

86. Jarow JP. Risk factors for penile prosthetic infection. J Urol 1996;156(2 Pt 1):402–4.

87. Knoll LD, Furlow WL. Corporeal reconstruction and prosthetic implantation for impotence associated with non-dilatable corporeal cavernosal fibrosis. Acta Urol Belg 1992;60(1):15–25.

88. Boyd SK, Martinns FE. Simultaneus ultrex penile prosthesis re-implantation and Gore-Tex grafting corporoplasty functional outcome of a surgical challenge. J Urol 1995;153(A):359–89.

89. Goldstein I, Nehra A, Werner M, et al. Technique and follow-up of sharp corporal tissue excision procedure for prosthesis implantation with bilateral severe diffuse corporal fibrosis. J Urol 1995;153.

90. Fishman IJ, Scott FB, Light JK. Experience with inflatable penile prosthesis. Urology 1984;23(5 Spec No):86–92.

91. Martínez-Salamanca JI, Mueller A, Moncada I, et al. Penile prosthesis surgery in patients with corporal fibrosis: a state of the art review. J Sex Med 2011;8(7):1880–9.

92. Carson CC, Noh CH. Distal penile prosthesis extrusion: treatment with distal corporoplasty or Gortex windsock reinforcement. Int J Impot Res 2002;14(2):81–4.

93. Diokno AC. Asymmetric inflation of the penile cylinders: etiology and management. J Urol 1983;129(6):1127–30.

94. Pathak AS, Chang JH, Parekh AR, et al. Use of rectus fascia graft for corporeal reconstruction during placement of penile implant. Urology 2005;65(6):1198–201.

95. Egydio PH, Kuehhas FE. Treatments for fibrosis of the corpora cavernosa. Arab J Urol 2013;11(3):294–8.

96. Knoll LD, Fisher J, Benson RC, et al. Treatment of penile fibrosis with prosthetic implantation and flap advancement with tissue debulking. J Urol 1996;156(2 Pt 1):394–7.

97. Palese MA, Burnett AL. Corporoplasty using pericardium allograft (tutoplast) with complex penile prosthesis surgery. Urology 2001;58(6):1049–52.

98. Shen J, Lee Z, Hagedorn JC, Wessells H. Corporal Excavation and Grafting for Inflatable Penile Prosthesis Implantation in Severe Corporal Fibrosis. Presented at the Annual Meeting of the Sexual Medicine Society of North America; October 27-30, 2022. Scottsdale, AZ 2021.

99. Jordan GH. Penile reconstruction, phallic construction, and urethral reconstruction. Urol Clin North Am 1999;26(1):1–13, vii.

Gender Affirmation Surgery, Transfeminine

Jason Elyaguov, MD[a],*, Jessica N. Schardein, MD[b,c], Joshua Sterling, MD[b,d],
Dmitriy Nikolavsky, MD[b,c]

KEYWORDS

- Gender dysphoria • Transgender • Gender affirmation surgery • Transfeminine • Vaginoplasty

KEY POINTS

- Vaginoplasty techniques include vulvoplasty, penile skin inversion vaginoplasty, peritoneal vaginoplasty, and enteric vaginoplasty.
- The majority of complications are minor, effectively treated with office-based procedures and local wound care. Major complications are rare and may require advanced reconstructive techniques.
- Patients should be advised to never stop self-dilations, even during the treatment of minor complications, to maintain patency of the neovagina.
- Sexual activity is shown to increase postvaginoplasty and orgasm is achievable with a sensate neoclitoris.

INTRODUCTION

Over the past 20 years, the health care community has slowly depathologized gender identity and seen a destigmatization of gender-variant behavior. This has led to improved societal visibility and acceptance of transgender individuals, as well as an acknowledgment in the medical community that gender dysphoria is not a rare condition.[1,2] In the United States, an estimated 0.7% of the population identify as transgender.[3] Overall, these figures likely underestimate the true prevalence of transgender individuals due to inconsistencies in patient self-reporting and electronic medical records unreliably capturing nonbinary genders.

The Affordable Care Act attributed to the growing accessibility of transgender health care, with a 390% increase in Medicare beneficiaries identifying as transgender from 2010 to 2016.[4] As a result, genital gender affirmation surgery (gGAS) is becoming increasingly common with approximately 50% of transgender females being interested in feminizing genital surgery and 20% to 25% of transgender males reporting an interest in masculinizing genital surgery.[5]

Though earlier examples of patients undergoing surgical excision of healthy organs to alleviate gender dysphoria have been described, the modern concept of gender affirming surgery for transgender females, whereby a patient on hormone therapy undergoes orchiectomy, penectomy, and vaginoplasty, starts after WWII.[6] The goal of feminizing gGAS is to remove the patient's natal sex organs and create genitalia that is aesthetically pleasing and indistinguishable from cisgender female genitalia, while also accomplishing the patient's functional goals of receptive penetrative sexual intercourse, adequate sensation, ability to achieve orgasm, and normal continent voiding. The timing of procedures can differ from patient to patient.

a Department of Urology, Westchester Medical Center-New York Medical College, Valhalla, NY, USA;
b Department of Urology, SUNY Upstate Medical University, Syracuse, NY, USA; c Department of Urology, Upstate University Hospital, 750 East Adams Street, Syracuse, NY 13210, USA; d Department of Urology, Yale School of Medicine, 333 Cedar Street, PO Box 208028, New Haven, CT 06520-8058, USA
* Corresponding author. Department of Urology, New York Medical College, 40 Sunshine Cottage Road, Skyline 1S-B50, Valhalla, NY 10595, USA
E-mail address: j.elyaguov@gmail.com

Urol Clin N Am 49 (2022) 437–451
https://doi.org/10.1016/j.ucl.2022.05.001
0094-0143/22/© 2022 Elsevier Inc. All rights reserved.

PREOPERATIVE COUNSELING AND PREPROCEDURE PLANNING

The current World Professional Association for Transgender Health (WPATH) standards of care state that patients who desire gGAS have[7]

1. Persistent, well-documented gender dysphoria.
2. Capacity to make a fully informed decision and to consent to treatment.
3. Age of majority in a given country.
4. Any significant medical or mental health concerns must be reasonably well controlled.
5. Twelve continuous months of hormone therapy as appropriate to the patient's gender goals (unless the patient has a medical contraindication or is otherwise unable or unwilling to take hormones).
6. Twelve continuous months of living in a gender role that is congruent with their gender identity.

In the context of gGAS specifically, WPATH requires two letters of support from qualified mental health professionals to corroborate the patient's stable transition and ability to make sound clinical decisions. Although not an explicit criterion, it is recommended that these patients also have regular visits with mental health or other medical professionals.

It is very important to discuss in detail patient goals in terms of aesthetic and functional outcomes, especially with respect to desired vaginal depth. The new genitalia is created from the skin and tissue of the existing male organs. A thorough penile and scrotal examination should be conducted in conjunction with this discussion to assess the amount of skin available to create the new vaginal lining. These discussions may direct the type of vaginoplasty performed as well as the order and timing of surgical procedures.

Preparation for Surgery

Patients should be medically optimized before surgery. Patients with diabetes should have HbA1c checked and referred to an endocrinologist for better glycemic control if necessary. HIV-positive patients should have an undetectable viral load and adequate T-cell count at the time of surgery. Tobacco use has been associated with worse surgical outcomes and cessation is recommended 4 weeks before surgery.[8] Obesity is a comorbidity that may have implications in any surgery. Some surgeons will advocate for strict BMI cutoffs before proceeding with surgery, but BMI has not been shown to significantly impact vaginoplasty outcomes.[9,10] Instead of strict parameters,

surgeons should have a discussion with the patient about what a realistic and achievable weight loss goal is.

Preoperative hair removal of the genital skin is recommended to prevent malodorous secretions, infections, hairballs, discomfort, and dyspareunia. Several modalities to achieve hairless skin exist including laser hair removal and electrolysis. Laser hair removal has been shown to have significantly less pain and discomfort.[11] It may take 6 to 12 months to achieve adequate hair removal so the patient and surgeon should plan accordingly.

The preoperative process is lengthy, and some patients may elect to have an orchiectomy before vaginoplasty. Before undergoing bilateral orchiectomy, fertility preservation should be discussed and offered. Currently, the only option for transgender females is sperm cryopreservation. It should be noted that while cessation of hormone therapy is recommended before procuring the sample for preservation, it is NOT necessary.[12] The benefits of upfront orchiectomy are a notable reduction in gender dysphoria, a decrease in estrogen dose by up to 50%, and ability to discontinue antitestosterone medications.[13,14] Some have argued that early orchiectomy can result in shrinkage and atrophy of the scrotal skin and penis, but the timing of orchiectomy has not been shown to alter vaginoplasty outcomes.[15] In fact, others have argued that orchiectomy should routinely be offered as a bridge to vaginoplasty given the lengthy preoperative process.[14]

These risks and benefits should be discussed with the patient as a part of surgical planning. If the orchiectomy is going to be performed as a standalone procedure, patients need to meet the WPATH requirements already described, and the location of the incision should not impede the ability to complete a vaginoplasty in the future.[7,16] Surgery should include opening the tunica vaginalis, dissecting the spermatic cord to the level of the external ring, and ligating the spermatic vessels and vas deferens to complete transection, with both specimens being sent for histopathologic examination.[17] High ligation of spermatic cords at the external inguinal ring avoids patients feeling remnant cord stumps. In patients that may pursue vaginoplasty, care should be taken not to remove any skin or fat. Alternatively, in patients that do not want a future vaginoplasty, scrotal skin and tissue can be altered based on individual patient desires.[13]

PREP AND POSITIONING

1. Surgery is usually performed with general anesthesia. Although, it is possible to complete this

procedure under spinal or epidural anesthesia, especially if only a perineal incision is used.

2. Patients are placed in the dorsal lithotomy position. Care is taken to pad all pressure points and not hyperflex the hips. Arms can be secured at the patient's sides.

3. Given the length of procedure and position, mechanical and chemical DVT prophylaxis is recommended.

VAGINOPLASTY TECHNIQUES
Zero-Depth Vaginoplasty or Vulvoplasty

A zero-depth vaginoplasty, or vulvoplasty, is the preferred method for transgender patients who are not interested in vaginal intercourse and wish to avoid invasive surgeries that require lifelong dilation and cleaning. The goal of the procedure is to remove the erectile tissue of the penis and testicles, and create a clitoris out of the glans of the penis, inner and outer labia from the penile and scrotal skin, a shortened urethra and repositioned meatus, and a vaginal introitus. This is conducted by folding the skin flap that would otherwise be used for the posterior neovagina and securing it to the urethral stump instead.[18] Though vulvoplasty is less common, with studies reporting 8% to 17% of cohorts opting for it, the satisfaction rate is very high, and most of the patients elect for it regardless of contra-indications to vaginoplasty.[15,19]

Vulvoplasty is a less invasive procedure compared with vaginoplasty and thus serious complications are rare.

Penile Skin Inversion Vaginoplasty

The penile skin inversion technique for vaginoplasty was first described by plastic surgeons Drs Gillies and Millard in 1957.[20] Since then, penile skin inversion vaginoplasty (PSIV) has been popularized as the most common vaginoplasty performed today.[21]

This single-stage procedure inverts the penile skin, and if present foreskin, to fashion the neovaginal canal. The depth and caliber of the neovaginal canal depend on the dimensions of the available penile skin. The neovagina should be similar to the average cis female vagina in length at 9.6 cm (range, 6.5–14.8 cm) and width at 2.7 cm (range, 2.4–6.5 cm).[22] Additional skin grafting is most commonly derived from the scrotum, though full-thickness nongenital skin grafts may be used if there are insufficient genital skin[23] (**Figs. 1–3**)

- Skin graft or flap for the lining of the neovagina is harvested.

- Once scrotal skin is discarded, or harvested for additional use, the testicles can be excised with the previously described technique.

- The penis is then degloved superficial to Buck's fascia down to the pubic bone via a circumcising incision. Penile skin is saved to form the vaginal introitus.

- The bulbospongiosus and ischiocavernosus muscles of the urogenital triangle are then transected.

- Penile disassembly is then performed . The pendulous urethra is dissected free from the bulbospongiosum and corpora cavernosa. The glans or neoclitoris with its associated neurovascular bundle is separated from the corpora. The corpora are then transected just distal to their insertion at the pubis minimizing the potential for bulky, occlusive tissue in the vagina during arousal and penetrative intercourse.

- The space for the neovagina is then dissected. The cavity is established via dissection anterior to Denonvillier's fascia in the rectoprostatic space. Rectal injury is avoided by dissecting along the prostatic capsule up to the seminal vesicles until the peritoneal reflection is met.[24]

- The dissection between the prostate and rectum can also be achieved transperitoneally with robotic assistance .

- The glans is reduced with careful preservation of dorsal neurovasculature to form the sensate neoclitoris. Clitoroplasty involves suturing the glans to the corporal base.

- The urethra is then fully separated off the corpora spongiosum, shortened to the level of the bulb, distal to the urinary sphincter, and over-sewn in place. A Y-shaped urethral flap can be created wherein the neoclitoris can be embedded within the two short arms of the "Y" to improve sensitivity by ensuring a moist mucosal environment.[25]

- At this point, the vagina can be fashioned by inverting the penile skin flaps with or without a graft, and filling the tubularized canal with packing to maintain shape. The neovaginal fixation can be facilitated robotically if the dissection between the prostate and rectum was performed with robotic assistance (see **Fig. 3**).

- The neoclitoris and urethra are brought through an incision made in these flaps. Careful attention should be made to deliver and situate the urethral meatus two-thirds the distance from the introitus to the clitoris, mirroring the cis female urogenital anatomy.

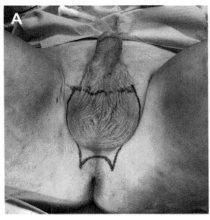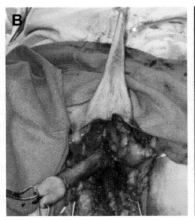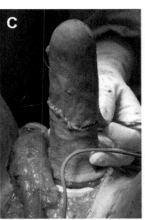

Fig. 1. Penile skin inversion vaginoplasty (PSIV) with scrotal graft. (*A*) Markings for removal of scrotal skin.[78] (*B*) Penile skin flap marked with an asterisk[79,] (*C*). Scrotal skin graft secured distally to the inverted penile skin flap.[78] (*From* Li JS, Crane CN, Santucci RA. Vaginoplasty tips and tricks. and Sigurjonsson H, Rinder J, Lindqvist EK, Farnebo F, Lundgren TK. Solely penile skin for neovaginal construction in sex reassignment surgery. Plastic and reconstructive surgery Global open. 2016;4(6).)

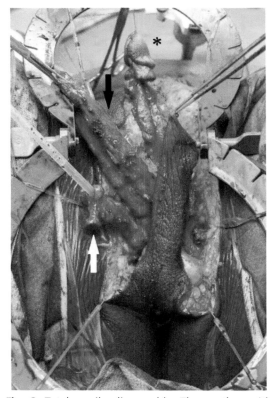

Fig. 2. Total penile disassembly. The urethra with indwelling Foley catheter is denoted by the white arrow. The black arrow denotes the corpora cavernosa, which have been sharply separated from the glans or neoclitoris and neurovascular bundle (*asterisk*).

- The clitoral hood and labia minora are subsequently created using redundant flap anteriorly. The labia majora are finally established as the scrotal skin is sutured to the original incision's skin edges and mons pubis.
- Vaginal packing is then sutured in place to reinforce the canal shape during early healing.
- Patients stay in the hospital for 3 to 7 days postoperatively.
- The vaginal packing is removed at 5 to 7 days postoperatively with the urethral catheter, which can be conducted prior to discharge or in the office depending on when the patient is discharged.

Modifications to the PSIV technique have been developed and can be substituted during the surgery. A double skin flap technique that uses a scrotal flap in addition to a penile flap has been proposed and utilized to avoid the complications that can be associated with a graft.[26,27] The creation of such a flap is seen in **Fig. 4**. **Fig. 5** shows the neovaginal anatomy following vaginoplasty.[28]

Peritoneal Vaginoplasty

The peritoneal vaginoplasty was first described by Russian gynecologist S.N. Davydov in patients with Mayer–Rokitansky–Kurster–Hauser Syndrome.[29] Originally considered in vaginal agenesis and other disorders of sexual dysfunction, use of the pelvic peritoneum can otherwise be offered to those with limited natal external genital tissue. It provides augmented depth to the standard PSIV while foregoing the more morbid use of

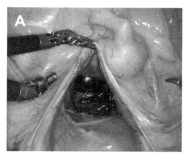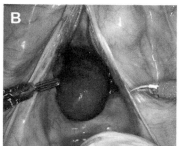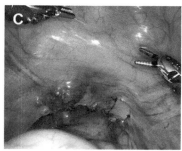

Fig. 3. Robotic assisted dissection and flap fixation. (*A*) Creation of vaginal cavity. (*B*) Neovaginal fixation. (*C*) Closure of peritoneum.

intestinal segments or extragenital skin grafts. Today, peritoneal vaginoplasty is feasible by robotic laparoscopy with a dissection akin to that of the transperitoneal radical prostatectomy (**Fig. 6**).[30,31] Both multi-port and single-port access techniques have been successfully attempted. This alternative approach begins with the classic PSIV and then identifies the peritoneum intraabdominally.

- Steps of the classic PSIV are followed until developing the space between the prostate and rectum.
- The peritoneum is incised over the rectovesical pouch, and dissection continues beneath the seminal vesicles until Denonvillier's fascia is met. Here, the same space for the neovaginal canal is developed in congruence with the extracorporeal perineal dissection.

- The anterior and posterior peritoneal flaps are developed which then become the apex of the neovagina as their borders are sutured to the inverted penoscrotal skin grafts. Intra-pelvic fixation sutures for the prevention of prolapse are optional as the neovagina is technically tethered to the abdominal wall via the peritoneal flaps.[31]
- The canal is then packed with or without a vacuum dressing.
- Postoperative course follows pathway for PSIV.

Enteric Vaginoplasty

Enteric vaginoplasty is a rarely employed technique in feminizing surgery, often considered for transgender women with insufficient external genital skin or who require revision vaginoplasty.

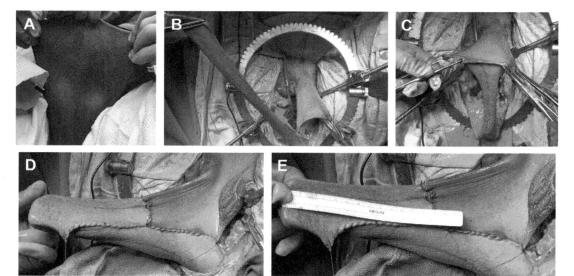

Fig. 4. Double skin flap technique. (*A*) Scrotal skin prior to incision. (*B*) Scrotal skin and penile skin shown separately and (*C*) together. (*D, E*) All edges sutured together for flap creation of adequate depth.

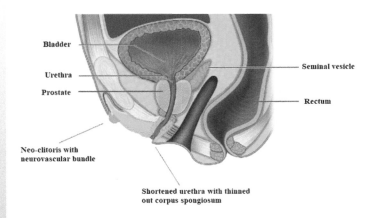

Fig. 5. Neovaginal anatomy following vaginoplasty.

Intestinal vaginoplasty was first described by Baldwin with the use of ileum.[32] Today, the most common bowel type used is rectosigmoid colon, and open, laparoscopic, hand-assist, and robotic approaches are all feasible.[33–35]

As the neovaginas are lined with a natural mucosa, the surface more closely mimics cisgender female vaginas. The bowel offers natural lubrication from mucus secretions, though not necessarily during arousal. Consequently, excessive mucosal secretion is the most common complaint; however, this usually resolves within 6 months of surgery.[36] If it is feasible to interpose a shorter segment of bowel, the smaller intestinal surface area would limit the potential for bothersome secretions.[37]

- Steps follow peritoneal vaginoplasty with intestinal harvest instead of using peritoneal flaps.

- An 8 to 15 cm pedicled segment of bowel is harvested and interposed with either a detubularization-retubularization method or a side-to-side reanastomosis pouch technique.[33,37] Intestinal continuity is then typically restored by way of conventional anastomotic stapling.
- A tension-free coloperineal anastomosis is fashioned to complete the neovagina (**Fig. 7**). To prevent prolapse, the proximal enteric end of the neovagina may be pexed to several pelvic structures such as the sacral promontory.[33]
- Postoperative course follows pathway for PSIV.

Complications of higher concern are those associated with bowel harvestings such as anastomotic leaks, fistulae, colitis, peritonitis, hernias, ileus, and bowel obstruction making this the

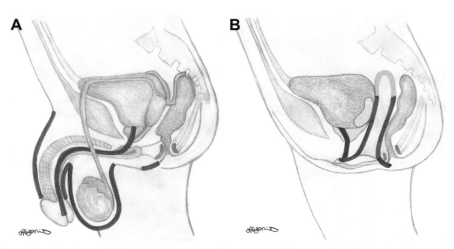

Fig. 6. Peritoneal vaginoplasty. (*A*) Preoperative cis-male anatomy (*blue*–penile skin, *red*-urethra, *green*–scrotal skin, *yellow*-peritoneum, *purple*–perineal skin). (*B*) The neovaginal canal is formed using peritoneal flaps, scrotal and penile skin, and perineal skin. (*blue*–penile skin, *red*-urethra, *green*–scrotal skin, *yellow*-peritoneum, *purple*–perineal skin).

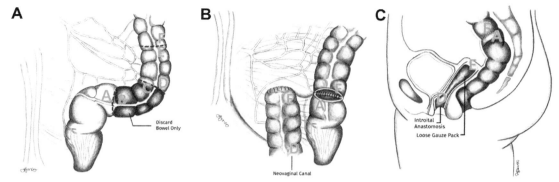

Fig. 7. Colon vaginoplasty. (*A*) markings for canal harvest, discard segment, and bowel-bowel anastomosis. (*B*) After the completion of bowel work. (*C*) final schematic after anastomosis of neovaginal canal to the vaginal introitus.

more morbid option for vaginoplasty.[38] In considering the neovagina, introital stenosis, prolapse, mucoceles, neuromas, bowel-bladder dysfunction and potentially increased susceptibility to sexually transmitted infections have all been described.[39] Overall reported complication rates are 6.4% for the sigmoid neovagina and 8.3% for the ileum neovagina.[33]

Vaginal Molds in Vaginoplasty

As it becomes more common for adolescents or prepubertal transgender patients to start gender affirmation hormone therapy, penile and scrotal skin may no longer provide the necessary coverage of the neovaginal canal. Several different biocompatible materials have been described as alternatives to scrotal skin grafts for neovaginal augmentation. These are all small case series and thus will not be discussed in detail in this forum. The surgical technique involves creating the space for the neovagina as already described.[24] Then the neovaginal lining is constructed around the outside of a malleable vaginal mold, which is inserted into the dissected space and sutured into place.[40] The mold is removed after 1 week. Depending on the biologic material used, multiple mold applications may be required.[40] Biocompatible materials that have been successfully used to create neovaginal lining include: meshed buccal mucosa, Nile Tilapia skin, human amniotic membrane, and Interceed which is a regenerated cellulose tissue.[40–42]

COMPLICATIONS AFTER VAGINOPLASTY

Complication rates vary from study to study with limitations in standardizing how they are measured. A meta-analysis of 13 studies found an overall complication rate of 32.5% and a

reoperation rate of 21.7% for nonesthetic reasons.[43] Poor cosmesis is the most common reason for reoperation; such revisions are often patient-driven and planned secondary interventions that are usually outpatient surgeries.[44–46] Overall, complications following vaginoplasty fall into three main categories: those managed with office procedures, those needing outpatient surgical correction, and those requiring complex reconstructive procedures.

Immediate/Early Complications

The majority of early postoperative complications are related to wound healing (infections, formation of granulation tissue, tissue necrosis, dehiscence, and bleeding) and most can be addressed in the office. Granulation, which may be an indicator of infection, can occur in 7% to 26% of patients.[46,47] Beyond antibiotic treatment, silver nitrate application can help mitigate fibroblast production in granulation.[48] Tissue necrosis is rare at 1% to 4% and can either affect the neovagina or the neoclitoris.[43,45] Conservative local wound care is recommended as well as smoking cessation and cardiovascular optimization preoperatively.[43] Wound dehiscence, most commonly in areas of increased tension such as the introitus or labia majora, has a higher incidence of 5% to 33%.[45,48] Office-based wound care will often suffice, though formal surgical debridement may be required in instances of greater tissue loss. Compliance with regular dilations is necessary even in patients with wound dehiscence to maintain the integrity of the neovaginal canal (**Fig. 8**).

Hemorrhage occurs in 3% to 12.5% of patients, with less than 1% requiring transfusions.[43,45,49] The corpus spongiosum surrounding the urethra is the most common source of bleeding, thus our recommendation would be to secure a tie-over

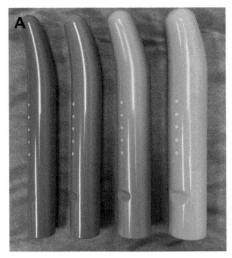
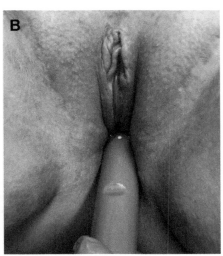

Fig. 8. (A) Sample dilators that can be used for (B) postoperative dilation to maintain the integrity of the neovaginal canal.

bolster or a wound vacuum over the spatulated strip of the remnant corpus spongiosum at the time of index surgery.[45] If hemorrhage recurs, the bolster or vacuum can be adjusted on the floor or in the office as needed. The bolster can be removed at the same time as the vaginal packing bolster.

Poor cosmesis is commonly the main reason for reoperation with patients electing for revision surgery at a rate of 20% to 54%.[50] It is encouraged to wait 3 months following vaginoplasty, once adequate wound healing is achieved, to properly assess the need for cosmetic revision.[46] Labiaplasty is most commonly performed (80%) followed by clitoral repositioning or hood reduction (20%).[50] Minor scar revisions or lipofilling of the labia majora can also be planned as office-based treatments. Importantly, aesthetic expectations should be reviewed extensively with the patient prior to vaginoplasty, during which planned secondary augmentation can be discussed.

Delayed Complications

Pelvic or genital pain has been reported in 1% to 20% of patients and can interfere with postoperative dilation, and sexual function.[45,47,51] Postoperative pain is one of the few complications associated with decreased quality of life.[52] Fortunately, this complication can be managed with office-based treatments including topical and oral analgesics, regional blocks, relaxation techniques, and physical therapy.[53–55] Patients that have preoperative or postoperative pain can benefit from working with a pain management specialist.[50]

Bothersome urinary symptoms can occur in 15% to 33% of patients, wherein 32% of complaints may be attributed to UTIs.[50,56,57] Conservative measures such as antibiotics, anticholinergics or pelvic floor physical therapy can abate most complaints. Though few ultimately seek surgery for stress incontinence, bladder neck bulking is considered a first-line operative intervention.[43,51] Additional outpatient procedures such as autologous/biological slings or bladder neck artificial urinary sphincter placements can be considered in refractory cases.[54] Divergent or spraying urinary stream (6%–33%) often resolves spontaneously, and rarely requires a secondary urethroplasty.[9,50] Bulky remnant corpus spongiosum may also change the angle of the urethra to protrude forward or upward.[51] Corrective surgery to resolve this involves resecting the residual erectile tissue and repositioning the urethra to establish a more ventral meatus[48] (**Fig. 9**).

Meatal or urethral stenosis can occur in up to 14% of patient cohorts.[43] Recent techniques involving spatulating the meatus, minimizing internal urethra manipulation, and anastomosing the urethra to the genitalia have improved incidences of meatal stenosis from 1% to 6% and urethral stenosis to 0% to 4%.[50] This is a critical complication to identify early as failure to address the stenosis may result in urethrovaginal fistula formation.[58] Urinary decompression via suprapubic or urethral catheterization is a necessary temporizing measure until more definitive dilation or urethroplasty can be performed.

Prolapse of the neovagina is relatively rare with an incidence of 1% to 2%, but can increase to

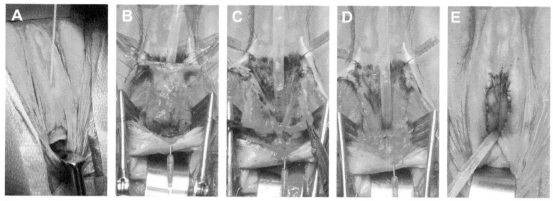

Fig. 9. Urethral shortening and debulking. (*A*) Q-tip demonstrating the upward direction of the urethra due to insufficient shortening and insufficient debulking of the corpus spongiosum. (*B*) Exposed remnant corpus spongiosum tissue after incision of neovaginal epithelium. (*C*) Proximal advancement of ventral urethrotomy. (*D*) Debulking of corpus spongiosum. (*E*) Repositioning of the urethral meatus to a more ventral opening.

6% at long-term follow-up[43,45,52] (**Fig. 10**). Sacrospinous ligament fixation of the neovagina during the index vaginoplasty reduces the risk of prolapse.[43,45] For patients that experience prolapse postoperatively an abdominal robotic or laparoscopic sacrocolpopexy is the most common repair.[54]

Inadequate neovaginal depth and stenosis of the introitus occur in up to 12% and 15% of transgender women, respectively.[50] Such outcomes are typically attributed to poor compliance with neovaginal dilation, though infections and compromised blood supply may contribute. Less invasive treatment includes gradual dilation, sometimes initially in the context of an exam under anesthesia. If the scarring is more extensive, revision techniques are recommended. Introital narrowing can be corrected with buccal mucosal augmentation grafts at the 3 and 9 o'clock positions of lateral vaginal walls[54] (**Fig. 11**). Reestablishing adequate depth by way of skin grafts or enteric revision vaginoplasty is feasible with equally successful outcomes.[59]

Neovaginal fistula formation is a serious complication that is more likely to occur in patients that have unrecognized injuries, postoperative infections, or pre or posttransition BPH procedures.[54] The overall incidence of fistula formation following vaginoplasty is 1% to 2% and can be separated into three categories: rectoneovaginal fistula, urethroneovaginal fistula, and vesiconeovaginal fistula.[43,45]

Rectovaginal fistula

Rectovaginal fistulae are the most common, occurring in approximate 1% of patients that undergo primary vaginoplasties and in up to 6% of patients that required a revision vaginoplasty.[45,58] This complication is usually the result of an unrecognized rectal injury at the time of vaginoplasty or failed repair of a recognized injury. Rectal injuries are reported in approximately 4% of

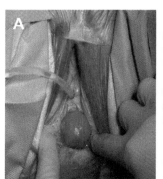
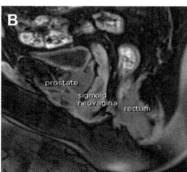
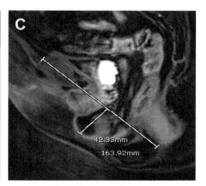

Fig. 10. Neovaginal prolapse of a sigmoid neovagina. (*A*) Prolapsing neovagina. (*B*) MRI show the reduced neovagina without Valsalva and (*C*) prolapsing neovagina with Valsalva.

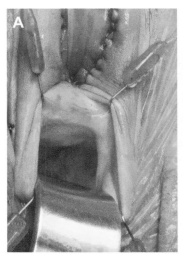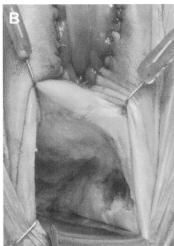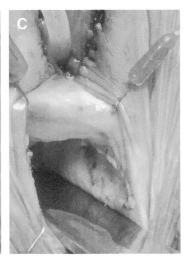

Fig. 11. Revision vaginoplasty with buccal mucosal graft (BMG). (*A*) Preoperative image showing neovaginal stenosis. (*B*) Lateral neovaginal incision demonstrated at 3 o'clock with subsequent (*C*) BMG fixation. Another incision was completed at 9 o'clock with subsequent BMG fixation (not pictured).

vaginoplasties.[45] If recognized at the time of surgery, primary repair and short-term low-residue diet will prevent any further complications in 80% to 85% of cases.[58,60] All patients with intraoperative repair of a rectal injury will need close monitoring postoperatively for signs of fistula formation. Diagnosis of a rectoneovaginal fistula is generally based on physical findings with patients reporting foul smell and stool in the neovaginal vault. Endoscopy or imaging studies (CT or MRI with rectal contrast) can confirm a diagnosis but are rarely required. While there are case reports of a rectoneovaginal fistula resolving with conservative management, it is not recommended because conservative management is unsuccessful in the overwhelming majority of patients.[58] Instead, we recommend definitive repair wherein fecal diversion may initially be required along with ceasing dilation for an extended period of time, carrying the potential for loss in the neovaginal canal depth. Repair can be accomplished via an open perineal or laparoscopic/robotic abdominal approach, depending on surgeon preference. Surgical repair follows the principles of any fistula repair: excision of the fistula tract, closure in layers with nonoverlapping suture lines, and interpositioning of tissue flaps including peritoneal, omental, rectus abdominus or gracilis.[61,62] Following repair, the authors of this review often place vaginal packing or stenting for a total of 4 weeks, which can be exchanged in the clinic weekly. This allows the neovaginal canal to stay patent without having patients self-dilate across a fresh suture line.

Urethroneovaginal fistula

Incidence of urethroneovaginal fistula is reported to be approximately 1%.[60] **Fig. 12** shows an example of a prostate-neovaginal fistula in a post-vaginoplasty patient who had a prior transurethral resection of the prostate.[63] Similar to rectoneovaginal fistula, the etiology of this complication is likely unrecognized urethral injury or breakdown of urethral injury repair.[60] In treating urethral fistulae, urinary diversion by way of suprapubic catheterization can be considered. Patients with distal fistulae can be left alone if not bothersome to the patient or can be treated by excising the distal bridge of tissue creating a more recessed meatus.[61] Patients with more proximal fistula can be repaired via a transvaginal approach. Repair involves separating the neovaginal and urinary structures, and closing both the urethral and neovaginal defects in multiple layers with interposition of healthy uninvolved tissue when possible.[54,56,58] Vaginal packing or stent may be placed and exchanged weekly to maintain patency of the neovaginal canal if there is concern the patient's self-dilation regimen will disrupt the repair.

Vesiconeovaginal fistula

Reported incidence of vesiconeovaginal fistula is under 1% and is usually the result of an unrecognized intraoperative injury.[46,64] Conservative management with just bladder decompression may resolve small fistulae. If conservative management fails, a formal repair is required and the authors recommend a laparoscopic or robotic abdominal approach with an omental interposition, using

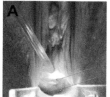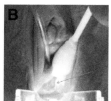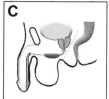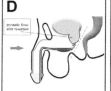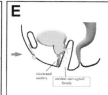

Fig. 12. Prostato-neovaginal fistula. (*A, B*) The fistula is denoted by the blue arrows. (*C*) Diagram showing the perineal dissection plane with a dashed line. (*D*) Diagram showing the thinned capsule of the prostatic fossa in close proximity to the dissection plane. (*E*) Urethroneovaginal fistula resulting postvaginoplasty due to the violation of the thinned capsule of the prostatic fossa. (Sager* R, Kaefer D, Ginzburg N, Nikolavsky D. V07-06 PROSTATO-NEOVAGINAL FISTULA REPAIR IN A PATIENT WITH PRIOR TRANSURETHRAL RESECTION OF THE PROSTATE. The Journal of Urology. 2020;203(Supplement 4):e644-e645.)

techniques described above.[61] There are otherwise case reports of successful transneovaginal repairs.[65]

OUTCOMES
Sexual Function

Sexual function is a major consideration of an individual seeking gGAS as a means to significantly enhance the quality of life. There are several components to ensuring satisfactory sexual function following the creation of a neovagina including desire, arousal, sexual activity, lubrication, dyspareunia, and orgasm. Libido may be markedly weakened in transgender women following the initiation of hormone therapy.[66,67] Feminizing gGAS has been shown to have a positive effect on spontaneous sexual desire as gender dysphoria is addressed and the majority of transgender women do not report distress over libido.[68] Conversely, supplementary androgen therapy aimed to restore testosterone to physiologic levels of cisgender women can be offered to increase desire.[69]

Sexual activity is shown to increase postvaginoplasty for the majority of patients promoting higher levels of sexual satisfaction.[70–72] Achieving orgasm postvaginoplasty is a variable outcome reported, but can be seen as high as 100%.[66,73] The neoclitoris plays a critical role in sexual stimulation and arousal wherein a sensate clitoris promotes successful orgasm in over 80% of transgender women.[68] Orgasm is best achieved via masturbation over penetrative activity, and can result in ejaculation during the climax in 52% to 76% of patients considering sustained prostatic and seminal vesicle function.[68,70]

Though the preservation of the bulbourethral (Cowper's) glands while creating the neovagina may promote secretions during episodes of arousal, this is insufficient to fully lubricate the neovagina. Ultimately, supplementary lubrication is always recommended when engaging in penetrative activities, be it dilation or intercourse. Dyspareunia may otherwise be attributed to pelvic floor dysfunction wherein the pelvic diaphragm is hyper-spastic. Once proper healing of the reconstructed area is achieved within 3 to 6 months, pain during intercourse is often reported to resolve on its own.[18,74]

Patient-Reported Outcome Measures

Several patient-reported outcome measures (PROMs) offer standardized methods for objectively assessing the quality of life as it relates to sexual function. The Female Sexual Function Index (FSFI) has historically been relied on for sexual function assessment postvaginoplasty, but, it was validated in cisgender heterosexual women so offers limited credibility in evaluating transgender women.[75]

Currently, two questionnaires have been formally validated for transgender women postvaginoplasty. Though the authors of this review recommend the preferred terminology "transfeminine," the operated Male-to-Female Sexual Function Index (oMtFSFI) is a 3-domain structure measuring sexual dissatisfaction, sexual pain, and genital self-image.[76] The AFFIRM similarly includes 3 domains that broadly gauge appearance, urologic and gynecologic areas of focus.[77] The AFFIRM is particularly reliable as it includes 33 questions of interest guided by both direct patient input and multidisciplinary expert opinion. The authors further demonstrated that scores significantly differ in the shorter term (within 6–12 months) postsurgery compared with later, stressing the importance of proactively counseling and managing expectations to improve satisfaction and subjective success.

SUMMARY

Feminizing gGAS for transgender women is a feasible and fulfilling intervention in alleviating gender dysphoria. Several techniques in neovaginal creation can be offered, though the PSIV is most commonly performed. Complication rates are low and often managed conservatively. Favorable sexual function outcomes indicate high satisfaction rates.

CLINICS CARE POINTS

- WPATH guidelines should be followed prior to offering feminizing genital surgery.
- Vaginoplasty techniques include vulvoplasty, penile skin inversion vaginoplasty, peritoneal vaginoplasty, and enteric vaginoplasty.
- The majority of complications are related to wound healing and can be effectively treated with office-based procedures and local wound care.
- Secondary operations for cosmetic revisions are common and often planned outpatient procedures.
- Major complications are rare but can be devastating. They include fistulae and complete obliteration of the neovaginal canal, requiring advanced reconstructive techniques.
- Patients should be advised to NEVER stop self-dilations, even during the treatment of minor complications.
- In situations where self-dilation might compromise a major complication's surgical repair, vaginal packing or a vaginal stent should be employed to maintain patency of the neovagina until self-dilating regimen can be resumed.
- Sexual activity is shown to increase postvaginoplasty and orgasm is achievable with a sensate neoclitoris.
- The oMtFSFI and AFFIRM questionnaires offer reliable assessments of postvaginoplasty outcomes specific to transgender women.

DISCLOSURE

J. Elyaguov; J.N. Schardein; J. Sterling have nothing to disclose. D. Nikolavsky Disclosures (receive honorarium) include (1) Contributor to UpToDate; (2) Co-editor of Springer Nature textbook "Urologic Care for Transgender Patients".

REFERENCES

1. Beek TF, Cohen-Kettenis PT, Kreukels BP. Gender incongruence/gender dysphoria and its classification history. Int Rev Psychiatry 2016;28(1):5–12.
2. Zucker KJ. Epidemiology of gender dysphoria and transgender identity. Sex Health 2017;14(5):404–11.
3. Flores AR, Brown TN, Herman J. Race and ethnicity of adults who identify as transgender in the United States. Williams Institute, UCLA School of Law Los Angeles, CA; 2016.
4. Ewald ER, Guerino P, Dragon C, et al. Identifying medicare beneficiaries accessing transgender-related care in the era of ICD-10. LGBT Health 2019;6(4):166–73.
5. Nolan IT, Dy GW, Levitt N. Considerations in Gender-Affirming Surgery: Demographic Trends. Urol Clin North Am 2019;46(4):459–65.
6. Meyerowitz J. How sex changed: a history of transsexuality in the United States. Harvard University Press; 2004.
7. Coleman E, Bockting W, Botzer M, et al. Standards of care for the health of transsexual, transgender, and gender-nonconforming people, version 7. Int J Transgenderism 2012;13(4):165–232.
8. Pluvy I, Garrido I, Pauchot J, et al. Smoking and plastic surgery, part I. Pathophysiological aspects: update and proposed recommendations. Ann Chir Plast Esthet 2015;60(1):e3–13.
9. Ives GC, Fein LA, Finch L, et al. Evaluation of BMI as a risk factor for complications following gender-affirming penile inversion vaginoplasty. Plast Reconstr Surg Glob Open 2019;7(3):e2097.
10. Brownstone LM, DeRieux J, Kelly DA, et al. Body mass index requirements for gender-affirming surgeries are not empirically based. Transgend Health 2021;6(3):121–4.
11. Zhang WR, Garrett GL, Arron ST, et al. Laser hair removal for genital gender affirming surgery. Transl Androl Urol 2016;5(3):381–7.
12. Sterling J, Garcia MM. Fertility preservation options for transgender individuals. Transl Androl Urol 2020;9(Suppl 2):S215–26.
13. van der Sluis WB, Steensma TD, Bouman MB. Orchiectomy in transgender individuals: a motivation analysis and report of surgical outcomes. Int J Transgend Health 2020;21(2):176–81.
14. Hehemann MC, Walsh TJ. Orchiectomy as bridge or alternative to vaginoplasty. Urol Clin North Am 2019; 46(4):505–10.
15. Jiang D, Witten J, Berli J, et al. Does depth matter? factors affecting choice of vulvoplasty over vaginoplasty as gender-affirming genital surgery for transgender women. J Sex Med 2018;15(6):902–6.
16. Washington S, Bayne D, Butler C, et al. 215 bilateral orchiectomy for transgender patients: an efficient surgical technique that anticipates future

vaginoplasty and is associated with minimal morbidity. J Sex Med 2017;14(2):e91–2.

17. Matoso A, Khandakar B, Yuan S, et al. Spectrum of findings in orchiectomy specimens of persons undergoing gender confirmation surgery. Hum Pathol 2018;76:91–9.

18. Garcia MM. Sexual function after shallow and full-depth vaginoplasty: challenges, clinical findings, and treatment strategies- urologic perspectives. Clin Plast Surg 2018;45(3):437–46.

19. Ferrando CA. Adverse events associated with gender affirming vaginoplasty surgery. Am J Obstet Gynecol 2020;223(2):267 e1–6.

20. Gillies H, Millard DR. The principles and art of plastic surgery. Boston: Little, Brown; 1957.

21. Pan S, Honig SC. Gender-affirming surgery: current concepts. Curr Urol Rep 2018;19(8):62.

22. Safa B, Lin WC, Salim AM, et al. Current concepts in feminizing gender surgery. Plast Reconstr Surg 2019;143(5):1081e–91e.

23. Hage JJ, Karim RB. Abdominoplastic secondary full-thickness skin graft vaginoplasty for male-to-female transsexuals. Plast Reconstr Surg 1998; 101(6):1512–5.

24. Shoureshi P, Dy GW, Dugi D 3rd. Neovaginal canal dissection in gender-affirming vaginoplasty. J Urol 2021;205(4):1110–8.

25. Ongaro L, Garaffa G, Migliozzi F, et al. Vaginoplasty in Male to Female transgenders: single center experience and a narrative review. Int J Impot Res 2020; 33(7):726–32.

26. Nijhuis THJ, Ozer M, van der Sluis WB, et al. The bilateral pedicled epilated scrotal flap: a powerful adjunctive for creation of more neovaginal depth in penile inversion vaginoplasty. J Sex Med 2020; 17(5):1033–40.

27. Namba Y, Sugiyama N, Yamashita S, et al. Vaginoplasty with an M-shaped perineo- scrotal flap in a male-to-female transsexual. Acta Med Okayama 2007;61(6):355–60.

28. Nikolavsky D, Blakely SA. Urological care for the transgender patient: a comprehensive guide. Springer Nature; 2021.

29. Davydov SN. [Colpopoeisis from the peritoneum of the uterorectal space]. Akush Ginekol (Mosk) 1969;45(12):55–7. Operatsiia kol'popeza iz briushiny matochno-priamokishechnogo prostranstva.

30. Jacoby A, Maliha S, Granieri MA, et al. Robotic davydov peritoneal flap vaginoplasty for augmentation of vaginal depth in feminizing vaginoplasty. J Urol 2019;201(6):1171–6.

31. Acar O, Sofer L, Dobbs RW, et al. Single port and multiport approaches for robotic vaginoplasty with the davydov technique. Urology 2020;138: 166–73.

32. Baldwin JF. XIV. The Formation of an Artificial Vagina by Intestinal Trransplantation. Ann Surg 1904;40(3): 398–403.

33. Bouman MB, van Zeijl MC, Buncamper ME, et al. Intestinal vaginoplasty revisited: a review of surgical techniques, complications, and sexual function. J Sex Med 2014;11(7):1835–47.

34. Kwun Kim S, Hoon Park J, Cheol Lee K, et al. Long-term results in patients after rectosigmoid vaginoplasty. Plast Reconstr Surg 2003;112(1):143–51.

35. Kim C, Campbell B, Ferrer F. Robotic sigmoid vaginoplasty: a novel technique. Urology 2008;72(4): 847–9.

36. Kim SK, Park JW, Lim KR, et al. Is Rectosigmoid Vaginoplasty Still Useful? Arch Plast Surg 2017; 44(1):48–52.

37. Djordjevic ML, Stanojevic DS, Bizic MR. Rectosigmoid vaginoplasty: clinical experience and outcomes in 86 cases. J Sex Med 2011;8(12):3487–94.

38. Bizic M, Kojovic V, Duisin D, et al. An overview of neovaginal reconstruction options in male to female transsexuals. ScientificWorldJournal 2014;2014: 638919.

39. Hage JJ, Karim RB, Asscheman H, et al. Unfavorable long-term results of rectosigmoid neocolpopoiesis. Plast Reconstr Surg 1995;95(5):842–8 [discussion: 849-50].

40. Ávila JS, Mendes LC. Systematic review: the use of vaginal mold in current vaginoplasty surgeries-techniques and materials. Int J Adv Med Biotechnology-IJAMB 2020;3(2):34–42.

41. Rodriguez AH, Lima Junior EM, de Moraes Filho MO, et al. Male-to-female gender-affirming surgery using nile tilapia fish skin as a biocompatible graft. J Minim Invasive Gynecol 2020;27(7):1474–5.

42. Wu M, Wang Y, Xu J, et al. Vaginoplasty with mesh autologous buccal mucosa in vaginal agenesis: a multidisciplinary approach and literature review. Aesthet Surg J 2020;40(12):NP694–702.

43. Dreher PC, Edwards D, Hager S, et al. Complications of the neovagina in male-to-female transgender surgery: a systematic review and meta-analysis with discussion of management. Clin Anat 2018;31(2):191–9.

44. Boas SR, Ascha M, Morrison SD, et al. Outcomes and predictors of revision labiaplasty and clitoroplasty after gender-affirming genital surgery. Plast Reconstr Surg 2019;144(6):1451–61.

45. Horbach SE, Bouman MB, Smit JM, et al. Outcome of vaginoplasty in male-to-female transgenders: a systematic review of surgical techniques. J Sex Med 2015;12(6):1499–512.

46. Gaither TW, Awad MA, Osterberg EC, et al. Postoperative complications following primary penile inversion vaginoplasty among 330 male-to-female transgender patients. J Urol 2018;199(3):760–5.

47. Massie JP, Morrison SD, Van Maasdam J, et al. Predictors of patient satisfaction and postoperative complications in penile inversion vaginoplasty. Plast Reconstr Surg 2018;141(6):911e–21e.

48. Suchak T, Hussey J, Takhar M, et al. Postoperative trans women in sexual health clinics: managing common problems after vaginoplasty. J Fam Plann Reprod Health Care 2015;41(4):245–7.

49. Papadopulos NA, Zavlin D, Lelle JD, et al. Combined vaginoplasty technique for male-to-female sex reassignment surgery: operative approach and outcomes. J Plast Reconstr Aesthet Surg 2017;70(10):1483–92.

50. Hontscharuk R, Alba B, Hamidian Jahromi A, et al. Penile inversion vaginoplasty outcomes: complications and satisfaction. Andrology 2021;9(6):1732–43.

51. Ferrando CA. Vaginoplasty complications. Clin Plast Surg 2018;45(3):361–8.

52. Lawrence AA. Patient-reported complications and functional outcomes of male-to-female sex reassignment surgery. Arch Sex Behav 2006;35(6):717–27.

53. Krick M. Pain With Vaginal dilation in a patient following sexual reassignment surgery. J Women's Health Phys Ther 2015;39(1):10–6.

54. Schardein JN, Zhao LC, Nikolavsky D. Management of Vaginoplasty and Phalloplasty Complications. Urol Clin North Am 2019;46(4):605–18.

55. Rossi Neto R, Hintz F, Krege S, et al. Gender reassignment surgery–a 13 year review of surgical outcomes. Int Braz J Urol 2012;38(1):97–107.

56. Goddard JC, Vickery RM, Qureshi A, et al. Feminizing genitoplasty in adult transsexuals: early and long-term surgical results. BJU Int 2007;100(3):607–13.

57. Hoebeke P, Selvaggi G, Ceulemans P, et al. Impact of sex reassignment surgery on lower urinary tract function. Eur Urol 2005;47(3):398–402.

58. van der Sluis WB, Bouman MB, Buncamper ME, et al. Clinical characteristics and management of neovaginal fistulas after vaginoplasty in transgender women. Obstet Gynecol 2016;127(6):1118–26.

59. Van der Sluis WB, Bouman MB, Buncamper ME, et al. Revision vaginoplasty: a comparison of surgical outcomes of laparoscopic intestinal versus perineal full-thickness skin graft vaginoplasty. Plast Reconstr Surg 2016;138(4):793–800.

60. Chen ML, Reyblat P, Poh MM, et al. Overview of surgical techniques in gender-affirming genital surgery. Transl Androl Urol 2019;8(3):191–208.

61. Mann RA, Kasabwala K, Kim N, et al. The Management of Complications of Feminizing Gender Affirming Genital Surgery. Urology 2021;152:67–73.

62. Byrnes JN, Schmitt JJ, Faustich BM, et al. Outcomes of rectovaginal fistula repair. Female Pelvic Med Reconstr Surg 2017;23(2):124–30.

63. Sager* R, Kaefer D, Ginzburg N, et al. V07-06 prostato-neovaginal fistula repair in a patient with prior transurethral resection of the prostate. J Urol 2020;203(Supplement 4):e644–5.

64. Bryson C, Honig SC. Genitourinary Complications of Gender-Affirming Surgery. Curr Urol Rep 2019;20(6):31.

65. de Toledo LGM, de Jesus Moreira R, de Almeida Tosi L. Transneovaginal repair of vesiconeovaginal fistula in female transgender. Int Urogynecol J 2018;29(9):1407–9.

66. Holmberg M, Arver S, Dhejne C. Supporting sexuality and improving sexual function in transgender persons. Nat Rev Urol 2019;16(2):121–39.

67. Wierckx K, Elaut E, Van Hoorde B, et al. Sexual desire in trans persons: associations with sex reassignment treatment. J Sex Med 2014;11(1):107–18.

68. Schardein JN, Nikolavsky D. Sexual functioning of transgender females post-vaginoplasty: evaluation, outcomes and treatment strategies for sexual dysfunction. Sex Med Rev 2021;10(1):77–90.

69. Kronawitter D, Gooren LJ, Zollver H, et al. Effects of transdermal testosterone or oral dydrogesterone on hypoactive sexual desire disorder in transsexual women: results of a pilot study. Eur J Endocrinol 2009;161(2):363–8.

70. LeBreton M, Courtois F, Journel NM, et al. Genital sensory detection thresholds and patient satisfaction with vaginoplasty in male-to-female transgender women. J Sex Med 2017;14(2):274–81.

71. Zavlin D, Schaff J, Lelle JD, et al. Male-to-female sex reassignment surgery using the combined vaginoplasty technique: satisfaction of transgender patients with aesthetic, functional, and sexual outcomes. Aesthetic Plast Surg 2018;42(1):178–87.

72. Scheim AI, Bauer GR. Sexual inactivity among transfeminine persons: a canadian respondent-driven sampling survey. J Sex Res 2019;56(2):264–71.

73. Hess J, Hess-Busch Y, Kronier J, et al. Modified preparation of the neurovascular bundle in male to female transgender patients. Urol Int 2016;96(3):354–9.

74. Bouman MB, van der Sluis WB, van Woudenberg Hamstra LE, et al. Patient-reported esthetic and functional outcomes of primary total laparoscopic intestinal vaginoplasty in transgender women with penoscrotal hypoplasia. J Sex Med 2016;13(9):1438–44.

75. Syed JS, Honig S. Sexual metrics in transgender women: transitioning from international index of erectile function to female sexual function index. Sex Med Rev 2021;9(2):236–43.

76. Vedovo F, Di Blas L, Perin C, et al. Operated male-to-female sexual function index: validity of the first questionnaire developed to assess sexual function after male-to-female gender affirming surgery. J Urol 2020;204(1):115–20.

77. Huber S, Ferrando C, Safer JD, et al. Development and validation of urological and appearance domains of the post-affirming surgery form and function individual reporting measure (AFFIRM) for transwomen following genital surgery. J Urol 2021; 206(6):1445–53.

78. Li JS, Crane CN, Santucci RA. Vaginoplasty tips and tricks. Int Braz J Urol 2021;47(2):263–73.

79. Sigurjonsson H, Rinder J, Lindqvist EK, et al. Solely penile skin for neovaginal construction in sex reassignment surgery. Plast Reconstr Surg Glob open 2016;4(6):e767.

Gender Affirmation Surgery, Transmasculine

Wai Gin Lee, MBChB, PhD, FRACS (Urol)[a,b,*], A. Nim Christopher, MBBS, MPhil, FRCS (Urol)[a,b],
David J. Ralph, MBBS, MS, FRCS (Urol)[a,b]

KEYWORDS

- Genital gender affirmation surgery • Gender incongruence • Phalloplasty • Metoidioplasty
- Urethral lengthening • Shared decision making • Functional outcomes

KEY POINTS

- The goal of genital gender affirmation surgery (GAS) is to align an individual's genital appearance more closely with their experienced gender identity with the least morbidity.
- The radial forearm free flap is the most used flap for phalloplasty.
- Metoidioplasty creates a small penis by lengthening the hypertrophied clitoris following testosterone stimulation.
- Adjunctive procedures including urethral lengthening, scrotoplasty, hysterectomy, and bilateral oophorectomy, vaginectomy, clitoral transposition, and insertion of an erectile device and testicular prosthesis can be offered depending on individual choice.
- Most transmasculine individuals are satisfied with the functional and esthetic outcomes of penile reconstruction.

INTRODUCTION

The field of transgender health care and gender affirmation surgery (GAS) has evolved and grown rapidly over the recent decades with improvements in the acceptance of diverse gender identities, reconstructive techniques, and funding (public and private) for GAS. In Europe, there has been a 20-fold increase in the number of individuals referred for assessment at the gender identity clinic in Amsterdam between 1980 and 2015.[1] The rates of genital GAS have doubled from an average of 11 procedures a year before 2011 to an average of 22 procedures a year since 2015.[2] Individuals are also requesting GAS at an increasingly younger age[3] possibly because information on transgender identities has become much more accessible via the Internet.

In the US, the incidence of genital GAS increased from 72% of patients undergoing gender-affirming procedures (2000–2005) to 83.9% of patients (2006–2011). Federal and state funding for GAS has improved following Section 1557 of the Affordable Care Act which prohibited discrimination based on gender identity.[4] Private insurers are also expanding coverage for transgender individuals because it has been shown to be affordable and cost-effective.[5]

In parallel, publications in this field have proliferated, reflecting the strong interest of clinicians to improve techniques and outcomes for genital GAS. Despite that, there are no accepted guidelines or gold standard treatment options. The aim of this review is to highlight contemporary techniques, controversies, and innovations within this growing field of reconstructive urology. Gaps in

[a] University College London Hospital NHS Foundation Trust, 16-18 Westmoreland Street, London W1G 8PH, UK; [b] St Peter's Andrology Centre, London, UK
* Corresponding author.
E-mail address: waigin.lee@nhs.net

Urol Clin N Am 49 (2022) 453–465
https://doi.org/10.1016/j.ucl.2022.04.007
0094-0143/22/© 2022 Elsevier Inc. All rights reserved.

the literature and future directions for research are also addressed.

Definitions and terminology

Clinicians who intend to work within the field of genital GAS must have some understanding of the terminology that underpins inclusive care.[6] *Sex assigned at birth* (eg, assigned male at birth) refers to the sex assigned to a newborn by a clinician. *Gender identity* is one's psychological sense of one's gender (a spectrum between female, male, and "other"). "Other" includes *non-binary* individuals who may identify with both genders, a gender different from male or female, outside the gender binary, or as not having a gender altogether.[7]

Transgender is an umbrella term for individuals whose sex assigned at birth do not match their gender identity. This mismatch is termed *gender incongruence*, which may lead to psychological distress or *gender dysphoria*. Distinct to one's gender identity is *one's gender expression* (the outward presentation of one's gender) and the term *gender diverse* describes any who don't follow stereotypical gender norms.[6] *Sexual orientation* is a separate concept that refers to the type of person one is sexually and/or emotionally attracted to.

We define *transmasculine* as those who identify as being part of the male or masculine half of the spectrum and would, therefore, seek some form of masculinizing GAS.

ROLE OF SURGERY

Genital GAS improves the psychological functioning of transmasculine individuals.[8] Genital GAS further ameliorates gender dysphoria experienced while on gender-affirming hormone therapy (GAHT). Body satisfaction scores are higher following surgery and GAHT compared with GAHT alone.[9] Furthermore, individuals awaiting genital GAS were less satisfied compared with those who did not wish to have genital GAS.

Young transgender adults who have completed puberty blockers followed by GAHT and GAS reported progressive improvement in gender dysphoria and psychological functioning after each stage of their transition.[10] They were generally satisfied, and their well-being were comparable to (or better than) peers in the Netherlands. Therefore, patients may be more likely to lead a productive and fulfilling life if treatment is initiated early enough.

GOALS OF SURGERY

The goal of genital GAS is to align an individual's genital appearance more closely with their experienced gender identity with the least morbidity. Surgeons are increasingly cognizant of the need for individualized care while satisfying the World Professional Association for Transgender Health Standards of Care.[11]

The seminal article by Hage *and colleagues* reported that patients prefer an esthetic and sensate (tactile and erogenous) neophallus that allows standing micturition and penetrative intercourse while minimizing donor-site morbidity.[12] Recently, a more diverse cohort of individuals confirmed that the most important priorities remained preserving orgasm ability, tactile sensation, and the ability to void while standing.[13] However, the ability to have penetrative intercourse and minimizing donor-site morbidity was deemed "low priority." Interestingly, although standing micturition was the most important request for many, 19% of individuals scored it "less important" and 21% ranked it as the "least important."

Individualized care

Knowing this, penile reconstruction should be viewed as a series of procedures that together constitute genital GAS.[14] These procedures are "modular" and various options or combinations can be safely offered or omitted. Not all transmasculine individuals will want, require, or qualify for all types of procedures. Partial treatment options are increasingly desired by a significant proportion of transmasculine individuals (40.9%), more so than in the transfeminine population.[15]

The risk of morbidity and unsatisfactory results also plays a significant role in decision-making.[16] A third of transmasculine individuals declined penile reconstruction due to the potential risks.[17] Another study of transmasculine individuals found that 24% were waiting for better techniques or were apprehensive of the functional outcomes and risk of complications associated with currently available techniques.[18]

Shared decision making and decision aids

Recognizing the importance of shared decision making and individualized care has underscored the need for decision aids in genital GAS. Such a tool (developed in Amsterdam, The Netherlands) integrated holistic assessment of surgical outcomes with quality of life, the environment, sexuality, and beliefs of the individual. The tool helped prepare transmen for their consultation with the surgeon, reduce decisional conflict and improve decisional confidence.[19,20] The Genital Affirmation Surgical Priorities Scale (GASPS) is alternative decision aid using a 5-point Likert scale to help the surgeon elucidate patient expectations of genital GAS.[21]

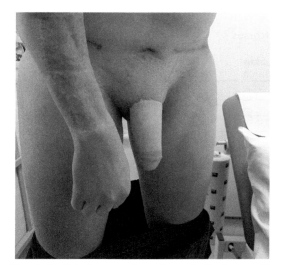

Fig. 1. Radial forearm free flap phalloplasty with donor site.

Table 1
Contemporary options for flap design based on the donor site

Donor Site	Flap Design		
	Tube-In-Tube	Phallus Only	Urethra Only
Radial forearm[23]	√	√	√
Anterolateral thigh[24]	√	√	
Abdomen[25]		√	
SCIP[26]	√	√	√
MLD[27]		√	√
Ulnar forearm[28]			√

Abbreviations: MLD, musculocutaneous latissimus dorsi; SCIP, superficial circumflex iliac perforator.

PENILE RECONSTRUCTION
Phalloplasty

Modern phalloplasty techniques use local or distant tissue flaps to reconstruct a neophallus. Distant flaps can be free flaps that require microsurgical techniques, or pedicled flaps involving transfer while maintaining the native blood supply. The radial artery forearm free (RFF) flap transformed phalloplasty techniques by allowing a sensate, tube-in-tube design with integrated urethra[22] (**Fig. 1**). An integrated urethra is better vascularized than prelaminated techniques, reducing the rate of urethral complications within the neophallus from 75% to 43%.[23]

The RFF flap remains the most used flap for phalloplasty but the anterolateral thigh (ALT) (pedicled or free) flap, musculocutaneous latissimus dorsi (free) flap, and superficial circumflex iliac artery perforator (pedicled) flap are other alternatives (**Table 1**). In particular, the ALT flap is gaining in popularity because it is a pedicled flap (90%) despite the variable vascular anatomy (**Fig. 2**). Characteristics of common flaps are summarized in **Table 2**.

The abdominal (pedicled) flap continues to play a (small) role and is offered in many centers. The flap is ideal for those who prefer a phallus-only procedure with a shorter operative and recovery time. It should be considered in individuals with multiple comorbidities that may complicate free flap phalloplasty.

Donor site morbidity

Donor site morbidity is the primary disadvantage of the RFF flap (see **Fig. 1**). The donor site is usually resurfaced with a full or split-thickness skin graft with no difference in cosmesis between both techniques.[29] Alternatively, a free flap can be used to resurface the arm donor site with good esthetic and functional outcomes.[30,31] This technique is time and labor-intensive requiring a third surgical team. Dermal matrices are expensive and currently have a limited role.[32]

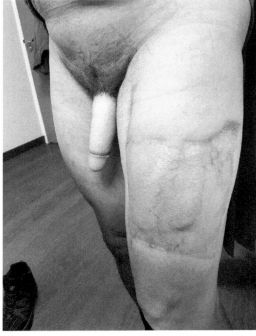

Fig. 2. Anterolateral thigh flap phalloplasty with donor site.

Table 2
Comparison of phalloplasty flap characteristics and outcomes

Flap	Sensation	Visible Donor Site Scar	Genital Skin Color Match	Urethral Segment Hair Removal	Bulky
RFF	Best	Yes	No	No	No
ALT	Yes	No	Yes	Yes	Yes
MLD	Poor	No	No	NA	Yes
SCIP	Yes[2]	No	Yes	No	Sometimes
AF	Variable	No	Yes	NA	Yes

Abbreviations: AF, abdominal; ALT, anterolateral thigh; MLD, musculocutaneous latissimus dorsi; NA, not applicable; RFF, radial forearm free; SCIP, superficial circumflex iliac perforator.

Donor site morbidity can be either functional or esthetic (**Table 3**). Detailed functional assessment showed a mild reduction in pressure sense but no changes in vibratory sense,[29] motor functioning, and grip sense.[33] One patient suffered a minor burn due to reduced temperature sense.[29] Esthetic concerns remain an issue, but most accept the tradeoff for a neophallus with good satisfaction reported (up to 75%).[29,34]

Composite phalloplasty

Donor site morbidity can be minimized by combining 2 smaller flaps. The radial[36] and ulnar forearm[28] free flap and SCIP[26] pedicled flap urethroplasty have been used for a 1- or 2-stage composite phalloplasty. Composite flaps (1-stage) pose a challenge because an extra surgeon and longer operating time are required. Monitoring the inner flap is difficult. The higher risk of flap or urethral complications[37,38] may be mitigated with a 2-stage approach.[39]

Metoidioplasty

Metoidioplasty is an alternative to phalloplasty. It is performed by lengthening the hypertrophied clitoris following testosterone stimulation to form a small penis (**Fig. 3**). We recommend at least 2 years of testosterone supplementation to achieve maximal hypertrophy of the clitoris before surgery.

Table 3
Summary of donor site complications following RFFF phalloplasty

Study Author	Type of Complication	Incidence (%)	Type of Skin Graft	Mean Follow-Up (Months)
Selvaggi et al,[29] 2006	Partial graft loss	4.8	STSG + FTSG	43
	Lymphedema	5.6		
Garaffa et al,[23] 2010	Partial graft loss	6.1	FTSG	26
	Lymphedema	1.7		
	Loss of sensation	8.7		
	Impaired function	1.7		
	Compartment syndrome	0.9		
Kuenzlen et al,[33] 2021	Partial graft loss	21.4	FTSG	21.5
	Partial graft loss	0	STSG + dermal matrix	
	Neuroma	10	STSG + FTFG	
Hage et al,[35] 1993	Partial graft loss	16.7	STSG	42
	Impaired function	16.7		

Abbreviations: FTSG, full-thickness skin graft; STSG, split-thickness skin graft.

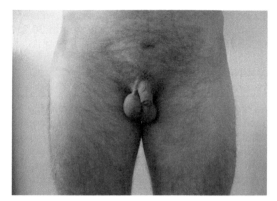

Fig. 3. Metoidioplasty with scrotoplasty and bilateral testicular prostheses.

The surgical principles to reconstruct a small penis were first described in 1973 by Durfee and Rowland.[40] The term "metoidioplasty" was coined several years later in 1989 by Laub and Lebovic from the Greek words "meta" (change), "aidion" (male genitalia), and "plasty" (formation).[41] The term "micropenis" has negative connotations and should be avoided.[20]

Notable techniques for metoidioplasty are summarized in **Table 4**. The Belgrade metoidioplasty forms the basis for most "full" metoidioplasty techniques today.

A metoidioplasty normally measures between 4.8 and 10.2 cm (mean 5.6 cm)[47] making it best suited for those of smaller build (body mass index $\leq$ 25 kg/m^2) but the extensive technique may achieve 6 to 12 cm (mean 8.7 cm).[46] Most will be able to void while standing (87%–100%)[48] but many will continue to void in a cubicle (rather than at a urinal). Penetrative intercourse is possible in 70% following extensive metoidioplasty but it's not usually possible following Belgrade metoidioplasty. In a series of 813 cases, urethral fistulae and strictures occurred in 8.85% and 1.70%,

Table 4
Summary of advances in metoidioplasty techniques

Name of technique	Description of Technique	Neourethra
Laub et al,[42] 1989	"Simple" metoidioplasty involving release of the clitoris with no division of the urethral plate. Small and curved neophallus.	Yes
Hage et al,[43] 1996	Combined clitoral release with vestibular skin flap, labia minora, and anterior vaginal flap neourethra.	Yes
Belgrade et al,[44] 2009	Clitoral release with the division of clitoral ligaments and urethral plate. Dorsal buccal mucosa augmentation with labia minora and anterior vaginal flap. Later refinements included optimizing clitoromegaly using dihydrotestosterone topical gel and vacuum device.	Yes
Ring et al,[45] 2009	Ventral urethral plate is lengthened with a labial ring flap. Urethral lengthening with labia minora and anterior vaginal wall flap	Yes
Cohanzad,[46] 2016	Mobilization of the crura off their attachments to the pubic arch followed by approximation to maximize length. A penile traction device is used for $\geq$1 y.	Yes

respectively, while 99% of 655 individuals were satisfied with the cosmesis.[47]

Deciding for metoidioplasty

Transmasculine individuals may prefer a metoidioplasty for several reasons. A donor site is not required (with the inherent risk of morbidity and scarring) and there is less local scarring. In turn, postoperative recovery is usually faster (3 weeks off work compared with between 6 and 12 weeks for free flap phalloplasty). The cost is also lower given the shorter duration of surgery and hospitalization. The small penis usually retains full tactile and erogenous sensation with the ability for natural erections. Lastly, the risk of local complications is likely to be lower because the tissue is better vascularized than a free (or pedicled) flap.[49]

When compared with individuals who prefer phalloplasty, those who preferred metoidioplasty were less concerned about penetrating a partner, penis length, penis girth, and tactile sensation.[21] Those who preferred phalloplasty were more likely to want to void while standing and to have easier access to male bathrooms and showers.[50]

Secondary Phalloplasty Following Metoidioplasty

Some transmasculine individuals may request a phalloplasty following the completion of metoidioplasty (table 5). Briefly, the small penis is degloved and neo-urethra separated from the body of the metoidioplasty.[51] A neophallus is constructed and transferred to the site of the small penis. Anastomotic urethroplasty between the phallus urethra and urethra of the small penis is performed and the deepithelialized small penis is subsequently buried within the neophallus.

Outcomes following secondary phalloplasty are good (98.5% satisfaction).[51] One patient suffered total flap loss (1.2% rate) while another 3 required microvascular revision to salvage the flap. Partial

flap loss occurred in 19.5% of patients, whereas urethral fistulae and strictures occurred in 30.3% and 35.6%, respectively.

ADJUNCTIVE PROCEDURES
Urethral Lengthening

The native urethra and phallus urethra need to be joined ("urethral lengthening") to allow standing micturition. Standing micturition was the most important request for many but 19% of individuals scored it "less important" and 21% ranked it as the "least important."[13,50] Outcomes and satisfaction following genital GAS without urethral lengthening are good with a marked reduction in urethral complications.[52]

Local tissue flaps (labia minora) for urethral lengthening are augmented by an anterior vaginal flap in many centers. Several adjunctive techniques to reduce complications have been described but there are no prospective comparative studies (**Table 6**). A long anterior vaginal flap (elevated with robotic assistance at the time of hysterectomy and vaginectomy) that reaches the pubic symphysis has been described in a conference abstract.[53]

Urethral complications are common and occur in almost half (43.5%) of all individuals following urethral lengthening in a contemporary series.[58] Most reported estimates have varied with rates of up to 75% but these were in heterogenous cohorts with incompatible techniques for urethroplasty, flap design and anatomy.[59–62] Urethral strictures and fistulae are most common, and repair is approached in a similar fashion to those assigned males at birth.[63–65] Anastomotic and reduction urethroplasty is performed more commonly in GAS due to the gradual increase in laxity of the skin tube urethra.

Vaginectomy, Hysterectomy, and Oophorectomy

Vaginectomy refers to the excision or ablation of the vaginal mucosa, often performed with hysterectomy and oophorectomy. Transvaginal,[66] laparoscopic,[67] and robotically assisted[68] approaches have been described. Transvaginal and laparoscopic approaches may have equivalent outcomes but transvaginal is quicker and more cost-effective.[69]

Vaginectomy is mandated in some centers if urethral lengthening is requested because it may reduce the risk of urethral fistulae.[70] However, a significant number of individuals would decline vaginectomy given the opportunity. Over 60% of them are gay or bisexual. Two-thirds of these individuals engage in receptive vaginal intercourse.[71]

Table 5 Reasons for secondary phalloplasty following metoidioplasty (multiple reasons accepted)		
Reasons	**n**	**%**
Preferred larger neophallus	32	38.6
Ability to have penetrative intercourse	25	30.1
Planned first stage of 2-stage phalloplasty	17	20.5
To void while standing	15	18.1
Other/unknown	3	3.6

Table 6
Adjunctive technique to reduce fistula rate following urethral lengthening

Adjunctive technique	Retrospective Study	n	Integrated Urethra	Comparative Study	Fistula Rate	Follow-Up (Months)
Anterior vaginal flap[54]	Yes	53	Not reported	Yes	Reduced	153 [a]
Gracilis pedicled flap[55]	Yes	15	No	Yes	Reduced	14.1 (2.5–25.1) [a]
Martius fat pad[23]	Yes	84	Yes	No	N/A	26 (1–270) "
Bulbospongiosus flap[56]	Yes	224	Yes	Yes	Reduced	643 d (308) [b]
Pedicled labia minora flap[57]	Yes	16	Flap is urethra	No	N/A	14 (4–32)[c]

Abbreviation: N/A, not applicable.
 [a] Mean (range).
 [b] Mean (SD).
 [c] Median (range).

Laparoscopic hysterectomy must be performed if vaginectomy is requested. Some individuals request the preservation of these organs for future fertility reasons.[72]

Scrotoplasty

Scrotoplasty (neo-scrotum formation) is usually performed using labia majora flaps. The goal is to reconstruct a pouch-like scrotum that sits anteriorly in an anatomic position at the base of the neophallus while maintaining tactile and erogenous sensation from the ilioinguinal and genitofemoral nerves. Techniques vary but excess hairless labia minora not used for urethral lengthening is usually excised. The labia majora can then be joined in the midline to give a single sac-like appearance.[73] A bifid appearance is unavoidable if midline structures like clitoris or vagina are preserved (**Fig. 4**).

A V-Y plasty creates a more pouch-like scrotum that sits more cephalad to approximate the male perineum more closely. In London (UK) the labia majora flap is rotated medially and joined anteriorly to form a pouch without a bifid appearance.[23] Another technique (Ghent, Belgium) is to rotate the labia majora flap medially and superiorly to the phallus base.[74] This last technique may have a lower risk of testicular prosthesis extrusion when combined with a horseshoe-shaped, vascularized prepubic skin flap.[75] Scrotoplasty can also be complicated by hematomas, wound dehiscence and distal labial flap necrosis.[76]

Erectile device

The decision to insert an erectile device should be made on a case-by-case basis. Erectile devices have a high complication rate that may directly compromise the neophallus. Insertion should be deferred $\geq$ 6 months from the previous operation. A para-scrotal[77] or infrapubic[78] approach can be used and commercially available inflatable penile prostheses (IPP) are currently adapted for use in this cohort (**Fig. 5**).

Satisfaction with the erectile devices is good and most can engage in penetrative intercourse (>80%).[79] The most common reason for not engaging was the lack of a partner. However, rates of mechanical failure, device infection, and erosion

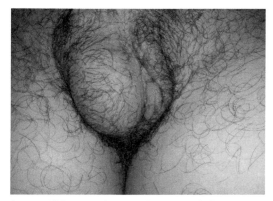

Fig. 4. Bifid scrotoplasty with unburied clitoris.

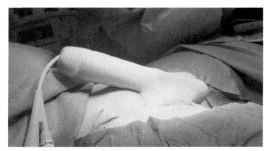

Fig. 5. Appearance following the insertion of erectile device and contralateral testicular prosthesis in radial forearm free flap phalloplasty.

are higher when compared with devices implanted within corpora cavernosa. The 5-year device survival was 78% in the UK.[79] Publications were all retrospective and should be compared with caution given the heterogenous patients (including the type of phalloplasty), devices, surgical techniques, and unvalidated assessment measures used.[78–81]

The first erectile devices customized for transmasculine individuals postphalloplasty (ZSI-475 FTM and ZSI-100 FTM, Zephyr Surgical Implants, Switzerland) are promising because they preclude the need for a cap and sock fashioned using either polyethylene, mesh or polytetrafluoroethylene.[82,83] However, numbers implanted, and reported outcomes (with short follow-up) are still limited, necessitating further studies. The devices are also not FDA-approved in the US.

Testicular Prosthesis

Staged testicular prosthesis can be considered $\geq$ 6 months following scrotoplasty. Only a single testicular prosthesis is inserted for individuals who request an IPP because the pump mimics a prosthetic testis on the contralateral side.

The surgical approach is either subinguinal or transscrotal, using previous incisions if possible. The size of prosthesis is dependent on the available space but is usually less than 4 cm in length (equivalent to a 16–21 cc implant).[75] One or both testicular prostheses were explanted in 20.8% of individuals due to infection or erosion while 15% required revision. Smoking and the type of scrotoplasty increased the likelihood of complications.[75]

Other Adjunctive Procedures

Further procedures can be performed to improve the functional and esthetic outcomes. Glans sculpting can be performed using a variation of the Norfolk technique[84] or the mushroom flap technique (glans is incorporated into the flap design).[85] The clitoris can be buried and transposed, if desired.

STAGING OF PHALLOPLASTY

The "staging" of genital GAS remains contentious. Staging relates to the decision to perform urethral lengthening at the time of phalloplasty in addition to the other adjunctive procedures. A 1-stage phalloplasty is when all the procedures are performed at the same time. An erectile device and testicular prosthesis are always inserted on a separate occasion.

A 1-stage phalloplasty is more convenient and cheaper for the patient and hospital (and insurance company).[86] Patients would only need to travel once to the hospital (that may be in another country), take one period off from work, and one period of convalescence. However, these benefits would only be realized if the surgical complication rate did not increase. Concerningly, the largest study to date reported a 19% flap-related complication rate and 43.1% rate of either urethral fistulae or strictures in 287 patients.[87]

A 2-stage approach may ameliorate these concerns. Flap (neophallus) complications can be treated independently from complications from the other procedures and would not be cumulative. They may heal spontaneously before the second stage, and if not, repaired at the time of the second stage without needing an additional operation. A smaller surgical team would be needed for the first stage of phalloplasty.

The 2-stage approach can be sequenced by neophallus formation followed by urethral lengthening, scrotoplasty, and the adjunctive procedures.[23] Alternatively, metoidioplasty with urethral lengthening and partial scrotoplasty can be offered first, followed by neophallus formation, transfer, and anastomotic urethroplasty.[88]

A systematic review comparing both approaches paradoxically found that a two-stage phalloplasty had a higher complication rate due to partial/total flap loss and urethral fistulae.[89] However, 2-stage phalloplasty was defined to include prelaminating the urethra. Prelaminated urethras have a higher complication rate, which would have negatively skewed the complication rate. Metoidioplasty was also misleadingly combined with phalloplasty even though it is not constructed from a tissue flap. The results should, therefore, be interpreted with caution.

Another systematic review pooled transmasculine and cis-gender patients in the analysis despite fundamental anatomic differences.[90] Cis-gender patients have a well-vascularized urethral segment, do not require urethral lengthening, and are more likely to have a 1-stage approach thereby biasing outcomes in favor of 1-stage phalloplasty.[90]

SURGICAL AND FUNCTIONAL OUTCOMES

Patient-reported outcomes measures (PROM) following transmasculine genital GAS are poorly evaluated and reported.[91] Most instruments are ad hoc (developed for a specific study) and have not been designed with rigor nor been validated.[92] Therefore, they lack validity and reliability and do not allow comparison between studies. There is an urgent need to design, test, and validate appropriate PROMs specific for transmasculine

Table 7
Categorization of regret according to Kuiper and Cohen-Kettenis[98]

Category	Feelings	Definition
Clear regret	Expressed	Openly expresses regret followed by role reversal (either detransition surgery or returning to former gender role).
Regret uncertain		Expresses regret and they would not have undergone GAS given a second chance or just regrets their decision to undergo GAS. Does not attempt gender role reversal.
Regret	Not expressed	No longer lives in previously desired role (for practical or social reasons) but does not express regret. They may even say they are happy with their decision and still consider themselves as transgender.
Regret assumed by others		Does not express regret nor return to their previous gender role. Unfavorable psychosocial issues (suicide attempts, psychiatric problems, or feeling lonely) suggest to others that the feelings of regret are present.

Abbreviation: GAS, gender affirmation surgery
   Data from Kuiper, A. J., & Cohen-Kettenis, P. T. (1998). Gender role reversal among postoperative transsexuals. International Journal of Transgenderism, 2(3).

individuals. Different PROMs should be developed for individuals at different "stages" of their journey and for different forms of penile reconstruction. There is little utility in questioning a transmasculine individual on their satisfaction with penetrative intercourse when they have not had penile reconstruction.

Noting these constraints, a narrative summary of the surgical and functional outcomes following genital GAS follows.

Satisfaction Following Phalloplasty

Satisfaction is high following phalloplasty despite the significant risk of postoperative complications (45% urethral complication rate[93]). Between 63% and 100% of individuals are satisfied with the esthetic appearance of their neophallus.[39,52,94–96] Satisfaction following phalloplasty was not correlated with partner sexual satisfaction, suggesting that the operation primarily provides personal satisfaction to the individual themself.[97]

Sexual Function

Almost all transmasculine individuals were able to achieve orgasm following RFFF phalloplasty.[97] Orgasm by masturbation was experienced by 93%, whereas orgasm by sexual intercourse was achieved in fewer individuals (78.5%) mostly because there was no available partner (83%).

The frequency of sexual activity or satisfaction with their partner does not change following the insertion of an erectile device.[97] Also, rates of sexual dysfunction were similar between individuals with or without an erectile device.[18] Sexual dysfunction was broadly defined to include low sexual desire, aversion to sexual activity or seeking sexual contacts and pain during sexual intercourse.

POSTSURGICAL REGRET

Regret following GAS is an important consideration and has been classified by Kuiper and Cohen-Kettenis[98] as "clear regret," "regret uncertain," "regret," and "regret assumed by others" (**Table 7**). The expression of regret is an important distinction because some may find it difficult to express regret for their decision even though their behavior clearly points in that direction.

The pooled prevalence of regret following transmasculine GAS is estimated to be 1% (confidence interval <1% - <1%) in a total of 2479 individuals from 27 publications.[99] Clear regret was expressed in 35 individuals and 26 had uncertain regret, whereas only 1 person had regret, and none had regret assumed by others. Regret following transmasculine GAS was previously estimated to be 3%.[98]

SUMMARY

Transmasculine genital GAS continues to evolve, and new innovations are frequently advanced by centers of excellence. Key milestones include the advent of free and pedicled sensate flaps with integrated urethra and the development of a customized erectile device for the neophallus. Our understanding of why, when, and how we offer genital GAS continues to improve. Functional and esthetic outcomes are acceptable with minimal regret expressed following GAS. However, further advances in this field depend on improving the quality of studies by embracing standardization, classification systems, and the use of validated instruments in defined (and appropriate) cohorts of patients. Prospective comparative studies are also clearly needed.

CLINICS CARE POINTS

- Shared decision making and inclusive care is integral when providing gender affirmation surgery.
- A full size or small phallus can be offered depending on patient preference.
- The best outcomes for patients who wish a full size to void while standing is a free flap phalloplasty with integrated urethra followed by urethral lengthening.
- Sexual intercourse is possible after inserting a penile prosthesis though the risk of device loss is higher than in device implanted within corpora cavernosa.
- Surgical regret is rare following transmasculine gender affirmation surgery.

DISCLOSURE

The authors have no relevant conflicts of interest to disclose.

REFERENCES

1. Wiepjes CM, Nota NM, de Blok CJM, et al. The Amsterdam Cohort of Gender Dysphoria Study (1972-2015): Trends in Prevalence, Treatment, and Regrets. J Sex Med 2018;15(4):582–90.
2. Al-Tamimi M, Pigot GL, Elfering L, et al. Genital Gender-Affirming Surgery in Transgender Men in The Netherlands from 1989 to 2018: The Evolution of Surgical Care. Plast Reconstr Surg 2020;145(1): 153e–61e.
3. Aydin D, Buk LJ, Partoft S, et al. Transgender Surgery in Denmark From 1994 to 2015: 20-Year Follow-Up Study. J Sex Med 2016;13(4):720–5.
4. Baker KE. The Future of Transgender Coverage. N Engl J Med 2017;376(19):1801–4.
5. Padula WV, Heru S, Campbell JD. Societal Implications of Health Insurance Coverage for Medically Necessary Services in the U.S. Transgender Population: A Cost-Effectiveness Analysis. J Gen Intern Med 2016;31(4):394–401.
6. Turban JL, Ehrensaft D. Research Review: Gender identity in youth: treatment paradigms and controversies. J Child Psychol Psychiatry 2018;59(12): 1228–43.
7. Galupo MP, Pulice-Farrow L, Pehl E. There Is Nothing to Do About It": Nonbinary Individuals' Experience of Gender Dysphoria. Transgend Health 2021;6(2):101–10.
8. Wernick JA, Busa S, Matouk K, et al. A Systematic Review of the Psychological Benefits of Gender-Affirming Surgery. Urol Clin North Am 2019;46(4):475–86.
9. Van De Grift TC, Elaut E, Cerwenka SC, et al. Effects of Medical Interventions on Gender Dysphoria and Body Image: A Follow-Up Study. Psychosom Med 2017;79(7):815–23.
10. de Vries AL, McGuire JK, Steensma TD, et al. Young adult psychological outcome after puberty suppression and gender reassignment. Arch Dis Child 2014; c(4):696–704.
11. Coleman E, Bockting W, Botzer M, et al. Standards of Care for the Health of Transsexual, Transgender, and Gender-Nonconforming People, Version 7. Int J Transgenderism 2012;13(4):165–232.
12. Hage JJ, Bout CA, Bloem JJAM, et al. Phalloplasty in female-to-male transsexuals: What do our patients ask for? Ann Plast Surg 1993;30(4):323–6.
13. Jacobsson J, Andreasson M, Kolby L, et al. Patients' Priorities Regarding Female-to-Male Gender Affirmation Surgery of the Genitalia-A Pilot Study of 47 Patients in Sweden. J Sex Med 2017;14(6): 857–64.

14. Lee WG, Christopher N, Ralph DJ. Penile Reconstruction and the Role of Surgery in Gender Dysphoria. Eur Urol Focus 2019;5(3):337–9.

15. Beek TF, Kreukels BP, Cohen-Kettenis PT, et al. Partial Treatment Requests and Underlying Motives of Applicants for Gender Affirming Interventions. J Sex Med 2015;12(11):2201–5.

16. Rachlin K. Factors which influence individual's decisions when considering female-to-male genital reconstructive surgery. Int J Transgenderism 1999; 3(3).

17. Ruppin U, Pfafflin F. Long-Term Follow-Up of Adults with Gender Identity Disorder. Arch Sex Behav 2015;44(5):1321–9.

18. Kerckhof ME, Kreukels BPC, Nieder TO, et al. Prevalence of Sexual Dysfunctions in Transgender Persons: Results from the ENIGI Follow-Up Study. J Sex Med 2019;16(12):2018–29.

19. Mokken SE, Ozer M, van de Grift TC, et al. Evaluation of the Decision Aid for Genital Surgery in Transmen. J Sex Med 2020;17(10):2067–76.

20. Ozer M, Pigot GLS, Bouman MB, et al. Development of a Decision Aid for Genital Gender-Affirming Surgery in Transmen. J Sex Med 2018;15(7):1041–8.

21. Ganor O, Taghinia AH, Diamond DA, et al. Piloting a Genital Affirmation Surgical Priorities Scale for Trans Masculine Patients. Transgend Health 2019;4(1):270–6.

22. Chang TS, Hwang WY. Forearm flap in one-stage reconstruction of the penis. Plast Reconstr Surg 1984;74(2):251–8.

23. Garaffa G, Christopher NA, Ralph DJ. Total phallic reconstruction in female-to-male transsexuals. Eur Urol 2010;57(4):715–22.

24. Felici N, Felici A. A new phalloplasty technique: the free anterolateral thigh flap phalloplasty. J Plast Reconstr Aesthet Surg 2006;59(2):153–7.

25. Bettocchi C, Ralph DJ, Pryor JP. Pedicled pubic phalloplasty in females with gender dysphoria. BJU Int 2005;95(1):120–4.

26. Koshima I, Nanba Y, Nagai A, et al. Penile reconstruction with bilateral superficial circumflex iliac artery perforator (SCIP) flaps. J Reconstr Microsurg 2006;22(3):137–42.

27. Djordjevic ML, Bumbasirevic MZ, Vukovic PM, et al. Musculocutaneous latissimus dorsi free transfer flap for total phalloplasty in children. J Pediatr Urol 2006; 2(4):333–9.

28. Lee HB, Hur JY, Song JM, et al. Long anterior urethral reconstruction using a sensate ulnar forearm free flap. Plast Reconstr Surg 2001;108(7):2053–6.

29. Selvaggi G, Monstrey S, Hoebeke P, et al. Donor-site morbidity of the radial forearm free flap after 125 phalloplasties in gender identity disorder. Plast Reconstr Surg 2006;118(5):1171–7.

30. Rieger UM, Majenka P, Wirthmann A, et al. Comparative Study of the Free Microvascular Groin Flap: Optimizing the Donor Site After Free Radial Forearm Flap Phalloplasty. Urology 2016;95:192–6.

31. Chang KP, Lai CH, Liang WL, et al. Alternative reconstruction of donor defect of free radial forearm flap in head and neck cancer. Scand J Plast Reconstr Surg Hand Surg 2010;44(1):31–6.

32. Pabst AM, Werkmeister R, Steegmann J, et al. Is there an ideal way to close the donor site of radial forearm free flaps? Br J Oral Maxillofac Surg 2018; 56(6):444–52.

33. Kuenzlen L, Nasim S, Neerven SV, et al. Multimodal evaluation of donor site morbidity in transgender individuals after phalloplasty with a free radial forearm flap: a case-control study. J Plast Reconstr Aesthet Surg 2021;75(1):25–32.

34. Van Caenegem E, Verhaeghe E, Taes Y, et al. Long-term evaluation of donor-site morbidity after radial forearm flap phalloplasty for transsexual men. J Sex Med 2013;10(6):1644–51.

35. Hage JJ, Bouman FG, de Graaf FH, et al. Construction of the neophallus in female-to-male transsexuals: the Amsterdam experience. J Urol 1993; 149(6):1463–8.

36. Harrison DH. Reconstruction of the urethra for hypospadiac cripples by microvascular free flap transfers. Br J Plast Surg 1986;39(3):408–13.

37. van der Sluis WB, Smit JM, Pigot GLS, et al. Double flap phalloplasty in transgender men: Surgical technique and outcome of pedicled anterolateral thigh flap phalloplasty combined with radial forearm free flap urethral reconstruction. Microsurgery 2017; 37(8):917–23.

38. Namba Y, Watanabe T, Kimata Y. Flap Combination Phalloplasty in Female-to-Male Transsexuals. J Sex Med 2019;16(6):934–41.

39. Garaffa G, Ralph DJ, Christopher N. Total urethral construction with the radial artery-based forearm free flap in the transsexual. BJU Int 2010;106(8): 1206–10.

40. Durfee R, Rowland W. Penile substitution with clitoral enlargement and urethral transfer. In: Laub DR, Gandy P, editors. Proceedings of the second Interdisciplanary Symposium on gender dysphoria Syndrome. Palo Alto: Stanford University Press; 1973. p. 181–3.

41. Lebovic GS, Laub DR, Ozek G. Metoidioplasty. In: Ehrlich RM, Alter GJ, editors. Reconstructive and plastic surgery of the external genitalia. Philadelphia: WB Saunders Co; 1999. p. 355–60.

42. Laub D, Eicher W, Hentz V. Penis construction in female-to-male transsexuals. In: Plastic surgery in the sexually handicapped. Springer; 1989. p. 113–28.

43. Hage JJ. Metaidoioplasty: An alternative phalloplasty technique in transsexuals. Plast Reconstr Surg 1996;97(1):161–7.

44. Djordjevic ML, Stanojevic D, Bizic M, et al. Metoidio-plasty as a single stage sex reassignment surgery in female transsexuals: Belgrade experience. J Sex Med 2009;6(5):1306–13.

45. Takamatsu A, Harashina T. Labial ring flap: a new flap for metaidoioplasty in female-to-male transsex-uals. J Plast Reconstr Aesthet Surg 2009;62(3):318–25.

46. Cohanzad S. Extensive Metoidioplasty as a Tech-nique Capable of Creating a Compatible Analogue to a Natural Penis in Female Transsexuals. Aesthet Plast Surg 2016;40(1):130–8.

47. Bordas N, Stojanovic B, Bizic M, et al. Metoidioplasty: Surgical Options and Outcomes in 813 Cases. Front Endocrinol (Lausanne) 2021;12:760284.

48. Bizic MR, Stojanovic B, Joksic I, et al. Metoidio-plasty. Urol Clin North Am 2019;46(4):555–66.

49. Frey JD, Poudrier G, Chiodo MV, et al. A Systematic Review of Metoidioplasty and Radial Forearm Flap Phalloplasty in Female-to-male Transgender Genital Reconstruction: Is the "Ideal" Neophallus an Achiev-able Goal? Plast 2016;4(12):e1131.

50. van de Grift TC, Pigot GLS, Boudhan S, et al. A Longitudinal Study of Motivations Before and Psy-chosexual Outcomes After Genital Gender-Confirming Surgery in Transmen. J Sex Med 2017;14(12):1621–8.

51. Al-Tamimi M, Pigot GL, van der Sluis WB, et al. The Surgical Techniques and Outcomes of Secondary Phalloplasty After Metoidioplasty in Transgender Men: An International, Multi-Center Case Series. J Sex Med 2019;16(11):1849–59.

52. Pigot GLS, Al-Tamimi M, Nieuwenhuijzen JA, et al. Gen-ital Gender-Affirming Surgery Without Urethral Length-ening in Transgender Men—A Clinical Follow-Up Study on the Surgical and Urological Outcomes and Pa-tient Satisfaction. J Sex Med 2020;17(12):2478–87.

53. Weinberg A, Granieri M, Cohen O, et al. Robotic-As-sisted Vaginectomy, Mobilization of Vaginal Mucosa for Urethral Lengthening and a Gracilis Muscle Flap for Phalloplasty: A Novel Technique for Female-to-Male Genital Reconstruction. J Sex Med 2018;15(2):S13–4.

54. Hage JJ, Bouman FG, Bloem JJAM, et al. Construc-tion of the fixed part of the neourethra in female-to-male transsexuals: Experience in 53 patients. Plast Reconstr Surg 1993;91(5):904–12.

55. Salgado CJ, Nugent AG, Moody AM, et al. Immedi-ate pedicled gracilis flap in radial forearm flap phal-loplasty for transgender male patients to reduce urinary fistula. J Plast Reconstr Aesthet Surg 2016;69(11):1551–7.

56. Massie JP, Morrison SD, Wilson SC, et al. Phallo-plasty with Urethral Lengthening: Addition of a Vas-cularized Bulbospongiosus Flap from Vaginectomy Reduces Postoperative Urethral Complications. Plast Reconstr Surg 2017;140(4):551e–8e.

57. Al-Tamimi M, Pigot GL, Ronkes B, et al. The First Experience of Using the Pedicled Labia Minora Flap for Urethral Lengthening in Transgender Men Undergoing Anterolateral Thigh and Superficial Circumflex Iliac Artery Perforator Flap Phalloplasty: A Multicenter Study on Clinical Outcomes. Urology 2020;138:179–87.

58. Lee WG, Li V, Ralph D, et al. Novel classification of urethral complications in female to male gender affir-mation surgery. J Urol 2021;206(SUPPL 3):e542.

59. Veerman H, dRFP W, Al-Tamimi M, et al. Functional Outcomes and Urological Complications after Geni-tal Gender Affirming Surgery with Urethral Length-ening in Transgender Men. J Urol 2020;204(1):104–9.

60. Hu C-H, Chang C-J, Wang S-W, et al. A systematic review and meta-analysis of urethral complications and outcomes in transgender men. J Plast Reconstr Aesthet Surg 2021;75(1):10–24.

61.. Nassiri N, Maas M, Basin M, et al. Urethral compli-cations after gender reassignment surgery: a sys-tematic review. Int J Impot Res 2020;33(8):793–800.

62. de Rooij FPW, Peters FRM, Ronkes BL, et al. Surgi-cal outcomes and proposal for a treatment algorithm for urethral strictures in transgender men. BJU Int 2021;28:28.

63. Pariser JJ, Cohn JA, Gottlieb LJ, et al. Buccal Mucosal Graft Urethroplasty for the Treatment of Urethral Stricture in the Neophallus. Urology 2015;85(4):927–31.

64. Lumen N, Monstrey S, Goessaert AS, et al. Urethro-plasty for strictures after phallic reconstruction: a single-institution experience. Eur Urol 2011;60(1):150–8.

65. Verla W, Hoebeke P, Spinoit A-F, et al. Excision and Primary Anastomosis for Isolated, Short, Anasto-motic Strictures in Transmen. Plast Reconstr Surg – Glob Open 2020;8(2):e2641.

66. Nikkels C, van Trotsenburg M, Huirne J, et al. Vaginal Colpectomy in Transgender Men: A Retro-spective Cohort Study on Surgical Procedure and Outcomes. J Sex Med 2019;16(6):924–33.

67. Gomes da Costa A, Valentim-Lourenco A, Santos-Ribeiro S, et al. Laparoscopic Vaginal-Assisted Hys-terectomy With Complete Vaginectomy for Female-To-Male Genital Reassignment Surgery. J Minimally Invasive Gynecol 2016;23(3):404–9.

68. Groenman F, Nikkels C, Huirne J, et al. Robot-assis-ted laparoscopic colpectomy in female-to-male transgender patients; technique and outcomes of a prospective cohort study. Surg Endosc 2017;31(8):3363–9.

69. Jeftovic M, Stojanovic B, Bizic M, et al. Hysterec-tomy with Bilateral Salpingo-Oophorectomy in Female-to-Male Gender Affirmation Surgery: Com-parison of Two Methods. Biomed Res Int 2018;2018:3472471.

70. Al-Tamimi M, Pigot GL, van der Sluis WB, et al. Col-pectomy Significantly Reduces the Risk of Urethral Fistula Formation after Urethral Lengthening in Transgender Men Undergoing Genital Gender Affirming Surgery. J Urol 2018;200(6):1315–22.

71. Bauer GR, Redman N, Bradley K, et al. Sexual Health of Trans Men Who Are Gay, Bisexual, or Who Have Sex with Men: Results from Ontario, Canada. Int J Transgenderism 2013;14(2):66–74.

72. Brandt JS, Patel AJ, Marshall I, et al. Transgender men, pregnancy, and the "new" advanced paternal age: A review of the literature. Maturitas 2019;128:17–21.

73. Stojanovic B, Bizic M, Bencic M, et al. One-Stage Gender-Confirmation Surgery as a Viable Surgical Procedure for Female-to-Male Transsexuals. J Sex Med 2017;14(5):741–6.

74. Selvaggi G, Hoebeke P, Ceulemans P, et al. Scrotal reconstruction in female-to-male transsexuals: a novel scrotoplasty. Plast Reconstr Surg 2009; 123(6):1710–8.

75. Pigot GLS, Al-Tamimi M, Ronkes B, et al. Surgical Outcomes of Neoscrotal Augmentation with Testicular Prostheses in Transgender Men. J Sex Med 2019;16(10):1664–71.

76. Miller TJ, Lin WC, Safa B, et al. Transgender Scrotoplasty and Perineal Reconstruction With Labia Majora Flaps: Technique and Outcomes From 147 Consecutive Cases. Ann Plast Surg 2021;87(3):324–30.

77. Lee WG, Christopher N, Ralph D. IPP in Neophallus. In: Moncada-Iribarren I, Martinez-Salamanca JI, Lledo-Garcia E, et al, editors. Textbook of Urogenital prosthetic surgery. Editorial Médica Panamericana S.A.; 2020. p. 213–31.

78. Chen ML, Patel DP, Moses RA, et al. Infrapubic Insertion of Penile Implants in Transmen After Phalloplasty. Urology 2021;152:79–83.

79. Falcone M, Garaffa G, Gillo A, et al. Outcomes of inflatable penile prosthesis insertion in 247 patients completing female to male gender reassignment surgery. BJU Int 2018;121(1):139–44.

80. Neuville P, Morel-Journel N, Maucourt-Boulch D, et al. Surgical Outcomes of Erectile Implants After Phalloplasty: Retrospective Analysis of 95 Procedures. J Sex Med 2016;13(11):1758–64.

81. Hoebeke PB, Decaestecker K, Beysens M, et al. Erectile implants in female-to-male transsexuals: our experience in 129 patients. Eur Urol 2010;57(2):334–40.

82. Verla W, Goedertier W, Lumen N, et al. Implantation of the ZSI 475 FTM Erectile Device After Phalloplasty: A Prospective Analysis of Surgical Outcomes. J Sex Med 2021;18(3):615–22.

83. Neuville P, Morel-Journel N, Cabelguenne D, et al. First Outcomes of the ZSI 475 FtM, a Specific Prosthesis Designed for Phalloplasty. J Sex Med 2019;16(2):316–22.

84. Gilbert DA, Winslow BH, Gilbert DM, et al. Transsexual surgery in the genetic female. Clin Plast Surg 1988;15(3):471–87.

85. Morrison SD, Son J, Song J, et al. Modification of the tube-in-tube pedicled anterolateral thigh flap for total phalloplasty: the mushroom flap. Ann Plast Surg 2014;72(Supplement 1):S22–6.

86. Danker S, Esmonde N, JU Berli. Staging" in Phalloplasty. Urol Clin North Am 2019;46(4):581–90.

87. Monstrey S, Hoebeke P, Selvaggi G, et al. Penile reconstruction: Is the radial forearm flap really the standard technique? Plast Reconstr Surg 2009; 124(2):510–8.

88. JU Berli, Monstrey S, Safa B, et al. Neourethra Creation in Gender Phalloplasty: Differences in Techniques and Staging. Plast Reconstr Surg 2021; 147(5):801e–11e.

89. Huayllani MT, Boczar D, Saleem HY, et al. Single versus two-stage phalloplasty for transgender female-to-male patients: a systematic review of the literature. Ann 2021;9(7):608.

90. Remington AC, Morrison SD, Massie JP, et al. Outcomes after Phalloplasty: Do Transgender Patients and Multiple Urethral Procedures Carry a Higher Rate of Complication? Plast Reconstr Surg 2018; 141(2):220e–9e.

91. Andreasson M, Georgas K, Elander A, et al. Patient-Reported Outcome Measures Used in Gender Confirmation Surgery: A Systematic Review. Plast Reconstr Surg 2018;141(4):1026–39.

92. Aaronson N, Alonso J, Burnam A, et al. Assessing health status and quality-of-life instruments: attributes and review criteria. Qual Life Res 2002; 11(3):193–205.

93. Lee WG, Li V, Ralph D, et al. Novel classification of urethral complications in female to male gender affirming surgery. BJU Int 2020;125(Supplement 1):4.

94. Terrier M, Morel-Journel N, Carnicelli D, et al. Suprapubic phalloplasty in transmen: surgical results and critical review. Int J Impot Res 2020;33(7):754–61.

95. Jun MS, Pusica S, Kojovic V, et al. Total Phalloplasty With Latissimus Dorsi Musculocutaneous Flap in Female-to-male Transgender Surgery. Urology 2018;120:269–70.

96. Leriche A, Timsit MO, Morel-Journel N, et al. Long-term outcome of forearm flee-flap phalloplasty in the treatment of transsexualism. BJU Int 2008; 101(10):1297–300.

97. Wierckx K, Van Caenegem E, Elaut E, et al. Quality of life and sexual health after sex reassignment surgery in transsexual men. J Sex Med 2011;8(12): 3379–88.

98. Kuiper AJ, Cohen-Kettenis PT. Gender role reversal among postoperative transsexuals. Int J Transgenderism 1998;2(3).

99. Bustos VP, Bustos SS, Mascaro A, et al. Regret after Gender-affirmation Surgery: A Systematic Review and Meta-analysis of Prevalence. Plast Reconstr Surg – Glob Open 2021;9(3):e3477.

Management of Necrotizing Soft Tissue Infections (Fournier's Gangrene) and Surgical Reconstruction of Debridement Wound Defects

Bradley A. Erickson, MD, MS*, Kevin J. Flynn, MD

KEYWORDS

- Necrotizing soft tissue infection of the genitalia • Fournier's gangrene • Genitourinary reconstruction
- Split-thickness skin graft • Necrotizing fasciitis

KEY POINTS

- Necrotizing soft tissue infections of the genitalia (NSTIG), historically referred to as Fournier's gangrene, is a potentially life-threatening infection, often polymicrobial, that can originate from a genitourinary or gastrointestinal source and spreads rapidly along fascial planes, resisting treatment from systemic antimicrobials and requiring emergent tissue debridement to stop the infection's spread.
- The primary goal of genital reconstruction after debridement, usually occurring after an extended period of time in which the active infectious process has subsided, is to cover the exposed soft tissue with skin. Secondary goals of reconstruction that must also be considered, given the sensitive nature of the anatomy, are the preservation of function (eg, sexual functioning, urination, fertility), and cosmesis.
- Depending on the extent of the debridement, reconstruction often involves the need to cover the penis, perineum, scrotal contents, and/or the suprapubic region. Occasionally, the debridement will extend beyond the classic boundaries of NSTIG into the thigh, buttocks, and abdomen, in which case burn and plastic surgeons are often involved in the management.
- NSTIG wound closure often involves one or more of the following closure techniques (1) conservative closure by secondary intention ± negative pressure wound treatment (NPWT), (2) component separation primary closure (CSC), (3) split-thickness skin graft (STSG) and/or (4) pedicled fasciocutaneous flap based on perforators from the circumflex, femoral and/or pudendal vasculature.

EPIDEMIOLOGY

Necrotizing soft tissue infections of the genitalia (NSTIG) is a rare condition, mostly commonly found in men (50:1 male to female ratio). (Given the rarity of NSTIG in women, reconstructive principles and techniques discussed in this article will focus on males only. Notably, while NSTIG is less common in females, mortality may be higher[1–3]). While NSTIG is often difficult to differentiate from

Department of Urology, University of Iowa, Carver College of Medicine, 3233 RCP, 200 Hawkins Dr., Iowa City, IA 52242, USA
* Corresponding author.
E-mail address: brad-erickson@uiowa.edu
Twitter: @baerickson29 (B.A.E.)

Urol Clin N Am 49 (2022) 467–478
https://doi.org/10.1016/j.ucl.2022.04.008
0094-0143/22/Published by Elsevier Inc.

severe cellulitis and genital abscesses when using administrative data, the most current epidemiologic studies report an incidence of 1.6/100,000 males – the highest rates being in middle-aged men (3.3/100,000) and lowest being in boys (0.3/100,000).[4]

Mortality rates from NSTIG are likewise difficult to accurately determine. Historical rates are as high as 80%, with most being in the range of 20% to 40%.[5–13] However, these mortality rates have significant biases, as most come from large, single-institution referral centers, likely with higher acuity patients. More contemporary, population-based studies suggest mortality rates of less than 10%, which may represent both improved care and inclusion of less severe cases.[4]

Because NSTIG is strongly associated with conditions of metabolic syndrome (eg, morbid obesity, hypertension, diabetes) it has been presumed (though not confirmed) that as the rates of these associated conditions are increasing, the rate of NSTIG is also rising.[10,14–18]

Most debridements and reconstructions are happening in tertiary care centers, with the average number of cases per hospital being 0.6 and the median being 0 cases, ranging from 0 to 23. The shift of NSTIG to tertiary care hospitals with expertise in management may be leading to an overall decrease in mortality.[4]

PATHOPHYSIOLOGY

In all cases of NSTIG, there is a superficial point of bacterial entry into the subcutaneous tissues. These entries can be the result of external trauma (ie, surgical incision, traumatic laceration), perforated viscous organ (eg, diverticulitis), urethral stricture ± periurethral abscess, perirectal abscess and/or decubitus ulcers.[1,4,11,14,19]. (Anecdotally, is it becoming more frequent at our institution to obtain a patient history that starts with a genital sebaceous cyst, in which the patient attempts to drain the cyst from manual compression, but may instead be facilitating the seeding of bacteria below the superficial tissues).[20,21]

Not all bacteria that violate the superficial fascia will lead to NSTIG, most ending up as simple abscesses. It is hypothesized that for bacteria to progress to NSTIG, two factors must be present – (1) impaired host immunity and (2) synergy of multiple bacterial species (ie, polymicrobial infections – Type I necrotizing fasciitis) and their respective toxins and enzymes.[14,22] For example, when aerobic bacterial infection leads to local ischemia and microvascular thrombosis, anaerobic species present in the wound are then allowed to proliferate freely. In patients with impaired tissue defenses (most commonly those on immunosuppression medications, diabetes mellitus, cirrhosis/alcoholism), this proliferation can go unchecked – and because antimicrobials cannot reach areas without blood supply due to local thrombosis, spread will continue rapidly without surgical debridement. The tissue ischemia facilitating the spread is thought to be responsible for the pain experienced by many with the condition.[23]

ANATOMY OF DISEASE SPREAD

Once the bacteria have violated the protection of the epidermis and dermis, bacterial proliferation within Camper's fascia can occur and spread rapidly along/above Buck's fascia (penis), Colle's fascia (perineum), the Dartos fascia (scrotum), Scarpa's fascia (abdomen), and the Fascia Lata (thigh). The deep Buck's Fascia, the tunica albuginea, and the urogenital diaphragm are reliable barriers to deeper infectious spread, which mostly allows for organ preservation.

Notably, the skin and dermis above the necrotic fascia are often (initially) spared and can often be preserved for later reconstructive purposes.[24,25]

PATIENT EVALUATION AND CLASSIFICATION

It is thought that most men presenting with NSTIG have a significant prodromic period prior to clinically recognizable disease. The most common prodromic feature, differentiating it from cellulitis, is pain (likely an indicator of ischemia), often in the setting of swelling, erythema, and constitutional symptoms (eg, fever, chills).[2,23,26,27]

Necrotizing fasciitis infections can be classified into three types based on the responsible pathogens and location: Type I (polymicrobial; trunk/perineum), Type II (monomicrobial, Gram +), Type III (monomicrobial, Clostridium/Gram -) and Type IV (fungal). The treatment, surgical debridement, remains the same regardless of type, but a thorough history can help predict the NSTIG type, prior to the return of wound cultures, allowing for improved tailoring of empiric systemic therapies.[28]

NSTIG severity indices have been developed to help with the diagnosis and predict outcomes. The Fournier's gangrene severity index (FGSI) computes a score based on laboratory and vital sign values at presentation including temperature, heart rate, respiratory rate, serum sodium, serum potassium, serum creatinine, hematocrit, white blood cell count, and serum bicarbonate levels.[5,29,30] Points are given for each value, ranging from 0 (normal laboratory/vital sign value) to 4 (above or below normal) with a theoretic max value of 36. The FGSI score appears to be most useful in predicting mortality from NSTIG with a value > 9 being consistent in its ability to predict death from NSTIG, but is not as useful when attempting to differentiate FGSI from other nonnecrotic soft tissue infections. The Laboratory Risk Indicator for Necrotizing Fasciitis (LRINEC) was a tool designed to do just that, combining scores from C-Reactive Protein (CRP), total white blood cell count, hemoglobin, sodium, creatinine, and glucose to generate a score that ranges from 0 to 13, with a score ≥ 6 having a high sensitivity (>90%) for diagnosing NSTIG. However, when evaluating the score prospectively, it appears that the tool is most useful in ruling out NSTIG (ie, high negative predictive value; 90%) with positive predictive values of only 35%.[31]

In equivocal cases, +/− abnormal LRINEC findings, imaging is often employed, with CT scan findings or air ± fluid tracking along the fascial planes being the most diagnostic for NSTIG.[32] While MRI has been shown to be the most sensitive test (T2 hyperintensity of deep fascia), its clinical availability in emergent settings limits its usefulness.[33]

ACUTE INFECTION CONTROL

All cases of suspected NSTIG must undergo immediate surgical debridement to stop infection spread. Late recognition of NSTIG is associated with higher mortality, as is incomplete debridement.[20,34–36] At the time of initial debridement, broad-spectrum antibiotics should be started that cover gram positive and negative aerobic bacteria, and anaerobes, most commonly (and per infectious disease recommendations) piperacillin/tazobactam (Zosyn) and vancomycin.[37] These antibiotics should be continued for at least 72-hours postdebridement, and can become more focused once wound cultures return.[38]

Normalization of the white blood cell count, and wound inspection for the absence of persistent necrotic tissue, are common indicators of adequate disease control and should be monitored at least once daily. Notably, contemporary studies have also shown a high rate of fungal coinfection (Type 1/Type IV), suggesting that the addition of fluconazole to the empiric regimen may improve outcomes.[38]

Debridement should begin at the necrotic tissue, and then carried out laterally at the fascial level until vascularized tissue is encountered (to which antibiotics can now reach) (**Fig. 1**). While adequate debridement is crucial to infection control, we have found that the skin lateral to the

obviously necrotic tissue is often salvageable, with the disease mostly traveling along the deep fascial planes. Following the approach first described for necrotizing fasciitis of the extremities, acknowledgment of Zone 1 (necrotic), Zone 2 (inflamed epidermis/dermis without necrosis, though with underlying necrosis of soft tissue/fascia), and Zone 3 (normal skin without erythema/infection), can allow for the preservation of local skin flaps, which remain perfused by collateral blood flow from the dermal and subdermal plexus, increasing the likelihood of primary closure with STSG or fasciocutaneous flaps from the thigh.[25] (**Fig. 2**).

Notably, it is uncommon for testicles, spermatic cords, penile/erectile bodies, or urethra to require excision, as they are often protected from infection by a strong fascial layer, unless the respective organ is the origin of the NSTIG (eg, urethra, testicle).[2,39]

WOUND MANAGEMENT

Once infection control has been achieved, the aim of wound management should be to prevent secondary infection of the exposed soft tissue. This is most commonly achieved with simple wet-to-dry saline dressings, often augmented with 0.025% sodium hypochlorite solution (0.025% Dakins),[40] which debrides and recruits fibroblasts, and/or silver sulfadiazine (SSD 1%), which decreases bacterial load, often covered with a nonadherent mesh (eg, Xeroform , Adaptic , Mepitel).[41]

Biologic dressings, such as dermal regeneration templates (Integra) are being used more commonly in burn patients and may be useful augment after debridement to speed spontaneous healing, especially when skin grafting is being considered. Dressing changes should be performed one to two times daily (enough to manage exudate without disrupting epithelialization), with thorough wound inspection to ensure adequate granulation tissue formation and absence of persistent (or new) necrotic tissue, in which case secondary debridement should be performed.

Negative-pressure wound therapy (NPWT, aka wound-vac) is often employed at this stage. Unlike traditional topical dressings, NPWT dressings need to be changed every 72 to 96 hours, thereby minimizing the frequency of painful dressing changes with the added benefits of expedited wound closure and decreased local edema.[42–45] However, these advantages must be weighed against the negative of not being able to visualize the wound daily, which can be problematic if inadequate debridement is suspected, and the

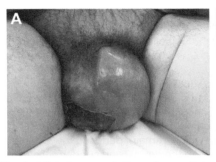
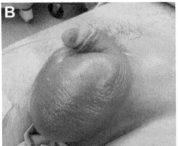
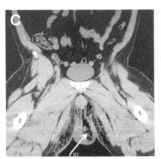

Fig. 1. (*A*) Late presentation of necrotizing soft tissue infection of the genitalia (NSTIG) with obvious necrotic skin. (*B*) Patient presenting with cellulitis and pain and unclear NSTIG risk. (*C*) Confirmatory CT scan showing area in scrotum and fluid along fascial layer.

anatomic awkwardness of the debridement wounds, which can make sealing of the NPWT dressings challenging. (We have found that the larger 3M Ioban dressings can be used in place of, or to augment, standard NPWT dressings to help minimize air leak.)

Simultaneous to local wound care, parental nutrition and electrolyte replacement should be employed to facilitate the healing process. The loss of protein from large open wounds can be > 10 g/d and is likely higher with the use of NPWT.[46,47]

The use of hyperbaric oxygen (HBO) therapy, when readily available, can improve local tissue oxygenation and theoretically improve healing. However, its benefits specific to NSTIG, relative to standard closure techniques below, have not been proven sufficiently to warrant routine use of this costly and timely treatment.[48,49]

WOUND CLOSURE TIMING

The optimal time to wound closure is unknown, but in general should not occur until the patient's systemic and local wound health are optimized. Many institutions, including our own, have employed a

wound closure philosophy that aims to close the wounds before the patient leaves the hospital. While there are many logistical reasons for adopting this policy (eg, arrangement of satisfactory outpatient wound and/or NPWT care can be challenging at best, detrimental at worst), it is mostly agreed upon that the historical practice of prolonged outpatient local care to ensure adequate infection control, even without obvious signs of persistence, prior to closure, is mostly unwarranted (some exceptions to the rule may be made in settings of severe malnourishment, in which care parenteral nutrition may be necessary to raise albumin levels).[25]

Normalization of the WBC after debridement and a minimum of 72 hours of culture-directed parenteral antibiotics, confirmation of granulation tissue covering the entire resection bed, and electrolyte/nutritional optimization, are clinical benchmarks that can help to ensure safe closure.

WOUND CLOSURE TECHNIQUES

NSTIG wounds are heterogeneous and each closure must be tailored to the individual's clinical

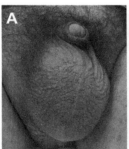
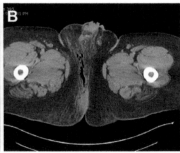
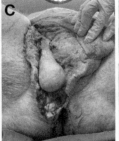
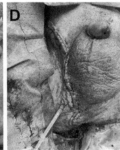

Fig. 2. (*A*) Patient presented with 2 days of testicular pain and swelling and equivocal physical examination findings. (*B*) CT scan is obtained to confirm the diagnosis of NSTIG. (*C*) Incision was made over right hemiscrotum with a skin-sparing approach to debridement. (*D*) After 5 days of culture-directed antibiotics, primary closure was easily performed over a drain using component separation principles and placement of the right testicle into the left hemiscrotum to prevent migration into the thigh/perineum.

situation and the condition, and quantity, of the healthy tissue lateral to the wound.

The primary objective of closure is to adequately cover all exposed soft tissue without the threat of trapping persistent infection under the closure. However, closure must also consider the preservation of the vital functions of the genitourinary system, including sexual functioning (ie, erections adequate for penetration with normal sensation and without pain), urination, and testicular function (ie, testosterone production and spermatogenesis).

We have found it to be useful to make our closure plan after first separating the wound by the anatomy, and anatomic extent, involved – namely anatomic extent of the (1) scrotum, (2) penis, (3) perineum and (4) suprapubic regions. (Notably, while NSTIG wounds can extend beyond these areas, for the purposes of this article, we will focus on closure in the genitourinary region, acknowledging that extension beyond these areas may alter closure techniques, especially as pertains to the use of split-thickness skin grafts (STSG)). Greater anatomic extent is associated with an increased need for STSG and flap use. However, because each of these four areas serves unique genitourinary functions, closure techniques must adapt accordingly.

SURGICAL RECONSTRUCTION

There are four commonly accepted techniques for NSTIG wound closure: (1) conservative closure by secondary intention ± NPWT, (2) component separation primary closure (CSC), (3) split-thickness skin graft (STSG) and (4) pedicled fasciocutaneous flap. Importantly, surgeons need not choose only one of these techniques for any given closure procedure and many closures may require two or more of these techniques depending on anatomic extent, if the primary objectives of coverage and function preservation are to be achieved (**Fig. 3**).

Secondary Intention

Debrided wounds will begin to granulate almost immediately, starting with an inflammatory phase which brings neutrophils, and then monocytes/macrophages, which begin the period of cell proliferation. Macrophages release VEGF and TGF-beta, among many other growth factors, which begin to create new (friable) blood vessels and collagen (Type III).[50]

Histologically, the wounds have a high percentage of fibroblasts, thin-walled capillaries, inflammatory cells, and a loose extracellular matrix, all of which protect the wound from secondary infection and aid in decreasing wound size by the contraction of the collagen.[50]

Wound closure by secondary intention minimizes the risk of secondary infection, assuming appropriate wound management. However, the length of time required for closure is proportional to the size of the wound and can range from weeks to many months.[25] In addition, prolonged closure time can negatively affect the quality of life and increase the risk of wound infection, if not cared for properly, which can be challenging as an outpatient.

Negative pressure wound therapy (NPWT) is often used to acutely manage the wound after debridement and as previously described, can decrease the need for painful dressing changes. NPWT can also be used as the primary means of closure. Though NPWT likely decreases the need for painful dressing changes, it remains a challenge to manage as an outpatient.

Component Separation (Delayed) Primary Closure

At the time of primary closure, most wounds ready to close have fully granulated. While granulation tissue is a necessary component to healing by secondary intention, if primary closure is to be attempted, the granulation tissue should be removed, as it will decrease tissue mobility, and is colonized with bacteria. While these bacteria are generally indolent and likely protect the granulating wound from harmful bacteria (eg, pseudomonas, e coli) that can delay healing, trapping these bacteria under a primary closure will increase the likelihood of postoperative wound infection.[51,52]

During closure, we prefer to remove granulation tissue with the Versajet II system using a 14 mm handset.[53] The healthy skin lateral to the wound is widely mobilized above the underlying deep fascia. Any exposed organs, most commonly the penis/corporal bodies and testicles/spermatic cords, are widely mobilized from the granulation bed. A reactive hydrocele is often present and if this impairs scrotal reconstruction, the tunica vaginalis is incised, the hydrocele is drained and then closed using interrupted 2 to 0 polyglactin suture behind the cord.

The deep tissues are then reapproximated over a 10 mm flat Jackson-Pratt closed drain when closure can be performed without tension using deep interrupted 2 to 0 polyglactin suture. The skin is then closed at approximately 1.5 cm intervals with 2 to 0 nylon suture in a horizontal mattress fashion.

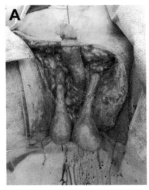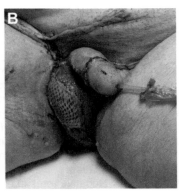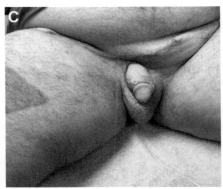

Fig. 3. (*A*) Wound after the debridement of case in **Fig. 1a**, leaving loss of 70% of scrotum, 100% of penile skin, and a significant loss of suprapubic skin. (*B*) Closure utilizing three reconstructive techniques. (1) component separation closure of the left hemiscrotum, (2) flap reconstruction of the suprapubic region utilizing a left medial thigh flap, and (3) split-thickness skin graft to the penis (0.18 in, unmeshed) and right hemiscrotum (0.18 in, meshed 1:1). (*C*) Wound appearance at 6 months.

Areas that cannot be closed without tension, or without compromising the function of the underlying tissue (eg, concern that closure will impair normal erections, lead to excessive tension on the spermatic cord and/or testicles), are either left to heal by secondary intention (+/− NPWT) or are grafted using a split-thickness skin graft (STSG) and/or a thigh-based fasciocutaneous flap.

Postoperative management: JP drains are removed when the serous output is < 20 cc/d. Sutures are removed at 14 days. Patients ambulate on POD 0 and are maintained on prophylactic subcutaneous heparin.

Postoperative complications: Minor wound separation is common and can be managed using the secondary intention principles discussed previously. Minimizing dead space under the skin during closure, as well as appropriate JP drain management, will decrease the risk of postoperative seroma and infection.

Split-Thickness Skin Graft (STSG)

Closure of NSTIG wounds with STSG should be reserved for wounds that are unable to be closed primarily without compromising urinary or sexual function.

Most STSG are harvested from the medial/lateral thigh, which is routinely prepped into the surgical field at the time of all closures. Alternative sites must be considered if infection has spread to the legs/thighs (abdomen/back).

Unlike primary closure cases, STSGs can be placed directly on granulation tissue as this is purported to increase the graft take, taking advantage of the neovascularization of the bed.

The use of dermal regeneration templates prior to grafting (eg, Integra, Matriderm) may improve the cosmesis of the STSG and decrease the contraction of the tissue. These dressings are used extensively in burn cases, especially with burns requiring a significant amount of graft tissue, serving both to stimulate granulation tissue and protect the wound from fluid loss. When dermal grafts are used, grafting is generally delayed for 3 to 4 weeks.[54,55]

A dermatome (Zimmer) set to 0.18-inch depth is used to harvest enough graft material to cover the exposed area, which is precisely measured prior to harvest. Grafts placed on the scrotum and suprapubic region are meshed (1:1). Grafts placed on the penis are not meshed which may improve postoperative cosmesis.

When placing graft, we prefer to staple the graft to the edges of the wound superiorly/proximally first, which allows for proper tailoring prior to formal securing of the graft to the wound. Once the template is set, we administer an aerosolized fibrin glue (ARTISS) to both the wound and to the underside of the graft, then cover the wound, again securing the remaining edges with staples. In areas where there is a higher potential for the graft to develop a seroma, we will place additional interrupted 4 to 0 polyglactin suture (eg, scrotal folds).

The graft is covered with a nonadherent perforated silicone dressing (Mepitel). When appropriate and feasible, we then prefer to place an NPWT dressing on the repair, set at a continuous rate of 125 mm Hg. (In difficult to seal wounds, we prefer to use large surgical loban dressings), which stays in place for 5 days. Once the NPWT dressing has been removed, coverage with petroleum-based gauze (Xeroform) and copious

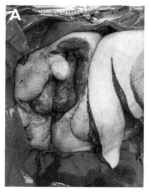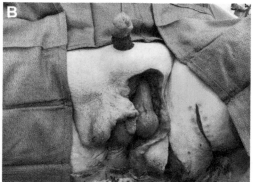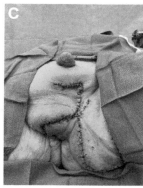

Fig. 4. (*A*) Large NSTIG debridement defect and preparation of the left medial thigh flap based on perforators from the femoral, circumflex, and pudendal vasculature. (*B*) Penis is brought through the mons tissue to allow inferior mobilization for the creation of neoscrotum. (*C*) Final closure appearance. (*Photos courtesy of* Dr Lee Zhao and Jamie Levine – New York University Departments of Urology and Division of Plastic Surgery)

petroleum-based antibiotic ointment (eg, bacitracin) is used to keep the wound moist.

Postoperative complications: Graft loss is uncommon, but generally dealt with using secondary intention principles stated above and/or revision STSG.

Pedicled Fasciocutaneous Flap

The most common fasciocutaneous flap utilized in NSTIG reconstruction comes from the medial thigh and is based on the femoral, circumflex, and pudendal vasculature (**Fig. 4**). Thigh flaps are most commonly used for scrotal reconstruction but can be fashioned to any desired shape for coverage of wound defects in the genital region.

The primary advantage of this flap is that it is has a reliable blood supply, does not require repositioning from lithotomy, and does not require dissection into the muscular tissue. The disadvantage is that the medial thigh is not always a reliable source of tissue as it is common for the disease to track down the thigh. Alternative flaps can come from abdominal or gluteal regions.[56]

Fasciocutaneous flap reconstruction of NSTIG has the potential to improve the cosmetic appearance of the region, especially in thin patients, relative to STSG or even primary closure. In our experience, however, the need for flaps is rare in the obese population most at risk for NSTIG.

CLOSURE CONSIDERATIONS BY ANATOMIC LOCATION
Scrotum

The scrotum is the anatomic region most commonly affected by NSTIG.[2] The primary function of the scrotum is to provide a safe habitat for the testicles that is sufficiently away from the body such that the temperature of the scrotal contents is approximately 2° Celsius lower than the body (35 v 37° C). Thus, closure techniques must attempt to reestablish this anatomic relationship without placing the testicles in potentially compromising positions (eg, in the perineum where one might sit directly on the testicles).

The scrotal skin is extremely elastic, allowing for movement, with the assistance of the underlying dartos m., in response to changes in ambient temperature. This elasticity can benefit the surgeon when attempting primary closure which can be attempted even in the setting of scrotal skin loss of greater than 50%.

Historically, placement of the testicles into temporary thigh pouches has been advocated. However, improved wound management options and a better understanding of STSG and CSC techniques have made the need for pouch creation mostly unnecessary.

For complete scrotal skin loss, we will graft directly onto the tunica vaginalis, often after the tunica from the testicles are sutured together to recreate a scrotal shape.[39] Importantly, the posterior portion of the testicles does not always require complete coverage as long as the testicles are not allowed to descend into the perineum (**Fig. 5**).

Perineal Closure

The perineal tissue extends from the base of the scrotum to the anus and is the area second most affected by NSTIG. Similar to the scrotum (especially in obese patients) primary closure is possible in most situations, often after the mobilization of the tissue lateral to the defect into the medial thigh.

In cases where primary closure is not possible, we have found the STSGs have poor outcomes given the difficulty of preventing shearing forces in the area. Secondary intention closure ± NPWT

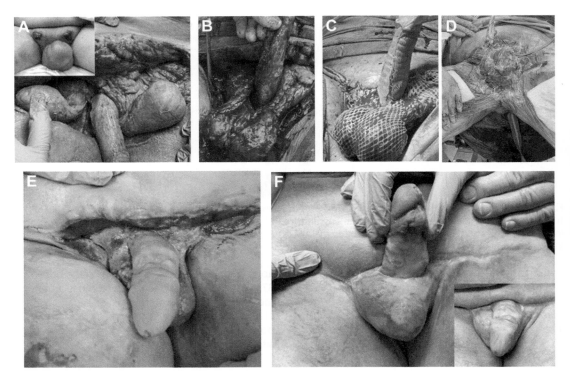

Fig. 5. (*A*) NSTIG wound defect after 5 days of postdebridement NPWT. (*B*) Debridement of granulation tissue with Versajet prior to reconstruction with suturing of the cut medial edges of the tunica vaginalis to each other to form a flat surface for grafting. (*C*) Grafting of penis (0.18 in, meshed 1:1) and scrotum (0.18 in, meshed 2:1) with primary CSC of the perineum and suprapubic regions. (*D*) Postclosure dressing with NPWT, placed at continuous 125 mm Hg. (*E*) Partial postclosure wound separation seen here at 1 month, managed with wet-to-dry dressing and Dakins. (*F*) Wound at 3 months. Patient noted bothersome swelling/edema of the unresected ventral mucosal collar tissue that required excision with primary closure at 6 months.

is our preferred method of management if CSC is not possible, followed by local flap closure with thigh flaps. Importantly, care must be taken to prevent pressure on an exposed urethra as erosion, and urethrocutaneous fistula formation, is inevitable without protection (**Figs. 6** and **7**).

PENILE CLOSURE

The penis is the third most-common area involved with NSTIG. Unlike the scrotum and perineum, aggressive maneuvers to perform CSC is not advisable given the critical importance of the penis

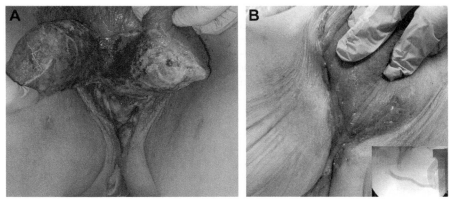

Fig. 6. (*A*) NSTIG wound after debridement and 10 days of wet-to-dry dressings. At 10 days, a proximal urethral erosion was noted (*white arrow*). (*B*) Primary component separation closure with urethroplasty was performed at 21 days after suprapubic tube placement at 10 days.

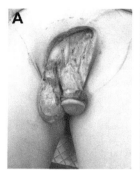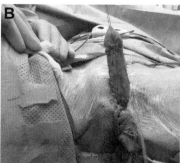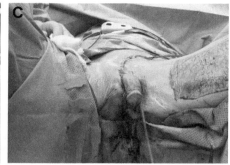

Fig. 7. (*A*) Postdebridement NSTIG wound secondary to epididymitis requiring orchiectomy. (*B*) Primary scrotal closure utilizing medial thigh tissue and (*C*) Advancement flap closure of the suprapubic region with split-thickness skin grafting of the penile shaft (0.18 in unmeshed).

for urination and sexual functioning. Advancement of scrotal tissue is sometimes possible for closure, but in general, defects of greater than 25% will require grafting.

We prefer to use unmeshed STSGs of 0.18-inch thickness to the penis. When possible, we also prefer to graft onto dartos m. and fascia, often mobilizing it from the scrotum when it has been removed with the original debridement. Grafting directly onto Buck's fascia is possible, but it will limit the expansion of the corpora with erections and can cause pain with intercourse. We have found Integra and Matriderm to be useful adjuncts when subcutaneous tissue to graft on is lacking and will allow it to mature for 3 to 4 weeks prior to grafting.

The mucosal collar is often preserved after debridement. However, caution should be taken when attempting to preserve this skin as the lymphatic drainage is often impaired and postclosure edematous swelling can develop.

Suprapubic/Mons Closure

The suprapubic area has the least functional importance of areas most commonly involved with NSTIG. Similar to the scrotum, primary closure is often possible, even with large defects, using rotational flaps that easily developed from the abdomen (see **Fig. 6**).

With exposed abdominal musculature and the inability to do CSC, we again prefer to use Integra prior to STSG placement. Notably, NSTIG debridements in the suprapubic region can extend up the abdominal wall along Scarpa's fascia. If debridement in the suprapubic region is progressing more superiorly than expected, consultation with general surgery is important as our experience has taught us that these are the patients that progress the most rapidly.

FUTURE DIRECTIONS

Given the nature of NSTIG, it is unlikely that debridements will ever be supplanted by medications. However, given the significant prodrome in this patient population, and a defined population of patients at risk for NSTIG development, earlier recognition and prevention are where we can make the most impact on this disease process.

Reconstructive options will continue to expand as the use of wound healing augments and alternatives to skin grafting become more widely available.

RELEVANT CPT CODES

- Debridement of genital skin for necrotizing fasciitis (CPT 11006)
- Complex scrotoplasty (CPT 55180)
- Adjacent tissue transfer (rotational/advancement flap) for the creation of scrotum (30–60 sq cm; CPT 14301)
- Split-thickness skin graft (100 sq cm; CPT 15120; > 100 sq cm; CPT 15121)
- Wound prep of genitalia (prior to grafting or CSC) (CPT 15002)
- Wound vac placement (CPT 97605)
- Hydrocelectomy (CPT 55040; bilateral CPT 55041)

CLINICS CARE POINTS

- NSTIG commonly presents with pain "out of proportion" to the physical examination, which may appear early on as simple scrotal swelling ± cellulitis.
- Genital pain, especially in patients at-risk for developing NSTIG (diabetics, obese, alcohol-

dependents) should thus warrant further scrutiny with imaging (usually CT scan) or laboratory testing to look for evidence of ischemia.

- The spread of NSTIG is dependent on local microvascular thrombosis, thought to be the source of the pain, which precludes antibiotics from reaching the area, necessitating emergent surgical debridement

- Primary closure of NSTIG surgical wounds is often possible with sufficient "separation of components" without compromising reconstructive goals.

- Closure of NSTIG can occur during their initial hospital stay, generally after a minimum of 72 hours of culture-directed antibiotics, clinical stability, and nutrition optimization. Surgeons must be prepared to use various closure techniques depending on the affected area if reconstructive goals are to be achieved.

DISCLOSURE

The authors have nothing to disclose.

REFERENCES

1. Hagedorn JC, Wessells H. A contemporary update on Fournier's gangrene. Nat Rev Urol 2017;14:205.
2. Beecroft NJ, Jaeger CD, Rose JR, et al. Fournier's Gangrene in Females: Presentation and Management at a Tertiary Center. Urology 2021;151:113.
3. Czymek R, Frank P, Limmer S, et al. Fournier's gangrene: is the female gender a risk factor? Langenbecks Arch Surg 2010;395:173.
4. Sorensen MD, Krieger JN, Rivara FP, et al. Fournier's Gangrene: population based epidemiology and outcomes. J Urol 2009;181:2120.
5. Arora A, Rege S, Surpam S, et al. Predicting Mortality in Fournier Gangrene and Validating the Fournier Gangrene Severity Index: Our Experience with 50 Patients in a Tertiary Care Center in India. Urol Int 2019;102:311.
6. Barupal SR, Soni ML, Barupal R. Factors Affecting Mortality Following Necrotizing Soft-Tissue Infections: Randomized Prospective Study. J Emerg Trauma Shock 2019;12:108.
7. Beyan C, Beyan E. Fournier Gangrene: Association of Mortality with the Complete Blood Count Parameters. Plast Reconstr Surg 2019;143:443e.
8. Demir CY, Yuzkat N, Ozsular Y, et al. Fournier Gangrene: Association of Mortality with the Complete Blood Count Parameters. Plast Reconstr Surg 2018;142:68e.
9. El-Qushayri AE, Khalaf KM, Dahy A, et al. Fournier's gangrene mortality: A 17-year systematic review and meta-analysis. Int J Infect Dis 2020;92:218.
10. Ersoz F, Sari S, Arikan S, et al. Factors affecting mortality in Fournier's gangrene: experience with fifty-two patients. Singapore Med J 2012;53:537.
11. Fernandez-Alcaraz DA, Guillén-Lozoya AH, Uribe-Montoya J, et al. Etiology of Fournier gangrene as a prognostic factor in mortality: Analysis of 121 cases. Actas Urol Esp 2019;43:557.
12. Tenório CEL, Lima SVC, Albuquerque AV, et al. Risk factors for mortality in fournier's gangrene in a general hospital: use of simplified founier gangrene severe index score (SFGSI). Int Braz J Urol 2018;44:95.
13. Wong R, Blachman-Braun R, Mann U, et al. Location of residence and mortality for patients diagnosed with Fournier's gangrene. Can Urol Assoc J 2020; 15(5):E267–71.
14. Czymek R, Hildebrand P, Kleemann M, et al. New insights into the epidemiology and etiology of Fournier's gangrene: a review of 33 patients. Infection 2009;37:306.
15. Madsen MB, Skrede S, Perner A, et al. Patient's characteristics and outcomes in necrotising soft-tissue infections: results from a Scandinavian, multi-centre, prospective cohort study. Intensive Care Med 2019;45:1241.
16. Raebel MA, Malone DC, Conner DA, et al. Health services use and health care costs of obese and nonobese individuals. Arch Intern Med 2004;164: 2135.
17. Sparenborg JD, Brems JA, Wood AM, et al. Fournier's gangrene: a modern analysis of predictors of outcomes. Transl Androl Urol 2019;8:374.
18. Yang JY, Wang T, Pate V, et al. Real-world evidence on sodium-glucose cotransporter-2 inhibitor use and risk of Fournier's gangrene. BMJ Open Diabetes Res Care 2020;8(1):e000985.
19. Zhenyu X, Shaowen K, Chaoqun H, et al. First characterization of bacterial pathogen, Vibrio alginolyticus, for Porites andrewsi White syndrome in the South China Sea. PLoS One 2013;8:e75425.
20. Abass-Shereef J, Kovacs M, Simon EL. Fournier's Gangrene Masking as Perineal and Scrotal Cellulitis. Am J Emerg Med 2018;36:1719.e1.
21. Gadler T, Huey S, Hunt K. Recognizing Fournier's Gangrene in the Emergency Department. Adv Emerg Nurs J 2019;41:33.
22. Dos-Santos DR, Roman ULT, Westphalen AP, et al. Profile of patients with Fournier's gangrene and their clinical evolution. Rev Col Bras Cir 2018;45:e1430.
23. Kawahigashi T, Kawabe T, Iijima H, et al. Beware of perianal pain: fournier gangrene. Am J Med 2020; 133:924.
24. Tom LK, Wright TJ, Horn DL, et al. A Skin-Sparing Approach to the Treatment of Necrotizing Soft-

Tissue Infections: Thinking Reconstruction at Initial Debridement. J Am Coll Surg 2016;222:e47.

25. Perry TL, Kranker LM, Mobley EE, et al. Outcomes in Fournier's Gangrene Using Skin and Soft Tissue Sparing Flap Preservation Surgery for Wound Closure: An Alternative Approach to Wide Radical Debridement. Wounds 2018;30:290.

26. Voelzke BB, Hagedorn JC. Presentation and Diagnosis of Fournier Gangrene. Urology 2018;114:8.

27. Nawijn F, Smeeing DPJ, Houwert RM, et al. Time is of the essence when treating necrotizing soft tissue infections: a systematic review and meta-analysis. World J Emerg Surg 2020;15:4.

28. Lancerotto L, Tocco I, Salmaso R, et al. Necrotizing fasciitis: classification, diagnosis, and management. J Trauma Acute Care Surg 2012;72:560.

29. Corcoran AT, Smaldone MC, Gibbons EP, et al. Validation of the Fournier's gangrene severity index in a large contemporary series. J Urol 2008; 180:944.

30. Laor E, Palmer LS, Tolia BM, et al. Outcome prediction in patients with Fournier's gangrene. J Urol 1995;154:89.

31. Tarricone A, Mata K, Gee A, et al. A systematic review and meta-analysis of the effectiveness of LRI-NEC score for predicting upper and lower extremity necrotizing Fasciitis. J Foot Ankle Surg 2021;61(2):384–9.

32. Bruls RJM, Kwee RM. CT in necrotizing soft tissue infection: diagnostic criteria and comparison with LRINEC score. Eur Radiol 2021;31:8536.

33. Kwee RM, Kwee TC. Diagnostic performance of MRI and CT in diagnosing necrotizing soft tissue infection: a systematic review. Skeletal Radiol 2021; 51(4):727–36.

34. Chen Y, Wang X, Lin G, et al. Successful treatment following early recognition of a case of Fournier's scrotal gangrene after a perianal abscess debridement: a case report. J Med Case Rep 2018;12(1): 193.

35. Hahn HM, Jeong KS, Park DH, et al. Analysis of prognostic factors affecting poor outcomes in 41 cases of Fournier gangrene. Ann Surg Treat Res 2018;95:324.

36. Louro JM, Albano M, Baltazar J, et al. Fournier's Gangrene: 10-Year Experience of a Plastic Surgery and Burns Department at a Tertiary Hospital. Acta Med Port 2019;32:368.

37. Stevens DL, Bisno AL, Chambers HF, et al. Practice guidelines for the diagnosis and management of skin and soft tissue infections: 2014 update by the Infectious Diseases Society of America. Clin Infect Dis 2014;59:e10.

38. Castillejo Becerra CM, Jaeger CD, Rose JR, et al. Microorganisms and Antibiogram Patterns in Fournier's Gangrene: Contemporary Experience from a Single Tertiary Care Center. J Urol 2020;204:1249.

39. Hayon S, Demzik A, Ehlers M, et al. Orchidopexy and Split-thickness Skin Graft for Scrotal Defects After Necrotizing Fasciitis. Urology 2021;152:196.

40. Crew JR, Thibodeaux KT, Speyrer MS, et al. Flow-through Instillation of Hypochlorous Acid in the Treatment of Necrotizing Fasciitis. Wounds 2016; 28:40.

41. Li S, Liu Y, Huang Z, et al. Efficacy and safety of nano-silver dressings combined with recombinant human epidermal growth factor for deep second-degree burns: A meta-analysis. Burns 2021;47:643.

42. Czymek R, Schmidt A, Eckmann C, et al. Fournier's gangrene: vacuum-assisted closure versus conventional dressings. Am J Surg 2009;197:168.

43. Franco-Buenaventura D, García-Perdomo HA. Vacuum-assisted closure device in the postoperative wound care for Fournier's gangrene: a systematic review. Int Urol Nephrol 2020;53(4):641–53.

44. Iacovelli V, Cipriani C, Sandri M, et al. The role of vacuum-assisted closure (VAC) therapy in the management of FOURNIER'S gangrene: a retrospective multi-institutional cohort study. World J Urol 2020; 39(1):121–8.

45. Syllaios A, Davakis S, Karydakis L, et al. Treatment of Fournier's Gangrene With Vacuum-assisted Closure Therapy as Enhanced Recovery Treatment Modality. In Vivo 2020;34:1499.

46. Hourigan LA, Hourigan L, Linfoot JA, et al. Loss of protein, immunoglobulins, and electrolytes in exudates from negative pressure wound therapy. Nutr Clin Pract 2010;25:510.

47. Graves C, Saffle J, Morris S, et al. Caloric requirements in patients with necrotizing fasciitis. Burns 2005;31:55.

48. Michalczyk L, Grabinska A, Banaczyk B, et al. Efficiency of hyperbaric oxygen therapy combined with negative-pressure wound therapy in the treatment strategy of Fournier's Gangrene -A Retrospective Study. Urol J 2021.

49. Feres O, Feitosa MR, Ribeiro da Rocha JJ, et al. Hyperbaric oxygen therapy decreases mortality due to Fournier's gangrene: a retrospective comparative study. Med Gas Res 2021;11:18.

50. Alhajj, M., Bansal, P., Goyal, A.: Physiology, Granulation Tissue. In: StatPearls. Treasure Island (FL), 2021. Available at: https://www.ncbi.nlm.nih.gov/books/NBK554402/.

51. Vanwijck R, Kaba L, Boland S, et al. Immediate skin grafting of sub-acute and chronic wounds debrided by hydrosurgery. J Plast Reconstr Aesthet Surg 2010;63:544.

52. Hirokawa E, Sato T, Fujino T, et al. Hydrosurgical debridement as an approach to wound healing: an animal thermal burn model. J Wound Care 2019; 28:304.

53. Chammas MF Jr, Gurunluoglu R, Carlsen SN, et al. Surgical debridement of mineral pitch and nonviable

penile tissue using water-jet power: a preliminary report. BJU Int 2009;103:974.

54. Phillips GSA, Nizamoglu M, Wakure A, et al. The use of dermal regeneration templates for primary burns surgery in a UK regional burns centre. Ann Burns Fire Disasters 2020;33:245.

55. Schneider J, Biedermann T, Widmer D, et al. Matriderm versus Integra: a comparative experimental study. Burns 2009;35:51.

56. Combs PD, Sousa JD, Louie O, et al. Comparison of vertical and oblique rectus abdominis myocutaneous flaps for pelvic, perineal, and groin reconstruction. Plast Reconstr Surg 2014;134:315.

Adult-Acquired Buried Penis Classification and Surgical Management

Kevin J. Flynn, MD[a], Alex J. Vanni, MD[b], Benjamin N. Breyer, MD, MS[c], Bradley A. Erickson, MD, MS[a],*

KEYWORDS

- Adult-acquired buried penis • Escutcheon • Mons pubis • Panniculectomy
- Split-thickness skin graft • Phimosis • Cicatrix • Lymphedema

KEY POINTS

- Adult-acquired buried penis (AABP) is an acquired condition where the shaft of the penis is partially or completely covered by the surrounding prepubic and suprapubic and/or scrotal skin and soft tissue.
- AABP occurs commonly in men with truncal obesity. However, men with clinically significant AABP are those who seek clinical care due to impaired sexual function, compromised hygiene, bothersome urinary symptoms, or cosmetic concerns. It is thus assumed that this condition is being undertreated and underappreciated.
- There are four areas of concern when surgically reconstructing AABP: (1) abdomen/pannus, (2) escutcheon, (3) penile skin, and (4) scrotal skin. Each area should be evaluated and managed separately to ensure a good clinical and cosmetic outcome.
- Recognizing the heterogeneity of the condition, we propose an AABP classification system to help standardize the way that clinicians and researchers communicate about surgical techniques and outcomes.
- Surgical techniques for AABP should differ by classification but also by patient expectations, which should be made very clear before reconstruction. Patient-centered, goal-directed surgical care is vital to ensuring successful "outcomes."

EPIDEMIOLOGY

The prevalence of adult-acquired buried penis (AABP) is unknown. However, given increasing trends in male obesity (38% of US men met criteria for obesity [BMI>30] in 2014 compared with 13% in 1960), AABP has become an increasingly common condition encountered by urologists.

PATHOPHYSIOLOGY

The pathophysiology of AABP in obese patients often begins with excess bulk of the prepubic soft tissue (escutcheon). With progressive weight gain, the escutcheon begins to fully cover the shaft of the penis, which is fixed in place inferiorly by the dermal attachment to the Scarpa's fascia (which is attached to the penile suspensory ligament),

a Department of Urology, University of Iowa, Carver College of Medicine, 3233 RCP, 200 Hawkins Dr., Iowa City, IA 52242, USA; b Department of Urology, Tuft University School of Medicine, Lahey Hospital and Medical Clinic, 41 Mall Road, Burlington, MA 01805, USA; c Department of Urology, University of California, San Francisco, UCSF ACC 6th Floor, 400 Parnassus Suite A610, San Francisco, CA 94143, USA
* Corresponding author.
E-mail address: brad-erickson@uiowa.edu
Twitter: @baerickson29 (B.A.E.)

Urol Clin N Am 49 (2022) 479–493
https://doi.org/10.1016/j.ucl.2022.04.009
0094-0143/22/© 2022 Elsevier Inc. All rights reserved.

urologic.theclinics.com

forming the pubic sulcus, and superiorly by the dermal attachment to the abdominal fascia, forming the abdominal sulcus. The increased bulk and heft of the escutcheon cause distal migration of the penile sulcus until the penile skin and escutcheon skin lose their definition. The ensuing telescoping of the penile shaft by overlying hypermobile skin serves as an additional mode of functional penile length loss.[1,2]

Once functionally buried in the surrounding tissue, a subsequent insult to hygiene can occur. Trapped urine and moisture initiate a progressive cycle of skin irritation, epidermal breakdown, and inflammation. Skin breakdown can lead to bacterial and fungal cutaneous infections, exacerbating a cycle of inflammation.[3] Permanent scarring in the form of lichen sclerosus can occur, and in some instances lead to a fibrotic/scarred ring of skin, a cicatrix, and completely prevent exposure of the penis even with compression of the surrounding tissue. Chronic lymphedematous changes of the scrotum and/or penile skin may also lead to AABP. Eventually, the health of the penile shaft skin is compromised. Comorbid conditions such as diabetes mellitus can worsen the inflammatory cycle.

There is also an iatrogenic element of AABP. In poorly selected patients, a circumcision to expose a partially buried penis can cause further loss of penile shaft skin and subsequent inward telescoping of the corporal bodies. The healing circumcision incision can scar into a cicatrix causing iatrogenic phimosis. This scar can preclude exposure of the penis and incite the trapped urine/inflammatory cycle detailed above.

Beyond the deleterious effects on the penile and surrounding skin, AABP can lead to irritative LUTS, urinary tract infections, sexual dysfunction with pain during erection due to the entrapped penis and significant detriment on psychological well-being and self-esteem.[4] Of note, the increase in penile cancer in the United States, even in the previously circumcised, which was thought historically to protect from men from penile cancer, is largely thought to be secondary to the increase in AABP, which can mimic the environment of an uncircumcised penis with a buildup of smegma and inflammation.[5–7]

Adult Scrotal/Genital Lymphedema

The lymphatic channels that drain the scrotum do not cross the midline. They then drain into the ipsilateral superficial inguinal nodes.[8] Lymphedema occurs when lymphatic drainage is compromised due to prior surgery, radiation, infectious disease, malignancy, or an autoimmune condition.[9] The impaired lymphatic drainage leads to swelling of the scrotum and associated skin changes specifically thickening of the scrotal wall. In the short term, the scrotal skin changes may be reversible with nonoperative management (eg, compressive dressings) and treatment of the underlying etiology.[10] When the lymphedema is isolated to the scrotum, the skin is healthy, the conservative measures have failed, and microvascular lymphatic surgery can also be used.[11] With prolonged edema, however, the skin will eventually thicken, leading to "woody" skin changes, which are irreversible and require surgical intervention/excision.

INITIAL PATIENT EVALUATION

Evaluation of a patient with AABP begins with a thorough history and physical examination with attention given to important comorbid conditions such as diabetes, autoimmune disorders, smoking, and nutritional status.[12] It is important to inquire about any prior urologic surgeries, specifically circumcision and prior inguinal or pelvic lymph node dissections.

We standardized our preoperative photos to help with surgical planning and disease classification (pictures are also critical when providing clinical justification for surgical reconstructive procedures when required for the insurance approval process).

1. Standing (AP)
2. Standing (AP) lifting pannus
3. Supine lateral view
4. Supine with escutcheon lifted, attempting to retract foreskin of the penis (**Fig. 1**).

Penile physical examination should evaluate for lichen sclerosus and determine if the penis is able to be exposed.[13–16] Once exposed, an assessment of the health of the penile shift skin is important for operative decision-making. Nonviable penile shaft skin commonly necessitates removal followed by split-thickness skin grafting (STSG). Other important findings include the status of the meatus, the presence of inguinal hernias (may require imaging), and presence/severity of scrotal and penile lymphedema.[10] The presence of a large overlying pannus that does not have a distinct boundary from the escutcheon may require assistance from a plastic surgeon for a simultaneous panniculectomy.[3]

Baseline urinary and sexual function should be established with validated questionnaires. Before surgical intervention for AABP, patients with bothersome lower urinary tract symptoms or other concerning signs/symptoms should be evaluated for urethral stricture disease. Fuller and colleagues

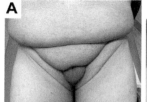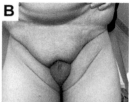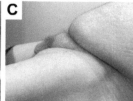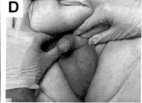

Fig. 1. Standardized physical examination for adult-acquired buried penis patients: (*A*) standing (AP), (*B*) standing (AP) with lifting of pannus, (*C*) supine lateral, and (*D*) retraction of escutcheon and exposure of glans penis.

identified a 31% rate of urethral stricture disease in patients undergoing surgical repair for AABP.[17] Lichen sclerosus is associated with both AABP and urethral stricture disease and likely accounts for the high rates of coexistent conditions.[13–16] It is adventitious to recognize urethral strictures before repair, but this is not always possible when the glans penis cannot be exposed preoperatively (management of AABP associated urethral strictures are discussed later in the article).

DISEASE CLASSIFICATION

AABP is a continuum of severity, the magnitude of which influences surgical decision-making. There are several published AABP classification systems. No one classification system is uniformly used, though three deserve further mention. A system reported by Tausch and colleagues used the viability of the penile skin at the time of surgery as a way to grade the disease process, acknowledging that AABP with nonviable skin and/or scrotal lymphedema increases surgical complexity given the need for skin grafting. Pariser and colleagues detailed a 5-category classification system for surgical complexity (though not the disease itself).[18] Patients were classified based on the highest category they qualified. A "complex" repair was defined as category ≥3. Most recently Hesse and colleagues published the Wisconsin Classification System for AABP which was the first to attempt classification of the disease process itself.[1] Of note, the group also provided the most common procedures associated with the AABP type, which validates the system for clinical utility. Although all three systems have merit, we believe that there is still a need for a system that is able to capture all of the diseases heterogeneity, especially if outcomes studies are to be interpreted collectively (eg, meta-analyses).

We present here our modified AABP classification system that uses the standardized photos listed above and description of seven anatomic landmarks listed in **Fig. 2**.

The Penis Abdomen Scrotum (PAS) classification system characterizes each clinically significant AABP component: Penile/Escutcheon Tissue (P), Abdominal/Pannus Tissue (A), and Scrotal Tissue (S) (**Tables 1–3**).

PENIS ABDOMEN SCROTUM CLASSIFICATION SCHEMA

The clinician should use the standardized AABP preoperative photos to classify using the PAS system. Analysis of the standard photos should allow the clinician to answer the following six questions using the definitions and examples provided below. This will then allow the clinician to follow the P, A, and S flowcharts in **Fig. 3**.

1. Is the pubic sulcus preserved?
   - Place the patient supine and palpate the dorsal penile skin at the junction with the escutcheon.
   - Maneuver the junction back to the pubic bone. If this significantly exposes the glans penis (or if there is significant phimosis preventing exposure), then the pubic sulcus is not preserved. If palpation does not expose more of the penile shaft, the sulcus is preserved (**Fig. 4**).
2. Is there an enlarged, contributory escutcheon?
   - Place the patient supine and assess the escutcheon relative to the glans penis. Does the escutcheon extend beyond the glans penis while on stretch? If yes, then it should be classified as a contributory escutcheon (note that although this designation does not necessitate its surgical removal at the time of AABP repair, we have found that when the escutcheon extends beyond the glans penis, postoperative wound management can be challenging if it is not removed, with higher reburying rates) (**Fig. 5**).
3. Is the penile skin reducible?
   - It is best to attempt penile skin reduction in the supine position (**Fig. 6**).
   - When the penile skin is unable to be reduced, the patient is classified as either P1x or P2x, depending on the escutcheon contribution.

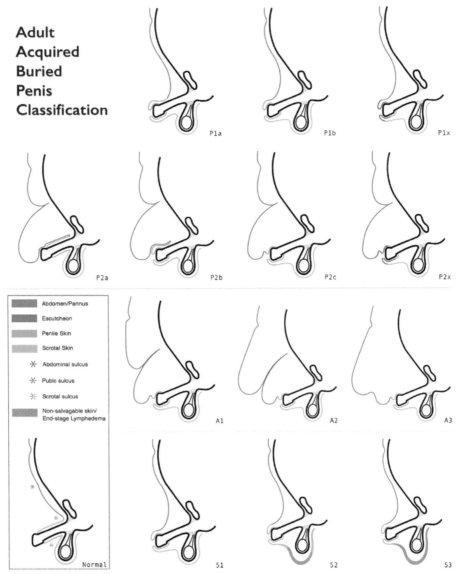

Fig. 2. Classification of AABP based on the status and health of seven anatomic features: (1) abdomen/pannus; (2) mons/escutcheon; (3) penile skin; (4) scrotal skin; (5) the presence/absence of the mons sulcus; (6) the presence/absence of the pubic sulcus; and (7) the presence/absence of the scrotal sulcus (penoscrotal angle).

- Once the skin is incised intraoperatively, the sufficiency of the penile skin can be determined and the AABP can be reclassified.
4. Is the penile skin sufficient for penile coverage?
  - Once the glans has been exposed, evaluate for any skin defects that can be closed using local skin flaps (eg, scrotal advancement flap, z-plasty) or will need to be covered with a skin graft.
  - If the skin is intact, one must still maneuver the pubic sulcus back to the pubic bone as was done in step 1. With the penis on stretch,

if reestablishing the pubic sulus does not allow for full penile stretch, then relaxing/circumcision incisions are likely needed (and will ultimately require coverage) (**Fig. 7**).
5. Is the abdominal pannus contributing to the buried penis (ie, will it need to be addressed at the time of surgery?).
  - Most abdominal panniculi will not need to be managed at the time of buried penis repair. However, if the panniculus hangs below the escutcheon/penis in the standing position, or if the pubic sulcus is absent (ie, no

Table 1
Penile/escutcheon (P) classification

	Reducible Penile Skin?	Penile Skin	Pubic Sulcus	Escutcheon
Buried Penis with Noncontributory Escutcheon				
P1a (Fig. S1)	Yes	Sufficient	Absent	Noncontributory
P1b (Fig. S2)	Yes	Insufficient	Absent	Noncontributory
P1x (Fig. S3)	No	NA	Absent	Noncontributory
Buried Penis with Contributory Escutcheon				
P2a (Fig. S4)	Yes	Sufficient	Present	Contributory
P2b (Fig. S5)	Yes	Sufficient	Absent	Contributory
P2c (Fig. S6)	Yes	Insufficient	Absent	Contributory
P2x (Fig. S7)	No	NA	Absent	Contributory

separation between escutcheon and panniculus tissue), then panniculectomy should be considered at the time of repair (**Fig. 8**).

6. Is irreversible lymphedema present?
   - Reversible lymphedema is often acute and the skin is compressible. Reversible lymphedema can occur in a patient with fluid overload (eg, heart failure) or after a groin lymph node dissection. In the case of the former, fluid management generally resolves the edema. In the latter case, mechanical compression, followed by microvascular lymph surgery, if without resolution, can be considered before resorting to excisional reconstruction.
   - Irreversible lymphedema is woody, noncompressible and has generally been present for many months to years. If present and contributing to the buried penis, it will likely need to be addressed at the time of surgery.
   - Lymphedema can occur anywhere in the genitalia, but most commonly affects the penile and/or scrotal skin (**Fig. 9**).

NONSURGICAL MANAGEMENT OF ADULT-ACQUIRED BURIED PENIS

Obesity is a driving factor in many patients with AABP. Weight loss and optimization of comorbid conditions such as diabetes before surgical intervention should be encouraged. However, weight loss alone is rarely a sufficient treatment of AABP because the cicatrix does not resolve, and the penis generally remains buried. Unfortunately, in patients who are successful in weight loss, a loosening of the escutcheon skin can actually exacerbate their buried penis sequelae.[19]

If present, the underlying cause of lymphedema should be sought. In developing countries, lymphedema caused by filarial disease should be treated with appropriate antimicrobial therapy.[10] Lymphedema caused by autoimmune disease can sometimes be effectively treated with steroids. Other conservative measures including scrotal compression or diuretic therapy can be effective. In appropriately selected patient's microsurgery anastomosing lymphatic channels to veins can prove successful.[11] This intervention requires the assistance of a surgeon trained in microvascular surgical techniques. Lymphedematous changes to the penis and scrotum eventually become permanent despite resolution of the underlying cause of lymphedema. Once permanent or woody edema develops management becomes surgical and follows the treatment plans outlined below.

Table 2
Abdominal/pannus (A) classification

	Abdominal Sulcus	Abdominal Pannus	Contributory Abdomen/Pannus
A0	Yes	Absent	No
A1 (Fig. S8)	Yes	Present	No
A2 (Fig. S9)	Yes	Present	Yes
A3 (Fig. S10)	No	Present	Yes

Table 3
Scrotal (S) classification

	Scrotal Sulcus	Scrotal Skin	Lymphedema
S0	Yes	Sufficient	Absent
S1 (Fig. S11)	No	Sufficient	Absent
S2 (Fig. S12)	No	Sufficient	Present
S3 (Fig. S13)	No	Insufficient	Present

SURGICAL MANAGEMENT OF ADULT-ACQUIRED BURIED PENIS
Perioperative

Weight loss before AABP repair should always be encouraged but is unlikely to significantly reverse the pathology. Medical management of comorbidities should be optimized, and diabetics should attempt to get their HgbA1c to less than 9% with assistance of an endocrinologist, when necessary. Anticoagulation and antiplatelet medications are held for a duration based on their respective half-lives.

Patient Positioning

- If scrotal work is being done (or if there is any chance of scrotoplasty being performed), we prefer to place the patient in low lithotomy position. Otherwise, supine with the bed flexed is our standard position for AABP repair.
- If the abdominal pannus is not being removed at the time of AABP repair, we will routinely retract this cephalad using specialized pannus retractors or surgical towels secured to the bed.

Surgical Goals

All cases of AABP are different, and goal-directed care is important in its management. For example, some patient's primary clinical concern may simply be improved genital hygiene, and thus, complicated surgical procedures using STSG and local flaps may be unnecessarily complex. All patients should be asked about their current urinary, sexual, and genital hygiene status before surgery, followed by their postoperative goals in each of these categories.[4] Surgical technique should then be altered as necessary.

Buried Penis Repair Surgical Principles

1. Exposure of the glans penis:
   - We start most cases of AABP repair start by exposing the glans penis. In P1x and P2x cases, the viability of the penile skin is still unknown until this step is performed. As many of our patients already have a dorsal

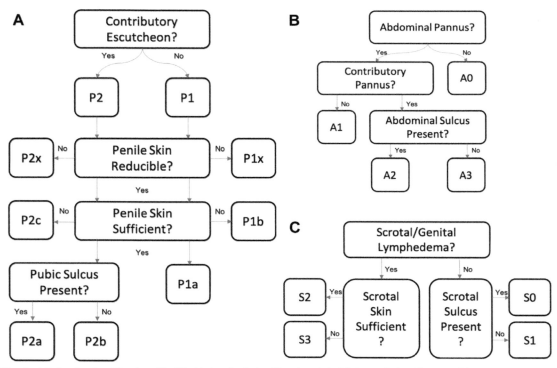

Fig. 3. (A) Penile classification (P). (B) Abdominal classification (A). (C) Scrotal classification (S).

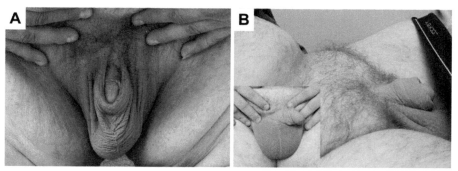

Fig. 4. (*A*) Patient with AABP but preserved pubic sulcus. (*B*) Patient with prior circumcision and AABP secondary to relaxation of the pubic sulcus. After manually reestablishing sulcus, penis unburies (note the minimal contribution from the escutcheon tissue).

skin deficiency, often the result of prior failed attempts at dorsal slit or revision circumcision, we will generally expose the phimotic penis using a dorsal incision of the phimotic band and/or the skin tube (though ventral or lateral incisions are also appropriate based on the operative findings of skin availability). Once the glans is out, a 2 to 0 nylon suture as then placed through the glans for traction, allowing for determination of penile skin sufficiency and the need for subsequent surgical steps (see **Fig. 7**).

2. Excision of nonviable penile skin
   • With the glans exposed, the skin viability is assessed. Not all "abnormal skin" must be removed as long as the abnormalities are superficial (see **Fig. 7**C). However, transdermal fibrotic skin should be excised, with care to preserve the underlying dartos when possible, which will improve its ability to support grafts and allow for movement of the skin with erections. Importantly,

edematous underlying tissue should be separate from dartos tissue and excised, as sub-graft edema can develop if this tissue is left in place.

3. Incision of phimotic rings
   • Even in situations in which the penile skin is reducible, phimotic bands should be incised. This will often leave a sizable defect which can then be covered with local tissue transfer and/or STSG (see **Fig. 7**C). Although the temptation is to perform a standard circumcision to remove all abnormal tissue, preservation of all useable skin is advisable, as it will likely be superior to any skin graft in the long-term (see **Fig. 7**D). (It is also useful for the native penile skin to be anchored to the penile base at the reestablished pubic sulcus to allow for STSGs to be placed on a flat surface.)

4. Excision of escutcheon
   • The escutcheon is the most commonly excised tissue superior to the penis during

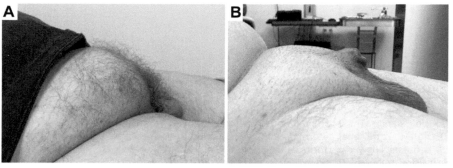

Fig. 5. (*A*) Patient with loss of pubic sulcus and escutcheon that extends well beyond the glans penis. (*B*) Patient with loss of pubic sulcus because of severe phimosis. However, the escutcheon does not extend beyond the penile skin tube (of note, although the escutcheon is noncontributory here, its removal can still be performed to improve definition of the pubic sulcus).

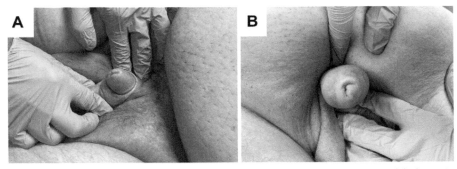

Fig. 6. (*A*) Reducible, though insufficient, penile skin after overly aggressive circumcision. (*B*) Phimotic penile skin of unknown sufficiency.

AABP repair. If the abdominal sulcus is intact, we will make our superior incision 1 cm inferior to the sulcus. Inferiorly, a mark is made 3 to 4 cm superior to the reestablished pubic sulcus (with the unburied penis on stretch) and then brought out laterally to meet the superior mark. The inferior line will be longer than the superior line, but in most cases, this incision can be closed linearly, with any mismatch usually managed laterally (**Fig. 10**A).

- During excision, care must be taken to avoid damage to the bilateral cord structures/testicles, which are often isolated with penrose drains, and the corporal body/penis (**Fig. 10**C).
- We have found that a Ligasure device can improve intraoperative hemostasis, and we use it liberally (Anecdotally, we have found the Ligasure device decreases postoperative seroma formation and Jackson-Pratt (JP) drain outputs as well) (**Fig. 10**B).[20]

- After escutcheon excision, penetrating towel clamps are used to plan a tension-free closure that best exposes the shaft (**Fig. 11**A). A linear closure is most commonly used, though if the lateral scrotal tissue excision is significant, a double "T" closure can be necessary (**Fig. 12**A and B).
- A JP is placed in the deepest part of the incision after excellent hemostasis is achieved. Interrupted 2 to 0 Vicryl sutures are used to bring the deep tissue together in at least two separate layers. The skin is then brought together with either staples or interrupted horizontal mattress 2 to 0 Nylon sutures.
- *Excision of pannus (as needed)*
- If a panniculectomy is required, this should be marked out at the beginning of the case, along with any mons tissue requiring excision. (Although we will not describe the details of panniculectomy in this article, as this is generally performed by our plastic surgeons, we will emphasize the need for

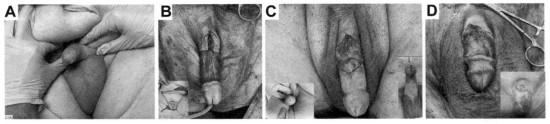

Fig. 7. (*A*) Reestablishing the pubic sulcus with palpation reveals sufficient penile skin for coverage (most of the time with reducible penile skin, it can be determined preoperatively whether a skin graft will be necessary. However, in (*B–D*), note that the final determination was not made until the glans had been fully delivered and untethered). (*B*) A dorsal slit was performed to expose the glans and then palpation revealed skin insufficiency. Circumcision incision reveals a significant defect. (*C*) Dorsal slit allowed for delivery of the glans penis. Note the significant dorsal defect present. Although the ventral skin seems to have evidence of lichen sclerosus, palpation reveals soft dermis and subdermis and we thus elected to preserve (and graft dorsally). (*D*) Circumcision incision reveals a significant skin deficiency (note our attempt at preserving the underlying dartos for grafting purposes.).

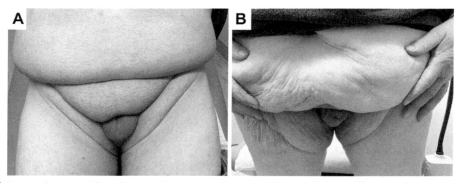

Fig. 8. (*A*) Pannus is present but does not hang over the mons tissue and the pubic sulcus is preserved (A1). (*B*) Large pannus is present and completely covers the underlying escutcheon (A2). Although panniculectomy is not mandatory (patient expectations should drive surgical technique), if the large overhanging pannus is left in situ, our experience had informed us of a high likelihood it will negatively affect postoperative healing.

escutcheon excision ± scrotal and penile skin rearrangement at the time of panniculectomy for AABP. In **Fig. 13**, note that two cases of panniculectomy for buried penis that resulted pathologic scrotal swelling [A] and escutcheon swelling [B].)

5. Reestablishing the pubic sulcus
   - Directly suturing the base of the penile skin to the fascia overlying the pubis to force the reestablishment of the pubic sulcus is not a necessary step during AABP repairs. Ideally, precise excision of escutcheon and scrotal tissue alone will reestablish the sulcus and prevent reburying. However, it is our experiences that in patients with a residual pannus or a large, protuberant abdomen, surgically reestablishing the pubic sulcus with sutures can improve postoperative cosmesis and functionality, as the mass of the abdomen, now in the absence of the escutcheon to provide support cephalad, can rebury the penis over time as attachments again loosen.
   - When used, we place three 2 to 0 PDS sutures on a CT needle to connect the penile skin dermis to the pubic fascia/periosteum. Similar tacking sutures can be placed lateral to the midline to help provide scrotal definition, as needed (**Fig. 11**C).

6. Scrotal excision/reconstruction
   - There are two primary reasons for needing scrotal excision during buried penis repairs. First, some patients simply have excess scrotal skin that can develop over time, often in the setting of morbid obesity (and often post-bariatric surgery) (see **Fig. 13**A).

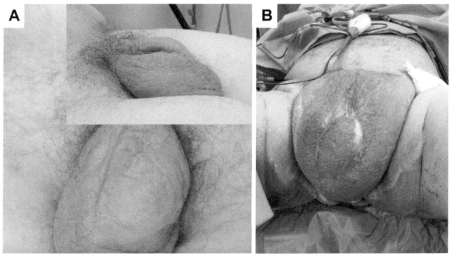

Fig. 9. (*A*) Scrotal lymphedema is present in the anterior/medial distribution. The lateral/posterior scrotal skin is preserved and can be used for reconstruction (S1). (*B*) End-stage large-volume scrotal lymphedema involving the entire scrotum and penis secondary to prior panniculectomy (S2).

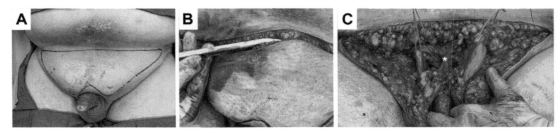

Fig. 10. Patient with P1xA1S0 buried penis. (*A*) Escutcheon marked out incorporating the lateral scrotal prominences. (*B*) Escutcheonectomy performed with aid of Ligasure. (*C*) Identification of bilateral spermatic cords, the erectile bodies (between surgeon fingers) and the suspensory ligaments (*asterisk*).

In these cases, simple scrotal reduction is necessary (when in line with patient goals). The second reason is for irreversible scrotal edema, which can develop iatrogenically or from chronic lymphatic obstruction secondary to morbid obesity (in developing countries, this is commonly from filariasis).

- The principles of reconstruction for scrotal/penile lymphedema are similar in both cases and require understanding of the normal scrotal lymphatic drainage.[8,9]

i. Lymphatic drainage from the scrotal does not cross over the midline (unilateral lymphedema can occur and this knowledge should direct the surgeon accordingly).

ii. The area of the median raphe and the 3 to 4 cm lateral to the median raphe contains the densest concentration of lymphatics. These lymphatics travel deep along the erectile bodies and then to the superficial inguinal nodes. Care

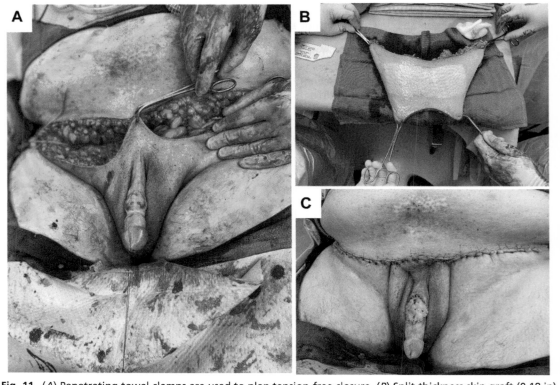

Fig. 11. (*A*) Penetrating towel clamps are used to plan tension-free closure. (*B*) Split-thickness skin graft (0.18 in) is harvested from the escutcheonectomy specimen after it has been removed. It is helpful to have the specimen on tension during removal as demonstrated. (*C*) Primary linear closure with deep 2 to 0 Vicryl sutures over a Jackson-Pratt drain and with superficial horizontal mattress 2 to 0 Nylon suture. Dorsal skin grafting performed with 4 to 0 Vicryl tacking sutures. Note the skin "dimples" superior to the penile shaft representing the reestablishment of the pubic sulcus using deep 2 to 0 PDS sutures.

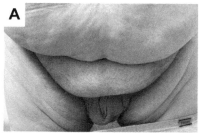 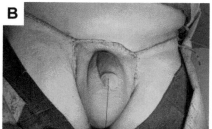 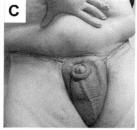

Fig. 12. (*A*) Patient with P2aA1S0 buried penis. (*B*) Escutcheonectomy performed with bilateral T closure using deep 2 to 0 Vicryl sutures over a Jackson-Pratt drain and superficial skin staples. (*C*) Patient at 2 weeks after staple removal (note the scrotal swelling medial to the T-closure. Patient was asked to compress the tissue twice daily to help removal of lymph as channels are reestablished).

must be taken to not completely disrupt this lymphatic tissue during escutcheonectomy so to prevent postoperative edema. (We have found that this can be accomplished with preservation of a continuous chain of deep fatty tissue extending from the scrotum to the inguinal region).

iii. The lateral scrotal tissue lymphatics and posterior/perineal lymphatics also (ultimately) drain into the superficial inguinal nodes, but lymph can travel via alternative routes (medial thigh, gluteal) bypassing the abdomen/mons. This alternative drainage helps to explain why idiopathic lymphedema is most commonly found medially, and why the lateral and posterior scrotal tissue is often preserved.

iv. Importantly, even with irreversible scrotal and penile edema, scrotal reconstruction can often be performed using the preserved posterior scrotal and medial thigh tissue (**Fig. 14**).

7. STSG to penis ± scrotum
- The skin grafting is often the last step of the AABP repair. If an escutcheonectomy is performed, we prefer to remove the skin graft from the excised escutcheon (**Fig. 11**B). In the setting of significant edema of the escutcheon, or if removal is not part of the AABP repair, the medial or lateral thigh is a reliable source for skin to cover the penis (Note that these areas are routinely prepped into the field in case escutcheon tissue is unusable).
- A Zimmer dermatome is used to harvest the skin graft at a depth of 0.18 in. If the graft is being used to cover the penis, it generally remains unmeshed. If the graft is used for scrotal reconstruction, a 1:1 mesh is used, which helps with drainage but also gives

the appearance of scrotal rugae after healing.
- All attempts are made after the delivery of glans and excision of the unhealthy penile skin to preserve native penile skin to establish the penile skin base. We have found that skin grafts do not do well in a deep pubic sulcus, and thus, we will secure the preserved skin, when present, to the corporal bodies to provide a flat surface for the distally placed graft (**Fig. 15**).
- Artis fibrin sealant can be used to fix the graft to the underlying dartos m. or Buck's fascia. We will also routinely place multiple 4 to 0 Vicryl taking sutures ("pie crust") to prevent fluid buildup under the graft, with care to avoid the neurovascular bundle dorsally (see **Figs. 11**C and **14C**).

8. Dressing placement
- If a STSG is used on the penile shaft, we place a compressive dressing for a minimum of 4 days. With tenuous closures involving multiple operative fields (eg, pannus, scrotum, penis), we will often place the patient on bed rest for 48 hours. However, if a small graft is being placed (see **Fig. 11**C), or if there is little risk of the dressing falling off, patients can ambulate on POD 1 and can even be discharged with a catheter and JP drain if their pain is sufficiently controlled.
- Negative pressure wound treatment (NPWT) is used with larger reconstructions (**Fig. 16**), set to continuous 125 mm Hg and kept in place for 4 days. When NPWT is used, Mepitel is placed directly on the graft and then covered with an appropriately tailored NPWT sponge, which is secured to the base of the penis with staples (note that if the NPWT device is having difficulty holding suction, we have found that a large Ioban surgical dressings can be helpful).

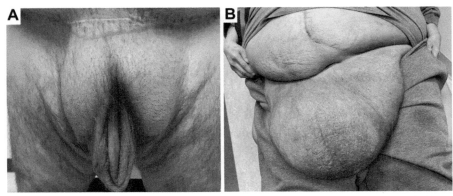

Fig. 13. (*A*) Patient with persistent bothersome buried penis after post-bariatric surgery panniculectomy. (*B*) Significant post-panniculectomy irreversible escutcheon and scrotal lymphedema.

- For more straightforward reconstructions in which the patient can be discharged to home, we prefer to use a dressing composed of Xeroform placed directly on the graft, then three 4 × 4 dressings (to prevent excessive compression), and finally a Coban compressive dressing, again secured to the base of the penis with staples (of note, there are multiple published techniques for dressing placement, all of which are likely sufficient as long as they maintain relative immobility of the reconstructed penis and compression of the graft onto the graft bed) (see **Fig. 14**E).

9. Urethral stricture management
   - The incidence of urethral stricture in patients with AABP has been reported to be as high as 30%.[17]
   - In general, we prefer to manage unrecognized meatal stenosis with a meatotomy at the time of the AABP repair. However, if the stricture extends more proximal (ie, S2c or S2b lichen sclerosus-related urethral stricture disease),[21] we will do a balloon dilation intraoperatively and then manage the LS stricture with intermittent catheterization, augmented with clobetasol, as was described by Hayden and colleagues.[22]
   - For isolated, unrecognized bulbar strictures (S1a/S1b), we will also dilate the stricture with a balloon intraoperatively, and then perform delayed urethroplasty if the stricture recurs.

10. Postoperative management:
   - Postoperative wound complications are common, reported to be as high as 50% to 80%.[18] Indeed, it is our practice to inform patients preoperatively that some degree of postoperative wound management should be expected (though most commonly superficial wound breakdown or minor graft loss).
   - Convalescence time after large AABP repairs can be expected to last up to 1 month and patients should be prepared for frequent return trips to the urologist for wound care.
   - We have found that it is absolutely critical that wounds are monitored on a weekly basis by the urology/reconstructive team. In the event of postoperative swelling (such as seen in **Fig. 12**C) that temporarily "reburies" the penis, the patient must be able to deliver the head of the penis multiple times per day to prevent graft loss or disease recurrence. Once the swelling has resolved, the penis with generally remain out—but if this is recognized late, repeat surgery is sometimes required.
   - Once incisions have healed, it is recommended to reassess patient goals and determine if surgical expectations have been met. Revision surgeries for minor cosmetic or functional concerns should be considered if expectations and outcomes are not matched.

11. Relevant CPT codes
   - Buried penis repair (14,040)
   - Complex scrotoplasty (CPT 55180)
   - Adjacent tissue transfer for creation of scrotum (30–60 sq cm; CPT 14301)
   - Harvest/placement of STSG (CPT 15120; > 100 cm 15,121)
   - Escutcheonectomy (CPT 15839)
   - Placement of wound vacuum (CPT 97606)

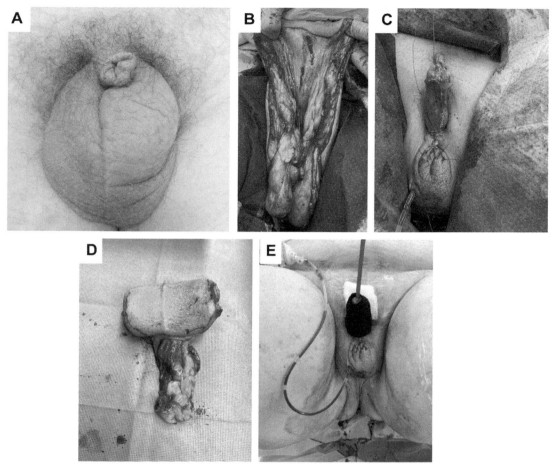

Fig. 14. (*A*) Idiopathic irreversible scrotal and penile lymphedema leading to a buried penis (note the preserved posterior scrotal tissue). (*B*) Excision of medial scrotal tissue and penile tissue after isolation of bilateral testicles. Note the dense network of abnormal scrotal vessels traveling along the corporal bodies. (*C*) Scrotal reconstruction using the preserved posterior scrotal and medial thigh tissue. (This will often come together in a lambda fashion with the apex of the posterior scrotal flap secured to base of the [now] unburied penis.) Split-thickness skin graft (0.18 in., unmeshed) harvested from the medial thigh placed onto the penile shaft with fibrin glue and 4 to 0 Vicryl tacking sutures. (*D*) Excised scrotal skin along with abnormal lymphatics. (*E*) Compressive dressing secured with staples at its based left in place for 4 days.

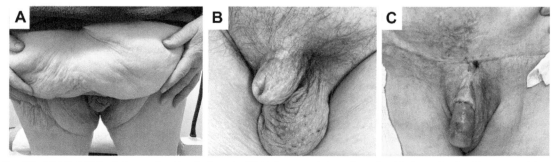

Fig. 15. (*A*) P2cA2S0 adult-acquired buried penis. (*B*) Unknown status of penile skin in patient with severe phimosis (P2x). After dorsal slit, patient noted to have insufficient penile skin (P2c). (*C*) Patient 1 month after buried penis repair in which panniculectomy and escutcheonectomy was performed. Note the penile skin was secured to the base of the penis and the unmeshed graft (harvested from the escutcheon) was placed distally.

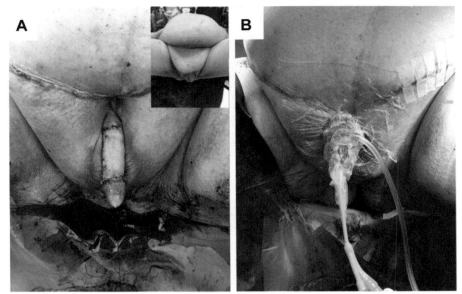

Fig. 16. (*A*) P2cA1S0 adult-acquired buried penis after escutcheonectomy and placement of split-thickness skin graft to the shaft. Note the preserved native penile skin proximally, allowing for placement of the graft on a flat surface. (*B*) NPWT placed onto the grafted penile shaft.

CLINICS CARE POINTS

- The incidence of adult-acquired buried penis (AABP) is increasing, in line with the increase in obesity and diabetes, which are significant risk factors for development.

- Men will seek care when their AABP significant affects genital hygiene (eg, recurrent phimosis and urinary tract infections), sexual functioning, and/or concern about genital appearance. However, given the sensitive nature of the condition, it is likely that the disease remains undertreated.

- Significant heterogeneity, both in AABP presentation and of the surgical goals in patients with AABP, means that many different types of repairs are required to adequately treat the condition.

- Postoperative management of minor wound concerns should be expected with convalescence often extending to a month. Patient satisfaction with the procedure is depends on early acknowledgment of the need for active wound management.

- When surgical outcomes are in line with surgical goals, the vast majority of patients report improvement in genital hygiene, urinary symptoms, and sexual functioning.

DISCLOSURE

"The authors have nothing to disclose."

SUPPLEMENTARY DATA

Supplementary data related to this article can be found online at https://doi.org/10.1016/j.ucl.2022.04.009.

REFERENCES

1. Hesse MA, Israel JS, Shulzhenko NO, et al. The surgical treatment of adult acquired buried penis syndrome: a new classification system. Aesthet Surg J 2019;39(9):979–88.
2. Rybak J, Larsen S, Yu M, et al. Single center outcomes after reconstructive surgical correction of adult acquired buried penis: measurements of erectile function, depression, and quality of life. J Sex Med 2014;11(4):1086–91.
3. Fuller TW, Theisen KM, Shah A, et al. Surgical management of adult acquired buried penis. Curr Urol Rep 2018;19(3):22.
4. Voznesensky MA, Lawrence WT, Keith JN, et al. Patient-reported social, psychological, and urologic outcomes after adult buried penis repair. Urology 2017;103:240–4.
5. Alzubaidi AN, Hahn AE, Gellhaus PT, et al. Circumcision, buried penis and obesity in a contemporary cohort of patients with penile cancer. Urol Pract 2019;6(4):243–8.

6. Pekala KR, Pelzman D, Theisen KM, et al. The prevalence of penile cancer in patients with adult acquired buried penis. Urology 2019;133:229–33.

7. Manwaring J, Vourganti S, Nikolavsky D, et al. Pannus is the new prepuce? penile cancer in a buried phallus. Case Rep Urol 2015;2015:403545.

8. Kavoussi P. Scrotum lymphatic drainage. In: Wein AJ, Kavoussi LR, Meredith F, editors. Campbell-walsh-wein urology. 10th ed. Philadelphia, PA: Elsevier Saunders; 2012. p. 67.

9. Pastor C, Granick MS. Scrotal lymphedema. Eplasty 2011;11:ic15.

10. Rusilko PJ, Fuller TW, Burks F. Textbook of male genitourethral reconstruction. In: FEMe al, editor. Textbook of male genitourethral reconstruction. Springer Nature; 2020. p. 737–48.

11. Phan R, Seifman MA, Dhillon R, et al. Use of submental and submandibular free vascularized lymph node transfer for treatment of scrotal lymphedema: report of two cases. Microsurgery 2020;40(7): 808–13.

12. Smith-Harrison LI, Piotrowski J, Machen GL, et al. Acquired buried penis in adults: a review of surgical management. Sex Med Rev 2020;8(1):150–7.

13. Fergus KB, Lee AW, Baradaran N, et al. Pathophysiology, clinical manifestations, and treatment of lichen sclerosus: a systematic review. Urology 2020;135:11–9.

14. Erickson BA, Tesdahl BA, Voznesensky MA, et al. Urethral lichen sclerosus under the microscope: a survey of academic pathologists. Can J Urol 2018; 25(3):9328–33.

15. Osterberg EC, Gaither TW, Awad MA, et al. Current practice patterns among members of the american urological association for male genitourinary lichen sclerosus. Urology 2016;92:127–31.

16. Erickson BA, Elliott SP, Myers JB, et al. Understanding the relationship between chronic systemic disease and lichen sclerosus urethral strictures. J Urol 2016;195(2):363–8.

17. Fuller TW, Pekala K, Theisen KM, et al. Prevalence and surgical management of concurrent adult acquired buried penis and urethral stricture disease. World J Urol 2019;37(7):1409–13.

18. Pariser JJ, Soto-Aviles OE, Miller B, et al. A simplified adult acquired buried penis repair classification system with an analysis of perioperative complications and urethral stricture disease. Urology 2018;120:248–52.

19. Ho TS, Gelman J. Evaluation and management of adult acquired buried penis. Translational Androl Urol 2018;7(4):618–27.

20. Siegel JA, Zhao L, Tachibana I, et al. Rapid excision of massive localized lymphedema of the male genitalia with vessel sealing device. Can J Urol 2016; 23(3):8291–5.

21. Erickson BA, Flynn KJ, Hahn AE, et al. Development and Validation of A Male Anterior Urethral Stricture Classification System. Urology 2020;143:241–7.

22. Hayden JP, Boysen WR, Peterson AC. Medical Management of Penile and Urethral Lichen Sclerosus with Topical Clobetasol Improves Long-Term Voiding Symptoms and Quality of Life. J Urol 2020;204(6): 1290–5.

Robotic Ureteral Reconstruction

Thomas W. Fuller, MD[a], Adam M. Daily, MD, MS[a], Jill C. Buckley, MD[b],*

KEYWORDS

- Robotics • Ureter • Upper tracts • Minimally invasive • Reconstruction

KEY POINTS

- Robotic ureteral reconstruction is safe, effective, and decreases patient pain and length of stay compared with open surgery.
- Indocyanine green allows ureteral identification when administered intraluminally and ureteral perfusion when given intravenously.
- TilePro multi-image display with simultaneous ureteroscopy allows identification of the ureter and localization of ureteral stenosis.
- Robotic reconstruction of the ureter below the pelvic brim is addressed nearly universally with a robotic approach.
- Buccal graft ureteroplasty with omental flap is an emerging alternative for enteric interpositions and autotransplant for long-segment mid and proximal ureteral strictures.

 Video content accompanies this article at http://www.urologic.theclinics.com.

INTRODUCTION

Robotic-assisted ureteral reconstruction has progressed beyond studies evaluating equivalency with laparoscopic or open approaches. Large retrospective series have shown comparable success rates for index procedures, such as pyeloplasty and ureteral reimplant. Adequately powered randomized studies are unlikely in the future because equivalency with open surgery is widely accepted, lengths of stay are shorter, and pain scores are reliably better in laparoscopic and robotic surgery.

Robotic-assisted surgery is particularly well suited for ureteral reconstruction. Robotics allow access to the deep pelvis and retroperitoneum. Precision in mucosal-to-mucosal anastomosis is facilitated by the stability of movement, robotic wrist degrees of freedom, and the magnification provided by the robotic camera. New adjunctive technologies and robotic platforms are particularly useful in ureteral reconstruction.[1] Simultaneous image display allows prompt ureteral identification in difficult surgical fields when a robotic approach is combined with concurrent ureteroscopy. Indocyanine green (ICG) delineates vascularized tissue. Both technologies can help accurately identify the location and extent of ureteral stenoses. A single site surgical system has been brought to market that minimizes pain and disfigurement with surgery.

There has been a recent rapid expansion of ureteral reconstructive techniques. Collaborative groups of robotic ureteral surgeons are combining experience to propel the field forward. Their collective experience is helping define optimal approaches and success rates for rare procedures.

[a] Virginia Mason Franciscan Health, 1100 9th Avenue, C7-UroSeattle, WA 98101, USA; [b] University of California San Diego, 9500 Gilman Drive, La Jolla, CA 92093, USA
* Corresponding author. 9500 Gilman Drive, La Jolla, CA 92093.
E-mail address: jcbuckley@health.ucsd.edu

Urol Clin N Am 49 (2022) 495–505
https://doi.org/10.1016/j.ucl.2022.05.002
0094-0143/22/© 2022 Elsevier Inc. All rights reserved.

NOVEL ROBOTIC PLATFORMS AND ADJUNCTS FOR URETERAL RECONSTRUCTION

Indocyanine Green

ICG fluoresces when exposed to near-infrared wavelengths. Photons produced by the excitation are detected by infrared high-definition cameras during robotic surgery. Intravenously delivered ICG can distinguish perfused from avascular tissue. Intraluminal ICG helps identify the ureter when delivered via a retrograde pyelogram or antegrade nephrostogram.

ICG for evaluation of tissue perfusion is delivered intravascularly. After reconstitution of 25 mg of ICG in 10 mL of saline or water, aliquots of ICG from 2 to 5 mg up to a full 25-mg dose are administered. It is usually visible with near-infrared imaging within 1 minute of injection.

ICG is particularly useful in robotic ureteral reconstruction to delineate avascular stricture or radiated ureteral tissue.[2] The most definitive evidence of this utility is in urinary diversion after cystectomy. The presumed cause of ureteroenteric stricture is poorly perfused tissue that is not clinically evident at the time of anastomosis. Retrospective series note a decreased stricture rate with the use of intravenous ICG to evaluate ureteral perfusion. In a single surgeon retrospective review of robotic ileal conduits, 5 of 31 patients were noted to have a ureteroenteric stricture versus only 1 out of 30 where ICG was used, and further ureteral resection was conducted as necessary.[3] A second retrospective series confirms this finding, noting a 10.6% stricture rate in 132 patients without ICG compared with no strictures in 47 patients with ICG.[4] In the latter series, the authors note that ICG administration often resulted in the decision to further resect the ureter to a more robustly perfused level.

Ureteral strictures are avascular or minimally vascularized and appear dark when ICG is administered intravascularly. High success rates have been shown for ureteral reconstruction with the use of ICG in this context. In a series of 42 upper urinary tract reconstructive procedures (pyeloplasty, 20; ureteral reimplant, 13; ureterolysis, 7; ureteroureterostomy, 2) there was a combined 95.2% success rate for reconstruction with ICG.[5] All failures in the series were with ureterolysis. Benefit over the standard (resection to visually well-vascularized bleeding tissue) has not been conclusively shown. It will be difficult to do so, considering the power required to show benefit in high success rate procedures, such as pyeloplasty and ureteral reimplant. The use of ICG to help identify viable ureteral tissue at the time of ureteral reimplantation or reconstruction is common practice and is common practice in high-volume upper tract reconstruction centers.

Intraluminal delivery of ICG expedites identification of the ureter in the difficult surgical field often encountered in ureteral reconstruction. Radiation, chemotherapy, prior surgical interventions, history of urine or bowel leaks, and primary retroperitoneal fibrosis are all associated with ureteral pathology and make ureteral identification and dissection more difficult. ICG is delivered either antegrade via nephrostomy or retrograde via a retrograde pyelogram to facilitate identification and dissection. The location of ureteral stricture or obliteration is evident by a cutoff or decrease in fluorescence (**Fig. 1**, Video 1).[6,7] Colorectal surgeons have also published their experience with retrograde ICG for ureteral identification and note the healthy ureter can still be identified with robotic infrared cameras up to 8 hours after instillation.[8] Ureteral fluorescence is extremely valuable to expedite ureteral identification and safe dissection especially after prior retroperitoneal dissection and/or injury to the ureter.

A typical protocol is reconstitution of 25 mg of ICG in sterile water or saline with antegrade, retrograde, or dual antegrade and retrograde administration of 10 to 15 mL. When administered antegrade, the nephrostomy is often capped for a period to allow the ICG to progress from the renal pelvis into the ureter up to the point of proximal obstruction. Caution should be taken with the amount of ICG instilled antegrade and duration of nephrostomy capping to avoid pyelovenous backflow and associated risk of bacteremia. Careful attention to appropriate preoperative antibiotics is necessary when using antegrade ICG with a long-standing colonized nephrostomy tube. If the ICG is given intraluminally to help identify the ureter, the ability to assess tissue vascularity is lost because the intraluminal fluorescence masks the fine ureteral vascularity.

ICG is currently Food and Drug Administration approved for intravenous use only and patients should be advised of the off-label use of the medication and poorly defined adverse event profile for intraluminal administration. Adverse events with intravenous ICG are rare. There are several reports of anaphylactic reactions associated with intravenous use.[9–11]

Multi-Image Display

White light from a ureteroscope is visible as bright green, like the appearance of ICG, when an infrared camera is used. TilePro, da Vinci Surgical System's multi-image display software (Intuitive

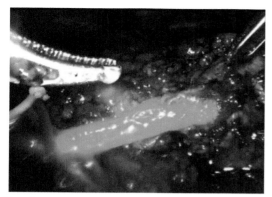

Fig. 1. Intraoperative identification of obliterated ureteral stricture in a redo pyeloplasty. Indocyanine green delivered via a retrograde pyelogram fluoresces up until the point of obstruction.

Surgical, Inc, Sunnyvale, CA), allows the surgical field and images derived from an endoscopic camera to be viewed simultaneously within the robotic console display. Common uses in ureteral reconstruction are integration of imaging from ureteroscopy and the robotic camera to identify the ureter in fibrotic fields and precisely identify the location and length of ureteral stenoses (**Fig. 2**, Video 2).[12] The ureteroscopic white light visualized with Firefly technology is a valuable tool to help identify the ureter in the reoperative or highly fibrosed ureteral reconstructive operative case.

Robotic-Assisted Single-Site Surgery

The da Vinci single port (SP) system allows single-site robotic ureteral reconstruction. It has not been widely adopted yet with limited small series on its merits in the literature. Feasibility has been demonstrated in small series of pyeloplasty and ureteral reimplantation.[13–15] The SP consists of a single 2.5-cm trocar passing three 6-mm arms and a 12-mm camera, all of which articulate to allow triangulation intracorporeally. The physical domain occupied outside the patient is significantly less than multiarm platforms allowing surgeons to work in tandem.[16,17] Other proposed benefits are cosmesis, decreased incisional morbidity, and decreased postoperative pain. Incisional hernia rates are higher and the range of dissection is limited.

The surgical field should ideally be 15 to 25 cm from the SP trocar. If the surgical field is less than 15 cm, the SP is used with a "floating dock" where the trocar is passed through a gel port coupled to a wound retractor incompletely secured to the skin. This creates a bridge that allows the trocar to hover further from the abdominal wall. The GelPoint system (Applied Medical, Rancho Santa Margarita, CA) is commonly used with AirSeal (ConMed, Utica, NY) (stable pneumoperitoneum platform with concurrent smoke evacuation) to counteract pneumoperitoneum loss with wound retractor interposition between fascia and the trocar.[16,18]

The SP system permits less traction on tissue than a multiport platform. Occasionally assistant ports, either through the GelPoint system or a second 5- to 8-mm port site, are necessary. Importantly, near infrared fluorescence imaging is not yet available with the da Vinci SP system.[17]

ROBOTIC URETERAL RECONSTRUCTION
Upper and Mid Ureter

Introduction
The appropriate technique for robotic reconstruction of the ureter above the pelvic brim depends on the cause, location, and length of obstruction (**Fig. 3**). Ureteropelvic junction obstructions are largely managed with a robotic pyeloplasty. More distal short strictures are addressed with ureteroureterostomy. Longer complex obstructions may require buccal augmentation, appendiceal onlay, or appendiceal interposition. Before techniques that require tissue transfer, it is advisable to remove ureteral stents and place a nephrostomy preoperatively to allow ureteral inflammation to resolve and the full extent of the stricture to declare itself. The longest and most complex obstructive processes can necessitate replacement of the ureter with ileum or obviating the ureter with an autotransplant.

Pyeloplasty and ureterocalicostomy
The gold standard treatment of ureteropelvic junction obstruction, either caused by a crossing vessel or an aperistaltic segment, is a dismembered pyeloplasty. Success rates across multiple single and multi-institutional retrospective cohorts for robotic pyeloplasty range from 95% to 98%.[19–22] This is equivalent to laparoscopic and open approaches in multiple meta-analyses.[23,24] Lengths of stays with laparoscopic and robotic approaches are considerably shorter than with an open approach. Complications with robotic surgery are minimal and many patients undergoing robotic-assisted pyeloplasty are discharged home the same day.

In the rare instance when a pyeloplasty is unsuccessful because of a recurrent ureteropelvic junction obstruction, studies note a good success rate in the redo setting. Blood loss, although still modest, is higher in redo surgery and operative times are longer. In the scarred redo field

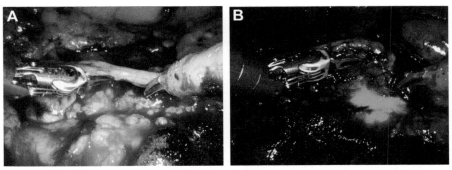

Fig. 2. Ureteral dissection for retroperitoneal fibrosis. (*A*) Dense fibrotic surgical field where ureter is not easily identified. (*B*) Ureter is easily identified in the same surgical field by simultaneous ureteroscopy where white light is seen as bright green with the infrared camera.

simultaneous ureteroscopy or injection of ICG can help identify the ureter and location of obstruction.[19,20,25]

In the case where there is an obliterated ureteropelvic junction and proximal ureter, a robotic-assisted renal pelvis flap and anterior buccal onlay flap with omental flap is used to salvage the renal unit and have a successful repair. We have had excellent patency rates with this technique. The ureter is identified and encircled as it crosses over the common iliac artery. It is mobilized proximally and transected. The renal pelvis is exposed, and an inverted U-flap is raised for reanastomosis

of the posterior wall of the ureter to the renal pelvis flap. A buccal graft is harvested to connect the anterior wall of the ureter to the pelvis. The omentum is tacked to the buccal graft to ensure a robust blood supply for survival. This is our preferred approach for a long obliterated ureteropelvic junction and proximal ureter.

When there is significant ureteral length loss where patent healthy ureter does not reach the renal pelvis and the renal pelvis cannot be adequately mobilized to the ureter, ureterocalicostomy is considered.[26] It requires transection of the lower pole of the kidney to expose the lower pole

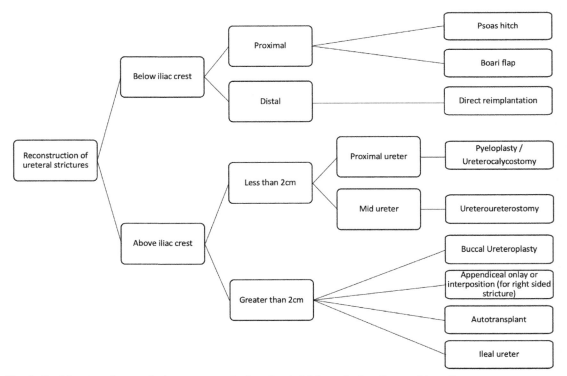

Fig. 3. Decision tree for surgical management of ureteral strictures by location and length.

calyx and provide a site for ureteral anastomosis. After clamping the renal artery, the lower pole is transected, including entry in the lower pole calyx. The location of the lower pole calyx is confirmed by ultrasound before clamping the renal artery. Before anastomosis of the ureter to the lower pole calyx, meticulous hemostasis is required over the transected lower pole with a renorrhaphy. This is similar in nature to hemostasis gained after robotic partial nephrectomy, which has been well described elsewhere. In a retrospective series of six patients undergoing robotic ureterocalicostomy all patients had successful outcomes at median follow-up of 15 months.[27] Ureterocalicostomy is rarely conducted and patient selection is critical to success.

Both interrupted and running anastomoses are commonly used in a pyeloplasty. Superiority of one technique over the other has not been shown. Our preference is interrupted sutures to provide redundancy should a suture break and to limit tissue ischemia. In either suturing technique, the key is attention to detail to create a wide lateral spatulation, followed by careful apposition of mucosa to mucosa to create a wide anastomosis. Critical to success is a dependent position of the new anastomosis. The need for a redo pyeloplasty is the result of a patent but poorly draining renal pelvis.

Stents are placed in an antegrade fashion at the time of the anastomosis with care taken to ensure the distal curl has coiled in the bladder. Alternative stent placement techniques, including preoperative retrograde approaches, are used and left to the surgeon's comfort. If there is any doubt intraoperative cystoscopy should be performed. Stents are typically maintained for 3 to 6 weeks postoperatively.

In contrast to variability in stent and drain management, there is general agreement that the ureter should be handled as little as possible with robotic instruments. This is especially true with crushing robotic instruments, such as needle drivers. Often a segment of ureter that will ultimately be discarded is left attached until the final anastomotic stitches are thrown. This segment of ureter acts as a handle to allow the ureter to be manipulated without compromising tissue that will ultimately be included in the anastomosis.

Patients are typically followed with renal ultrasounds and symptomatically. If there is a concern for drainage or the patient remains symptomatic, a diuretic renogram is performed.

Ureteroureterostomy

Ureteroureterostomy has limited utility. It is restricted to strictures less than 2 cm that are proximal enough to preclude reimplantation with a psoas hitch or Boari flap and distal enough to preclude pyeloplasty. The ureter typically cannot be mobilized enough to create a well-vascularized tension-free anastomosis if the stricture is longer than 2 cm when also performing a proper ureteral spatulation distally and proximally.

Surgery starts with circumferential dissection of the ureter. Stenotic tissue is excised. The ureter is spatulated distally and proximally for approximately 1 to 1.5 cm on opposing sides. A running or interrupted anastomosis is carried out. Stents are typically left for 3 to 6 weeks postoperatively. A surgical drain is not routinely left.

Strictures can be longer than noted on preoperative imaging. If the entire length of avascular strictured tissue is not excised there is a higher risk of recurrence. Surgeons should be facile with alternate techniques and prepared to transition to a different approach, such as a buccal ureteroplasty or appendiceal augmentation, in the event the stricture is longer than anticipated.

Buccal ureteroplasty

In the case of a ureteral stricture that is too long for a tension-free ureteroureterostomy, too proximal for a reimplant, and too distal for a pyeloplasty, buccal mucosa is used to augment the luminal diameter of the ureter. Robotic ureteroplasty with buccal mucosa graft is a new procedure but it is gaining traction. The Collaborative of Reconstructive Robotic Ureteral Surgery (CORRUS) has published the largest cohort to date using this technique. In the CORRUS experience of 54 patients they describe an 87% success rate at a median follow-up of 27.5 months. Within this cohort 18 patients had a prior attempt at ureteral reconstruction. Fourteen (78%) redo procedures were successful. There were three major postoperative complications including a port site hernia, hypercapnia necessitating reintubation, and gluteal compartment syndrome necessitating fasciotomy.[28]

There are two approaches to ureteroplasty with buccal mucosa depending on the underlying pathology. Stenotic segments are incised longitudinally, and a 10- to 18-mm-wide buccal mucosa graft is then circumferentially anastomosed to the defect using long-acting absorbable suture in an onlay fashion. The buccal mucosa requires a robust vascular flap for imbibition and inosculation. A circumferential omental wrap or a backing omental flap is used for neovascularization. The flap is secured to the graft using a series of quilting sutures (Video 3).

When there is an obliterative segment, an augmented anastomotic approach is needed. In this case the obliterated segment of ureter is excised, and a ureterotomy is made on the same side of the proximal and distal ureteral segments beyond any stenosis. A posterior plate of native ureter to native ureter is created with long-acting absorbable sutures. The buccal mucosa is then circumferentially anastomosed to the ureterotomy. The omentum is used as a vascular backing for the buccal mucosa.

In both techniques a double J stent is placed and maintained for 4 to 6 weeks postoperatively. A surgical drain is placed depending on the surgeon's comfort. Observation with interval renal ultrasounds and measures of glomerular filtration are advisable. Diuretic renogram is used for patients with pain discordant with imaging findings.

Appendiceal onlay and interposition

An alternative to buccal onlay or buccal augmented anastomotic ureteroplasty on the right side is an appendiceal onlay or interposition. In both procedures the right colon is mobilized along the white line of Toldt to the level of the hepatic flexure. The appendix is transected at the base and the distal tip of the appendix is excised and discarded. The appendix is left on a vascular pedicle containing the appendiceal artery. ICG is a useful adjunct to ensure perfusion of the transected and mobilized appendix.

In an appendiceal onlay the ureter is mobilized only on the anterior surface and incised longitudinally extending beyond the stenosis proximally and distally. The appendix is incised longitudinally on the antimesenteric border. The detubularized appendix is then anastomosed to the ureteral plate using running long-acting absorbable suture.

Appendiceal interposition maintains a tubularized appendix. It is typically used when there is a long right-sided obliterative ureteral stricture where an anastomotic augmented approach seems impossible or ill-advised. The stenotic segment of ureter is excised. The appendix and ureter are typically spatulated and two anastomoses are performed. In both techniques a stent is left for 4 to 6 weeks. A surgical drain may be left at the time of surgery.

Adequate mobility of the colon and appendix, satisfactory health and luminal diameter of the appendix, and the appearance of well-perfused tissue after transection is required for the technique. The appendix can appear several centimeters long with only 3 to 4 cm of patency for use. These characteristics are not obvious on preoperative imaging. Surgeons should have the flexibility and preparation to transition to an alternate technique. Patients should be informed of this possibility and the risks and benefits of alternate options.

There are several advantages with appendiceal onlay and interposition. The ureter does not have to be mobilized circumferentially preserving more native ureteral blood supply. The appendix has intrinsic vascularity from the appendiceal artery. In contrast to a buccal graft, there is no need for a vascularized omental flap and the risk of buccal graft loss. Additionally, there is no donor site morbidity from buccal mucosa graft harvest.

In 13 patients retrospectively reviewed by the CORRUS collaborative undergoing appendiceal ureteroplasty (onlay, 8; interposition, 5), there was a 92% success rate at a mean follow-up of 14.6 months. The mean stricture length treated with these techniques was 6.5 cm.[29–31]

There is not enough retrospective or prospective data to evaluate the long-term efficacy of buccal ureteroplasty versus appendiceal interposition. Given the scarcity of the pathology a multi-institutional effort is required to clarify an optimal approach.

Lower Ureter

Introduction

Ureteral obstruction below the pelvic brim is typically managed by ureteroneocystotomy (ureteral reimplant). Distal focal obstructions are approached by directly anastomosing the bladder with a transected ureter above the level of obstruction. Increasingly proximal disease requires adjunctive maneuvers for the bladder to reach above the point of obstruction (see **Fig. 3**). A psoas hitch elevates the bladder and deviates toward the obstructed side by securing the side of the bladder to the psoas tendon. A transverse incision on the bladder at the time of hitching provides additional bladder reach to the psoas muscle. For even more proximal obstruction a Boari flap is conducted in which an inverted U-flap of the anterior bladder is created to reach above the level of obstruction. More technically demanding pathologies to approach for ureteral reconstruction include robotic transplant ureteral reconstruction, ileal ureters, radiation-associated strictures, and ureteroenteric strictures.

Psoas hitch

When the transected ureter does not reach the bladder in its anatomic location during a ureteral reimplant, a psoas hitch can help bridge the distance. The bladder is mobilized from the anterior abdominal wall down to the level of the endopelvic fascia. The contralateral bladder pedicle is partially or entirely divided to gain extra length. The bladder can then be deviated toward the side of ureteral injury and secured to the psoas tendon in a

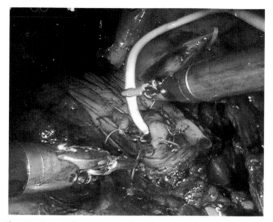

Fig. 4. Boari flap ureteral reimplant. The Boari flap has been secured to the psoas tendon with interrupted absorbable suture. The ureter has been spatulated anteriorly and brought through the flap. An interrupted anastomosis has been completed with absorbable suture. The ureter is being stented in a retrograde fashion.

position for the transected ureter to reach without tension.

The bladder is filled and opened transversely or slightly angled to the side of ureteral injury to allow the bladder to be easily secured to the psoas tendon. In cases where the bladder is very large the bladder may not need to be opened to hitch it. Detrusor muscle and serosa of the bladder are secured to the psoas tendon with three interrupted long-acting absorbable sutures. Care must be taken to avoid injury to the genitofemoral nerve. The ureter can then be reimplanted in a standard fashion. Our preferred location is posterior and lateral to allow for natural lie of the ureter.

Keys to successful ureteral reimplant with a psoas hitch are an adequately mobilized bladder, resection beyond all stenotic avascular ureteral tissue, and a widely spatulated ureteral tension-free anastomosis with meticulous mucosa-to-mucosa apposition.

Boari flap

When the level of stenosis is higher than can be bridged with a psoas hitch, a Boari flap is useful. Several techniques for Boari flap have been described. Classically an anterior bladder inverted U-flap is created and secured to the psoas tendon in a similar fashion to a psoas hitch. A length to width ratio of 2:1 for the bladder flap ensures adequate vascularity. Alternatively, a long transverse Heineke-Mikulicz incision of the bladder is effective for reaching high ureteral injuries. When performing a bladder elongation psoas hitch approach a transverse cystotomy is made and it

is then closed longitudinally in two layers to lengthen the bladder allowing it to be secured higher on the psoas and reach more proximal ureteral injuries.

After the bladder has been secured to the psoas tendon the ureter is anastomosed in one of two fashions. The ureter is spatulated on the posterior surface, secured to the apex of the flap, and then included as part of a longitudinal bladder closure. Alternatively, the ureter is spatulated anteriorly, brought through the bladder pedicle, and secured circumferentially (**Fig. 4**, Video 4). In either technique, a stent is placed and maintained postoperatively for 4 to 6 weeks. The bladder is closed longitudinally in two layers with running long-acting absorbable suture. Omentum or a peritoneal flap is wrapped around the reimplanted ureter to maximize vascular supply to the region. We routinely cover all ureteral reconstructions with a local tissue flap (omentum or peritoneal flap). The bladder closure and anastomosis is tested by retrograde filling the bladder with 150 to 200 mL of saline to evaluate for a leak. Limited small case series support the feasibility and success of robotic-assisted Boari flap.[32]

Transplant ureter

There is an approximate 2% to 10% risk of ureteral stricture after renal transplantation generally attributed to ischemia. Attempts are made at endoscopic balloon dilation for short strictures but ischemic strictures respond poorly. Strictures greater than 2 cm are unlikely to have a successful endoscopic outcome. Short strictures refractory to endoscopic intervention and longer strictures should be offered operative revision if the patient is a safe surgical candidate.[33]

The reconstruction required is determined by location and extent of the transplant ureteral stricture. Short distal strictures are often amenable to redo reimplantation. More proximal strictures may require a bladder flap to reach patent proximal ureter. If healthy native ureter remains in situ it may be used for ureteroureterostomy or anastomosis to the graft pelvis. Panureteral transplant strictures require a pyelovesicostomy.

Preoperatively a nephrostomy tube is placed, and stents are removed to allow the stricture to mature. A combination of antegrade nephrostogram and cystogram can determine the extent of the stenosis.

By the nature of the surgery, it is always a redo surgical field and there is often dense fibrosis. The position of the ureter is far more variable than for the native ureter. ICG delivered via nephrostomy and antegrade nephroscopy with TilePro can help identify the transplant ureteral pelvis

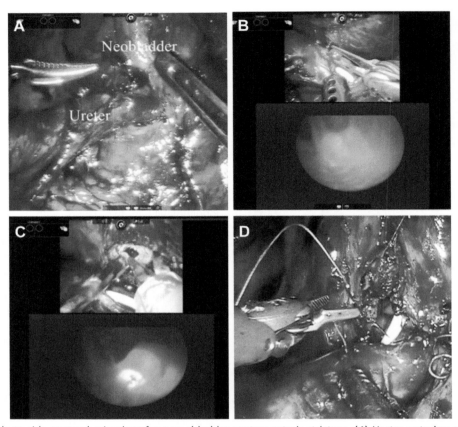

Fig. 5. Side-to-side ureteral reimplant for a neobladder ureteroenteric stricture. (*A*) Ureter entering a dense region of fibrosis near the neobladder. (*B*) Longitudinal ureterotomy with simultaneous TilePro cystoscopic image showing site for reimplant. (*C*) Enterotomy into neobladder with TilePro cystoscopic observation. (*D*) Side-to-side stented interrupted anastomosis with absorbable suture.

and proximal ureter. Care must be taken not to confuse the transplant ureter with other tubular structures in the area, such as the native ureter, vas deferens, vascular structures, round ligament, or medial umbilical ligament.

Once identified the ureter can either be transected and anastomosed to the bladder or incised longitudinally for side-to-side anastomosis. The latter minimizes ureteral dissection and devascularization. A stent is left for 4 to 6 weeks postoperatively. The patient is maximally drained with a nephrostomy tube, ureteral stent, and urethral catheter in the acute recovery phase. When a pyelovesicostomy is conducted or there is a widely refluxing anastomosis, a catheter is typically maintained for 7 to 10 days. Because the transplant kidney is the only functioning renal unit, patients require careful monitoring with transplant renal ultrasounds and intermittent evaluation of creatinine and glomerular filtration rate.

In two independent series of five patients undergoing robotic transplant ureteral stricture reconstruction there was a 100% success rate at short follow-up (median follow-up, 79 days and 97 days, respectively).[34,35]

Ureteroenteric strictures

Strictures after urinary diversion often do not respond to endoscopic interventions and are challenging to repair because of the dense desmoplastic reaction to the region of the urinary diversion and ureteroenteric anastomosis. ICG delivered antegrade via a nephrostomy catheter or antegrade ureteroscopy help to expedite identification and dissection of the obstructed ureter. It also helps identify a suitable site for redo anastomosis. The stricture region has minimal fluorescence and helps define the extent of ureteral resection.

The typical revision for ureteroenteric stricture is ureteral transection and anastomosis. A side-to-side anastomosis to a nearby section of the urinary diversion precludes the necessity of mobilization in the most densely fibrotic region around the anastomosis and minimizes ureteral mobilization and devascularization (**Fig. 5**).[36] Small retrospective cohorts describe noninferiority of a robotic approach to ureteroenteric stricture repair compared with open surgery.[37] In our high-volume robotic reconstructive center, all ureteral reconstruction is completed robotically including ureteroenteric strictures.

Ileal ureter

Robotic ileal ureter is an advanced robotic reconstructive procedure. Port placement and access from the renal hilum to the bladder are important. This is more easily facilitated with the da Vinci Xi System, which is designed for multiquadrant access. Once the renal pelvis and bladder are prepared for the ileal anastomosis a 15- to 20-cm segment of ileum is harvested intracorporal based on the measured distance. ICG is used to ensure adequate blood supply to the ileal segment and the bowel is anastomosed proximally and distally with absorbable sutures. A ureteral stent, Foley catheter, and a nephrostomy tube (if the patient had one preoperatively) are left for maximal drainage. In a retrospective series of seven patients that underwent robotic total intracorporal ileal ureteric replacement, one patient required prolonged stenting for pyeloileal anastomosis insufficiency but otherwise there were no major complications or recurrence at short follow-up of 3 months.[38] These technically demanding cases are successfully performed at robotic referral reconstructive centers and likely need multicenter collaboration to report long-term outcomes.

Radiation-associated strictures

Ureteral strictures as a result of radiation are poorly vascularized and tend to be in densely fibrotic surgical fields. The ureter can be inseparable from nearby structures. Mobilization over the iliac vessels is particularly hazardous.

As with all ureteral reconstruction, the radiated ureteral stricture is reattached to the bladder with either an end or side ureteral anastomosis to the bladder. Both are successful without a clear superior approach. The use of intravenous ICG is valuable to assess the blood flow to the distal aspect of the ureter. Identifying where the well-vascularized segment of ureter starts dictates not only which segment of the ureter to use but also the type of repair to ensure a tension-free anastomosis.

Recent innovation in the treatment of radiation-associated ureteral strictures is a robotic side-to-side anastomosis with the bladder. The ureter is only dissected on its anterior aspect, precluding the necessity to mobilize it from the iliac vessels, and then anastomosed circumferentially to a cystotomy of comparable size. The initial description of the technique by Slawin and colleagues[39] advocates for a long ureterotomy of 3 to 4 cm. A psoas hitch or Boari flap are often required to reach the proximal extent of the stricture. The theoretic benefits are maintenance of the native ureteral orifice, less morbidity from ureteral dissection in complex surgical fields, and decreased devascularization of the ureter with circumferential dissection.

In small retrospective series the technique has shown good success. The CORRUS collaborative included eight patients undergoing this technique in their broader evaluation of robotic ureteral reconstruction for radiation-induced ureteral strictures and noted no recurrences with the side-to-side technique.[40] The median follow-up for the broader cohort was 13 months. In a dedicated article to the technique from many of the same authors, 16 patients underwent the procedure (radiated and nonradiated).[39] Success, defined as clinical improvement in flank pain and decrease in hydronephrosis when imaging was performed, was 93.8%.

SUMMARY

The magnification, stability and range of motion, and ability to work in small remote surgical fields afforded by robotic platforms makes it ideal for the gamut of ureteral reconstruction. Robotic ureteral techniques are growing rapidly and have shown excellent results. Tissue transfer techniques, such as robotic-assisted buccal and appendiceal ureteroplasty, can address long-segment ureteral strictures often precluding the need for ileal ureter, autotransplant, or nephrectomy. The robotic platform enhances ureteral surgical technique and patient recovery and limits morbidity seen with more historical approaches. Collaborative multi-institutional research is needed to continue to compare the efficacy and durability of these low-volume procedures that are performed at referral reconstructive centers.

CLINICS CARE POINTS

- Indocyanine green improves the speed of ureteral identification in difficult surgical fields and helps identify the location of ureteral stenosis in expert opinions.

- Robotic pyeloplasty has equivalent success rates as open and laparoscopic approaches. Minimally invasive approaches are associated with less pain, shorter lengths of stay, and quicker recovery.

- Robotic ureteral reimplant is a safe, highly reproducible, and effective procedure to perform. Adjunctive maneuvers including robotic-assisted psoas hitches and Boari flaps are performed effectively.
- Buccal ureteroplasty and appendiceal ureteroplasty are new robotic reconstructive ureteral procedures with promising early results for stricture patency and a favorable safety profile. More research is needed to evaluate long-term outcomes.
- Feasibility of treating complex stricture disease of the transplant ureter and for ureteroenteric strictures has been successfully shown and is done at referral robotic reconstructive centers.

DISCLOSURE

The authors have no financial or commercial conflicts to declare.

SUPPLEMENTARY DATA

Supplementary data related to this article can be found online at https://doi.org/10.1016/j.ucl.2022.05.002.

REFERENCES

1. Patel SH, Fuller TW, Buckley JC. Why robotic surgery?. In: Stifelman MD, Zhao LC, Eun DD, et al, eds. Techniques of robotic urinary tract reconstruction. Cham: Springer; 2022. p. 3–9.
2. Elbakry AA, Pan MM, Buckley JC. Frontiers in post-radiation urologic reconstruction; robotic surgery and near-infrared fluorescence imaging: a narrative review. AME Med J 2021;0(0):0.
3. Doshi CP, Wozniak A, Quek ML. Near-infrared fluorescence imaging of ureters with intravenous indocyanine green during radical cystectomy to prevent ureteroenteric anastomotic strictures. Urology 2020;144:220–4.
4. Ahmadi N, Ashrafi AN, Hartman N, et al. Use of indocyanine green to minimise uretero-enteric strictures after robotic radical cystectomy. BJU Int 2019;124(2):302–7.
5. Bjurlin MA, Gan M, McClintock TR, et al. Near-infrared fluorescence imaging: emerging applications in robotic upper urinary tract surgery. Eur Urol 2014;65(4):793–801.
6. Lee Z, Moore B, Giusto L, et al. Use of indocyanine green during robot-assisted ureteral reconstructions. Eur Urol 2015;67(2):291–8.
7. Lee Z, Simhan J, Parker DC, et al. Novel use of indocyanine green for intraoperative, real-time localization of ureteral stenosis during robot-assisted ureteroureterostomy. Urology 2013;82(3):729–33.
8. Soriano CR, Cheng RR, Corman JM, et al. Feasibility of injected indocyanine green for ureteral identification during robotic left-sided colorectal resections. Am J Surg 2022 Jan;223(1):14–20.
9. Hope-Ross M, Yannuzzi LA, Gragoudas ES, et al. Adverse reactions due to indocyanine green. Ophthalmology 1994;101(3):529–33.
10. Chu W, Chennamsetty A, Toroussian R, et al. Anaphylactic shock after intravenous administration of indocyanine green during robotic partial nephrectomy. Urol Case Reports 2017;12:37–8.
11. Kim M, Lee S, Park JC, et al. Anaphylactic shock after indocyanine green video angiography during cerebrovascular surgery. World Neurosurg 2020;133:74–9.
12. Hockenberry MS, Smith ZL, Mucksavage P. A novel use of near-infrared fluorescence imaging during robotic surgery without contrast agents. J Endourol 2014;28(5):509–12.
13. Billah MS, Stifelman M, Munver R, et al. Single port robotic assisted reconstructive urologic surgery with the da Vinci SP surgical system. Transl Androl Urol 2020;9(2):870–8.
14. Kaouk JH, Garisto J, Eltemamy M, et al. Robot-assisted surgery for benign distal ureteral strictures: step-by-step technique using the SP ® surgical system. BJU Int 2019;123(4):733–9.
15. Buffi NM, Lughezzani G, Fossati N, et al. Robot-assisted, single-site, dismembered pyeloplasty for ureteropelvic junction obstruction with the new da Vinci platform: a stage 2a study. Eur Urol 2015;67(1):151–6.
16. Shakir NA, Zhao LC. Robotic-assisted genitourinary reconstruction: current state and future directions. Ther Adv Urol 2021;13:1–10.
17. Covas Moschovas M, Bhat S, Rogers T, et al. Technical modifications necessary to implement the da Vinci single-port robotic system. Eur Urol 2020;78(3):415–23.
18. Lenfant L, Kim S, Aminsharifi A, et al. Floating docking technique: a simple modification to improve the working space of the instruments during single-port robotic surgery. World J Urol 2021;39(4):1299–305.
19. Sivaraman A, Leveillee RJ, Patel MB, et al. Robot-assisted laparoscopic dismembered pyeloplasty for ureteropelvic junction obstruction: a multi-institutional experience. Urology 2012;79(2):351–5.
20. Mufarrij PW, Woods M, Shah OD, et al. Robotic dismembered pyeloplasty: a 6-year, multi-institutional experience. J Urol 2008;180(4):1391–6.
21. Gupta NP, Nayyar R, Hemal AK, et al. Outcome analysis of robotic pyeloplasty: a large single-centre experience. BJU Int 2010;105(7):980–3.

22. Hong P, Ding G, Zhu D, et al. Head-to-head comparison of modified laparoscopic pyeloplasty and robot-assisted pyeloplasty for ureteropelvic junction obstruction in China. Urol Int 2018;101(3):337–44.

23. Braga LHP, Pace K, DeMaria J, et al. Systematic review and meta-analysis of robotic-assisted versus conventional laparoscopic pyeloplasty for patients with ureteropelvic junction obstruction: effect on operative time, length of hospital stay, postoperative complications, and success rate. Eur Urol 2009; 56(5):848–58.

24. Light A, Karthikeyan S, Maruthan S, et al. Peri-operative outcomes and complications after laparoscopic vs robot-assisted dismembered pyeloplasty: a systematic review and meta-analysis. BJU Int 2018;122(2):181–94.

25. Dirie NI, Ahmed MA, Wang S. Is secondary robotic pyeloplasty safe and effective as primary robotic pyeloplasty? A systematic review and meta-analysis. J Robot Surg 2020;14(2):241–8.

26. Korets R, Hyams ES, Shah OD, et al. Robotic-assisted laparoscopic ureterocalicostomy. Urology 2007; 70(2):366–9.

27. Ramanitharan M, Lalgudi Narayanan D, Sreenivasan SR, et al. Outcomes of robot-assisted ureterocalicostomy in secondary ureteropelvic junction in adults: initial experience using da Vinci Xi system with near-infrared fluorescence imaging. J Laparoendosc Adv Surg Tech A 2020;30(1):48–52.

28. Lee Z, Lee M, Koster H, et al. A multi-institutional experience with robotic ureteroplasty with buccal mucosa graft: an updated analysis of intermediate-term outcomes. Urology 2021;147:306–10.

29. Sun JY, Granieri MA, Zhao LC. Robotics and urologic reconstructive surgery. Transl Androl Urol 2018;7(4):545–57.

30. Duty BD, Kreshover JE, Richstone L, et al. Review of appendiceal onlay flap in the management of complex ureteric strictures in six patients. BJU Int 2015;115(2):282–7.

31. Jun MS, Stair S, Xu A, et al. A multi-institutional experience with robotic appendiceal ureteroplasty. Urology 2020;145:287–91.

32. JU S, Rai BP, Do M, et al. Robot-assisted technique for Boari flap ureteric reimplantation: replicating the techniques of open surgery in robotics. BJU Int 2016;118(3):482–4.

33. Kumar S, Ameli-Renani S, Hakim A, et al. Ureteral obstruction following renal transplantation: causes, diagnosis and management. Br J Radiol 2014; 87(1044).

34. Abdul-Muhsin HM, McAdams SB, Nuñez RN, et al. Robot-assisted transplanted ureteral stricture management. Urology 2017;105:197–201.

35. Kim S, Fuller TW, Buckley JC. Robotic surgery for the reconstruction of transplant ureteral strictures. Urology 2020;144:208–13.

36. Lee Z, Sterling ME, Keehn AY, et al. The use of indocyanine green during robotic ureteroenteric reimplantation for the management of benign anastomotic strictures. World J Urol 2019;37(6): 1211–6.

37. Scherzer ND, Greenberg JW, Shaw EJ, et al. Robotic vs. open surgical management of ureteroenteric anastomotic strictures: technical modifications to enhance success. J Robot Surg 2020;14(4): 615–9.

38. Ubrig B, Janusonis J, Paulics L, et al. Functional outcome of completely intracorporeal robotic ileal ureteric replacement. Urology 2018;114:193–7.

39. Slawin J, Patel NH, Lee Z, et al. Ureteral reimplantation via robotic nontransecting side-to-side anastomosis for distal ureteral stricture. J Endourol 2020; 34(8):836–9.

40. Asghar AM, Lee Z, Lee RA, et al. Robotic ureteral reconstruction in patients with radiation-induced ureteral strictures: experience from the collaborative of reconstructive robotic ureteral surgery. J Endourol 2021;35(2):144–50.

Robotic-Assisted Lower Genitourinary Tract Reconstruction

Alex J. Xu, MD[a],*, Kirtishri Mishra, MD[a], Yeonsoo S. Lee, BS[b,1], Lee Cheng Zhao, MD[a]

KEYWORDS

- Robotic surgery • Lower tract • Reconstruction • Bladder • Urethra • Stricture • Urinary diversion

KEY POINTS

- Reconstruction of the lower urinary tract (LUT) is amenable to robotic approaches for several reasons including improved access to the deep pelvis, ability to perform concurrent procedures, and improved clinical outcomes while maintaining a minimally invasive approach.
- Several approaches have been described for robotic-assisted repair of complex posterior urethral strictures or bladder neck stenosis including Y-V plasty, buccal grafting, and Tanagho flap.
- While the learning curve for intracorporeal robotic-assisted urinary diversions is steep, mastery of the technique may lead to superior clinical outcomes.
- Various forms of robotic-assisted ureteral reimplantation and associated adjunct procedures produce durable results in both adults and children with minimal morbidity.
- Many of the previously described techniques for rectourethral fistula repair are amenable to a robotic approach, which facilitates both fistula takedown and harvesting/grafting of various flaps.

INTRODUCTION TO ROBOTIC-ASSISTED LOWER TRACT RECONSTRUCTION

Reconstruction of the lower urinary tract (LUT) poses unique challenges, such as narrow working spaces with limited mobility, poor blood supply to various parts of the urinary tract, and few reconstructive options based on disease pathology. Before the advent of laparoscopy, the LUT posed a therapeutic challenge, as our treatment algorithm was limited to endourologic or largely open surgical interventions.

Laparoscopy introduced a minimally invasive technique as an alternative to open reconstruction in challenging cases involving complex pathology. Robotic surgeries have been shown to decrease mortality, reduce postoperative pain, shorten hospital stay, and often have equivalent or improved clinical outcomes based on the pathology. The adoption of robotics has also led to tremor reduction, finer control, less blood loss, and shorter hospital stay.[1]

The most widely disseminated robotic-assisted surgical platforms to date are those using multiple instrument arms, and consequently multiple incisions for ports, such as the Intuitive da Vinci Si, X, and Xi devices. While multi-port architecture remains the most accessible and familiar to urologists across a variety of practice settings, limitations include the need to triangulate the ports strategically to maximize instrument range of motion and avoid collisions, especially in the narrow confines of the deep pelvis.

The da Vinci SP platform addresses some of these concerns by directing 3 double-jointed, independent arms through a 2.5 cm multichannel trocar from a single incision.[2] Further advantages

[a] Department of Urology, NYU Langone Health, 222 E 41st Street 11-12 Floor, New York, NY 10016, USA;
[b] Mayo Clinic Alix School of Medicine; Rochester, MN 55902, USA
[1] Present address: 222 East 41st Street 11-12 Floor, New York, NY 10016.
* Corresponding author.
E-mail address: Alex.xu@nyulangone.org

Urol Clin N Am 49 (2022) 507–518
https://doi.org/10.1016/j.ucl.2022.05.003
0094-0143/22/© 2022 Elsevier Inc. All rights reserved.

include the ability to rotate the entire system completely while docked, visual feedback on the surgeon console of the location of each arm, and the ease of performing concurrent procedures (eg, combined transabdominal and perineal dissection).[3] Apart from the immediate benefits of fewer required incisions, which correspond to less morbidity and improved cosmesis, as well as potentially more rapid convalescence, a variety of LUT pelvic pathology can be approached with the SP system.[4,5] The operating distance of 15 to 25 cm for the instrument arms to articulate is ideal for a transabdominal approach to the deep pelvis. In cases whereby the target anatomy is closer to the abdominal wall than this distance, a "floating dock" or "air dock" technique using a GelPoint Mini retractor and AirSeal can effectively create a surrogate for pneumoperitoneum (**Fig. 1**A).[6] Limitations of the SP platform include limited instrumentation relative to its multiport counterparts, in particular lacking a vessel sealer or near-infrared fluorescence (NIRF)-mode camera at the time of this publication. While the double-jointed instruments facilitate dissection and suturing in narrow confines, less force can be applied correspondingly with an individual arm. Due to the need to triangulate the instrument arms from a single trocar, countertraction can be problematic, potentially necessitating the placement of an assistant trocar or the use of external aids such as magnetic retractors.[7,8]

Novel platforms produced by an array of manufactures and industry-academic collaboratives are on the horizon for clinical deployment and may prompt a diversification of the current offerings, from which surgeons will undoubtedly benefit.[9] For instance, the recent development of the DaVinci SP Access Kit allows for improved integration of the assistant port, increased extracorporeal working space, and increased stability (**Fig. 1**B). Of particular note, the Virtuoso Surgical/Vanderbilt concentric tube technology prototype, allowing for the articulation of instruments from a fixed endoscope tip, is an exciting development that possesses striking implications for traditional LUT reconstruction owing to the potential for endoluminal surgery.[10] The data underpinning these novel techniques are eagerly awaited and herald a bright future for surgical innovation.

POSTERIOR URETHRA AND BLADDER NECK PATHOLOGY

Bladder neck reconstruction and posterior urethroplasty have posed a major challenge in surgical reconstruction for urologic surgeons. Often, these patients present with the previous history of radiotherapy or ablative interventions for other pathologies that have resulted in obstructive or devastated bladder necks with poor function. Previous study from the Cancer of the Prostate Strategic Urologic Research Endeavor database has cited the rate of BNC to be 8.4% and the Prostate Cancer Outcome Study has cited the rate to be 16% in patients undergoing radical prostatectomy.[11,12] Many patients present with symptoms 6 to 24 months after their index operation.[13] Often these patients are managed with an initial endoscopic intervention such as dilation or incision of the vesicourethral anastomosis (VUA).[14] These interventions are often short-lived and may be inapplicable in cases of complete urethral obliteration. Furthermore, they may exacerbate dense stricture and lead to recalcitrant situations requiring more involved surgical procedures to salvage urethral voiding and maintain quality of life.

Robotic-assisted approaches to recalcitrant posterior urethral stenoses were developed in response to the sheer technical difficulty of visualization and precise suturing in the deep pelvis, as well as the close proximity of critical structures including the external urinary sphincter, cavernous nerves, and rectum. Maneuvers such as pubectomy and combined abdominoperineal dissection may be required to facilitate anastomosis. The functional outcomes of open reconstruction, even when technically successful (as quantified by urethral patency), demonstrate a high rate of de novo stress urinary incontinence.[15] For this reason, it is critical to counsel the patient preoperatively on the possibility of requiring an Artificial Urinary Sphincter as an adjunct procedure to reestablish continence. Furthermore, extensive urethral mobilization and bulbar artery transection are independently associated with increased risk of AUS cuff erosion.[16,17] Collectively, the morbidity of these historical approaches may discourage providers from attempting definitive surgical management, and consequently patients may be deemed "unreconstructible," with the end-stage options of repeated endoscopic procedures, chronic catheter drainage, or cystectomy and urinary diversion.

In the past several years, novel techniques to address this pathology have been described. These procedures combine improved articulation and precision, with modalities such as NIRF imaging, to facilitate mucosal anastomosis with excellent short- and mid-term results.

Y-V Plasty

We start by first performing a cystoscopy to visualize the obstructed urethra and passing a wire

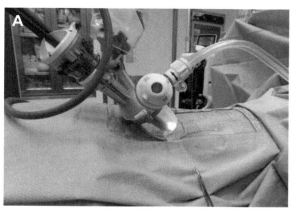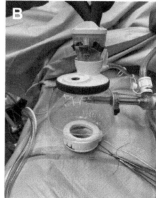

Fig. 1. Use of a "floating dock" technique with the SP robot via GelPoint Mini in a pediatric patient (*A*). DaVinci SP Access Kit with integrated assistant port (*B*).

into the bladder. If a wire cannot be passed, then the scope is left in the urethra at the point of obstruction and secured to the draping. The ports are placed similar to a robotic prostatectomy on the Xi system. With the SP robotic system, the port is docked in the midline, immediately above the umbilicus. The bladder is dropped from the anterior abdominal wall and mobilized. It is crucial to liberate the bladder on the anterior side to reach the distal-most segment. The proximal urethra is dissected and mobilized as distally as possible. At this point, the surrounding tissue and any sphincteric muscle is carefully dissected off the urethra. A Y incision is then made on the anterior side of the urethra and bladder: a longitudinal incision is made on the anterior urethra using scissors and carried past the point of obstruction. The Y limbs are made on the bladder, paying careful attention to the ureteral orifices. Next, the Y limbs are advanced to the apex of the urethral spatulation. We typically use a 3-0 Stratafix suture for this advancement to complete a watertight closure (**Fig. 2**). A foley catheter is placed at the end of the procedure and a drain is left in place. A 2018 study by Granieri and colleagues demonstrated well-preserved urinary function in a small series of patients with recalcitrant bladder neck contracture, and this operation has been well adapted by multiple other institutions for this pathology.[18]

Whereby the urethral lumen or vesicourethral orifice is completely obliterated, concomitant transrectal ultrasonography and flexible cystourethroscopy can facilitate circumferential dissection and excision of fibrotic tissue. For stenoses spanning the membranous urethra, combined robotic-perineal dissection to mobilize the distal urethra may be required.[19]

Buccal Graft Onlay/Interposition

A novel repair using buccal graft in the repair of posterior urethral fistulas involving the bladder neck or vesicourethral anastomoses greater than 2 cm in length was recently described in a small series with good outcomes.[20] A transvesical approach was used if there was a concern for significant abdominal adhesions with a large bladder capacity. A transabdominal approach is used if the abdomen is less hostile, with low-capacity bladders, or if flap interposition is anticipated. Sharp and electrocautery-assisted robotic dissection is performed into the urethra at the 9-o'clock position. Cystoscopy is used to assist with the initial robotic posterior dissection. After the BMG is passed into the surgical field, the anastomosis is created using 3-0 barbed polydioxanone sutures proximally at the level of the bladder neck. This is continued as far distally as feasible with the robot. The urethra is calibrated with a 22 French Bougie or foley catheter to ensure patency throughout the anastomosis. Distally, the graft is fixed to the mucosal edge with 5-0 absorbable monofilament and 4-0 absorbable braided sutures and quilted to the perivesical tissue using an 18-gauge hypodermic needle loaded with 4-0 absorbable biological monofilament suture and 3-0 absorbable barbed sutures via a "sewing machine" technique.

If necessary, adjacent tissue transfer is performed to bridge any defects in the repair, fill dead space, prevent fistulization, and bolster vascular supply, especially in areas of poor periurethral tissue quality (ie, patients with a history of radiation). A rectus abdominis, gracilis, or omental flap of the appropriate size is carefully

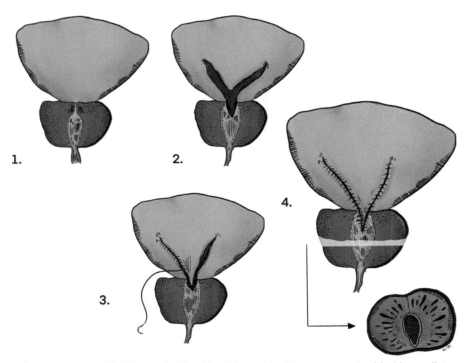

Fig. 2. Y-V plasty. Narrowed bladder neck (1) with Y-shaped incision on anterior bladder wall traversing the bladder neck to the proximal prostatic urethra (2). The Y limbs are advanced to the apex of the urethral spatulation and the cystotomy closed with running 3-0 Stratafix (3). A foley catheter is placed at the end of the procedure and a drain is left in place. The lumen of the bladder neck at the conclusion of the procedure is noted to be teardrop shaped (4).

dissected, translocated to the cavity, and sutured in place. A simple prostatectomy is performed to enhance the tissue to which the graft and anastomosis are sewn given there is no evidence of residual malignancy. An augmentation cystoplasty may also be performed in patients with low bladder capacity and high filling pressures evidenced by preoperative videourodynamics. Additionally, for longer strictures or additional distal strictures, concurrent perineal urethroplasty can be performed with or without buccal graft. In our technical case series of 9 patients with complex urologic histories undergoing a novel SP robotic-assisted posterior urethroplasty, we demonstrated 3 key findings: (1) the technique is effective with a urethral patency rate of 67% which is consistent with comparable open and robotic series, (2) the technique is safe, with no intraoperative complications and only 1 postoperative complication related to the technique itself, and (3) the technique is durable, with patency in 6 patients at a median follow-up of approximately 1 year.[20]

Tanagho Flap

A Tanagho flap can be used for bladder neck and posterior urethral reconstruction in cases whereby

there is severe dystrophic calcification of the bladder neck and poor bladder neck tissue for anastomosis. The robotic setup for the procedure is similar to those described above. If the prostate remains in situ, a posterior prostatic dissection is performed similar to a robotic prostatectomy: a peritoneal incision is made directly beneath the vas deferens and dissected toward the prostate. The prostate is elevated from the rectum down to the genitourinary diaphragm. Then the bladder is dropped from the anterior abdominal wall. Of note, if a suprapubic tube is present, then the tract must be transected. The dissection is carried to the apex of the prostate at which point the proximal urethra is visualized and dissected as distally as possible. Sometimes placing a stitch into the distal aspect of the urethra allows the surgeon to pull the distal urethra further into the field of operation to fully resect the stricture. Care must be taken to avoid damage to the sphincter to preserve continence.

There are instances when the stricture may span further than anticipated and may require a combined abdominoperineal approach. In these cases, the urethra is dissected through a midline perineal incision in a typical fashion and mobilized circumferentially to facilitate passage of the proximal limb. The robotic surgeon should be prepared to grab the mobilized urethra internally through the urethrotomy made previously. Once the urethrotomy and adequate spatulation is performed, the native bladder neck is closed primarily. If the preexisting suprapubic tube site is unable to reach the urethral stump for a tension-free anastomosis a Tanagho flap is used. An anterior bladder flap is created similar to a Boari flap; however, this flap is generated to drop downwards toward the urethra rather than upwards toward the ureter. A primary anastomosis is performed in a standard running fashion with a 3-0 Stratafix suture over a 16 or 18 French catheter. The catheter is left in place for 3 weeks for the anastomosis to heal. A drain may also be left in place anterior to the anastomosis.

This flap has been used previously in patients with complex voiding pathology and neurogenic bladders. The application in this instance is expanded from its original usage, and there is a lack of robust evidence and long-term follow-up on these patients at this point; however, in our experience, these patients do well and have a high satisfaction rate from the procedure.[21,22]

The aforementioned techniques are significantly easier to perform with the working space of the SP platform, which facilitates dissection and suturing under the pubic bone and allows for concurrent endoscopic or transperineal manipulation. In terms of patency and continence, the short and mid-term outcomes reported thus far are highly encouraging,[23] though these patients should be counseled on the possible need for adjunct procedures to restore continence including slings or artificial urinary sphincters. Crucially, if a perineal dissection can be avoided, long-term durability and continence may be improved.

A similar approach may be taken for adjacent disease processes including rectourethral fistulae, or if salvage prostatectomy is clinically indicated. In these situations, the versatility of the robotic platform lies not only in the technical benefits it offers, but also in terms of adjunctive procedures such as the feasibility of minimally invasive flap harvest for vascularized tissue coverage, and the possibility of multiple surgical approaches that are performed concurrently. Further comparative studies of the long-term durability of these techniques are needed, especially with respect to operating efficiency and potential cost.

A schematic of the technique is shown in **Fig. 3**.

INTRACORPOREAL URINARY DIVERSIONS

With the recent publication of the RAZOR randomized trial, in which robotic-assisted radical cystectomy was demonstrated to be noninferior to open radical cystectomy in terms of oncologic outcomes, the safety of the robotic approach was underscored.[24] Urinary diversion, however, was accomplished via an extracorporeal approach in this and other studies. The precision of robotic-assisted ureteroenteric anastomosis, as well as decreased blood loss, lower insensible fluid loss, and more prompt recovery are potential advantages of intracorporeal diversions.[25] Nevertheless, complete intracorporeal approaches have not been adopted widely to date, and ileal conduits constitute most of the intracorporeal diversions.[26] Learning curve is thought to account for some of the lack of widespread utilization. In a large single-center comparison of open, robotic extracorporeal, and intracorporeal diversion, the anastomotic stricture rate was greatest for patients undergoing intracorporeal diversion, but after 75 cases, this rate declined to 4.9% which is significantly less than either extracorporeal (11.3%) or open (9.3%) procedures.[27] While operative volume influences operative time and subsequent development of complications and readmissions, a reasonably high-volume robotic practice may have the appropriate infrastructure and personnel to support routine intracorporeal diversion.[28] This approach may be particularly applicable to the construction of orthotopic neobladder, as performing a tension-free, watertight urethroileal anastomosis may be a challenging step during open surgery. Multiple techniques have been described with the aim of maximizing intraoperative efficiency and teachability. The method first reported and consequently with the longest follow-up is from the Karolinska group, for which the urethroileal anastomosis is performed before bowel detubularization and reservoir creation.[29] However, several alternative orders of steps have been reported with similar short and mid-term data with respect to continence and stricture formation. Larger studies with longer follow-up are warranted to define ideal parameters for this technically demanding operation.

The SP platform may also have a role to play in the realm of urinary diversion, not only in terms of reconstruction following radical cystectomy, as has been reported by Kaouk and colleagues, but also in populations with neurogenic or end-stage bladder.[30] Grilo and colleagues report a series of 10 patients undergoing complete intracorporeal supratrigonal cystectomy with augmentation cystoplasty, in which median operative time was 250 min, hospital stay was 12 days, and 1 year functional and urodynamic outcomes were acceptable.[31] Conceivably, within a high-volume robotic surgical practice, as refinements of the

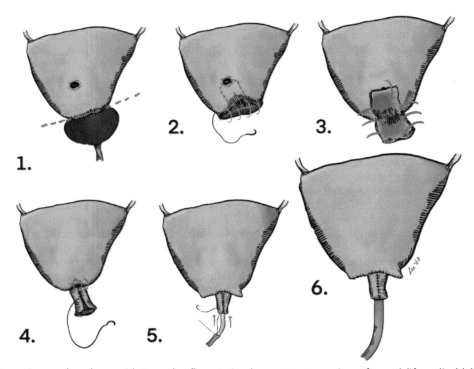

Fig. 3. Posterior urethroplasty with Tanagho flap. A simple prostatectomy is performed (if applicable) and the pre-existing suprapubic tube removed (1). The native bladder neck is closed (*green arrows*) (2). If the pre-existing suprapubic tube site is unable to reach the urethral stump to create a tension-free anastomosis, an anterior bladder flap is raised incorporating the prior cystotomy (*dashed blue line*) (2). The flap is then tubularized and the cystotomy closed (3, 4). The urethral stump is then anastomosed to the tubularized flap over a catheter with running 3-0 stratafix suture (5). The finished product is shown in 6.

technique accrue, the intracorporeal approach may fit into a niche that benefits both providers and patients. The complications of urinary diversions such as parastomal hernia may also be managed with a robotic approach as reported in a recent report of a small cohort of patients.[32]

URETERAL REIMPLANT

Robotic-assisted ureteral reimplantation and its associated adjunct procedures such as Boari flap, psoas hitch, and downward nephropexy have been studied and found to produce durable results in both adults[33,34] and children[35] with minimal morbidity.

For pathology of the distal ureter, the patient is placed in a low-lithotomy position with steep Trendelenburg and the robot is docked either between the patient's legs or at the patient's side. For pathology extending up to the mid-ureter, a lateral decubitus position can be used with the patient in the modified low-lithotomy position.

The peritoneum is incised longitudinally at the level of the iliac vessels, and the ureter is identified.

With the aid of concurrent ureteroscopy, the peritoneum is incised over the ureter distally to the insertion of the ureterovesical junction and proximally until healthy proximal ureter is encountered. For male patients, whereby fertility is not a concern, the vas deferens can be ligated to improve exposure. For female patients, the ovary and ovarian ligaments are retracted anteriorly to facilitate exposure.

The ureter is transected just proximal to the diseased segment of ureter and spatulated. For patients with ureteral malignancy, a clip is placed on the distal ureter before ureteral transection to avoid tumor spillage.

If sufficient ureter is removed such that a psoas hitch is necessary, the bladder is filled with saline and subsequently mobilized off the anterior abdominal wall. Absorbable suture is used to fix the posterior bladder wall to the psoas muscle tendon in a longitudinal fashion, taking care to avoid the genitofemoral nerve. The bladder may also be affixed to the side of the peritoneum to achieve a similar effect. Should further bladder mobilization be necessary to reach the psoas muscle, the bladder may be incised horizontally and then closed vertically in a Heineke–Mikulicz fashion to stretch the bladder vertically toward the psoas muscle. Furthermore, transection of the contralateral superior vesical pedicle may be performed, though this is rarely necessary. In the largest prospective series of robotic psoas hitch, all 12 patients who underwent treatment with distal ureteral reimplantation with psoas hitch had successful outcomes with no obstruction on postoperative MAG-3 scan or IV urography.[36]

Should a Boari flap be necessary, the bladder is filled with saline and a pedicle of bladder is created starting 3 cm proximal to the bladder neck and extended toward the dome to create a flap of tissue with its base wider than its apex. The flap is fixed to the psoas, tubularized, and anastomosed to the spatulated ureter[37,38] in an interrupted or running fashion. A ureteral stent is advanced in a retrograde manner up to the kidney before completing the anastomosis. The defect in the bladder is closed using barbed suture in a running fashion. In the largest series of robotic ureteral reimplantation with a Boari flap, all 11 patients had durable repair of their distal stricture at 15 months of follow-up.[38]

In the event that the above maneuvers are insufficient to complete bladder mobilization, downward nephropexy is performed after ureteral dissection and before ureteral reanastomosis. An intra-Gerotal dissection is performed such that the kidney is dissected free from surrounding attachments in a circumferential manner. At this point, the kidney is only attached to the renal hilum and ureter. The adrenal gland is completely detached from the upper pole of the kidney The posterior kidney capsule is affixed to the psoas fascia using absorbable suture. The suture is fixed twice more to securely fasten the kidney. Alternatively, this stitch may be secured by clipping a Weck Hem-o-loc clip.

To perform a refluxing extravesical reimplant, the bladder wall and mucosa of the dome are incised for 1 to 2 cm. The distal ureter is anastomosed to the bladder dome with running absorbable suture to create a water-tight anastomosis. A double-J stent is passed into this incision before its completion. The second layer of closure is performed to include the bladder serosa and ureteral adventitia.

When performing a nonrefluxing reimplant, an incision is made in the detrusor muscle and extended distally for 5 to 7 cm to create 2 detrusor flaps. This incision is directed away from the ureter. The detrusor flaps are used to create a submucosal tunnel. The ureter is anastomosed to the bladder at the most distal aspect of this tunnel with 2 running sutures. A ureteral stent is advanced in a retrograde manner before the completion of the anastomosis. A second layer closure of detrusor muscle is then performed with interrupted absorbable suture to create a nonrefluxing tunnel.

Once anastomosis is completed, the pelvic peritoneum is closed over the anastomosis.

At any time during anastomosis using any of the aforementioned techniques, intravenous indocyanine green (ICG) can be administered to ensure vascularity.

We recently described a nontransecting side-to-side anastomosis as an alternative method to ureteral reimplantation in cases whereby ureteral excision is nonmandatory (**Fig. 4**). The strictured ureter is first identified and a vessel loop placed around to aid dissection without directly grasping the ureter. As the blood supply of the distal ureter originates from a posterolateral direction, the distal ureter is not mobilized in this area. Intravenous indocyanine green may be administered to help identify vascularity. The bladder is freed from its attachments to the anterior abdominal wall and pelvis until it is adequately mobilized to allow for a tension-free anastomosis. If needed, a psoas hitch or Boari flap can be performed in the manner described above. A longitudinal ureterotomy is made proximal to the ureteral stricture while leaving the distal strictured ureter in situ. A long ureterotomy (∼3–4 cm) is preferred to ensure a widely patent anastomosis. A cystotomy is made in the posterolateral portion of the bladder. Anastomosis is performed using a running 4-0 absorbable suture. First, one wall of the anastomosis is completed in a running manner. Next, a double-J stent is placed in a retrograde manner into the ureterotomy and across the anastomosis. Once the stent is in position, the remaining portion of the side-to-side anastomosis is closed. After the anastomosis is complete, the bladder is filled with normal saline to ensure a watertight closure.

We reported on a series of 16 patients at 3 institutions who underwent robotic ureteral reimplant through nontransecting side-to-side anastomosis between 2014 and 2018. The median stricture length was 3 cm. The various etiologies for stricture development in our cohort were representative of the literature. Approximately one-third of patients had undergone previous endoscopic balloon dilation.

The median operative time and estimated blood loss were 178 minutes and 50 mL, respectively. Median length of stay was 1 day (IQR 1–2). No intraoperative complications or postoperative complications with Clavien score ≥3 were reported. A total of 15 of 16 (93.8%) patients were

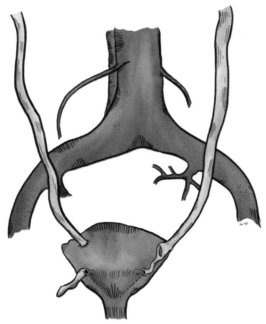

Fig. 4. A traditional transecting end-to-end ureteral reimplant is shown with the right ureter. A non-transecting side-to-side ureteral reimplant is shown with the left ureter.

found to have clinical success defined as the absence of flank pain, and 100% of patients with follow-up imaging had radiographic improvement at a median follow-up time of 12.5 months.[39]

RECTOURETHRAL FISTULA REPAIR

Rectourethral fistula (RUF) is an uncommon but devastating complication with significant deterioration in quality of life.[40,41] There are more than 40 different techniques described for RUF repair.[42] In the past, we preferred the da Vinci Robotic System Xi as it can more easily be side docked to better facilitate perineal access. More recently, we have shifted to the SP system as its narrow profile better facilitates access deep into the pelvis with less interference from the pelvic wall.

All cases begin with flexible cystoscopy. A guidewire or ureteral catheter is placed across the fistula. When feasible, the wire is grasped and externalized through the rectum for through-and-through access from urethra to anus. If the ureteral orifices are in close proximity to the fistula, it may behoove one to place ureteral stents at the beginning of the case.

The robotic dissection begins with a posterior approach. The vas deferens are identified and used to guide dissection to Denonvillier's fascia. Sharp dissection with judicious bipolar electrocautery is used to separate the rectum from the urinary tract. An EEA sizer can provide downward tenting of the rectum, aiding in the separation of rectum from bladder neck and prostate. If using the Xi system, the Firefly camera can aid in identifying the urethra as the white light of the cystoscope emits in the near-infrared spectrum, which penetrates a modest amount of tissue. As one nears the fistula, the assistant can perform a DRE to help guide the final approach. The fistula is then divided. One will see the wire, stent, or blue dye placed at the beginning of the case. The edges of the rectum are then freshened and closed primarily with barbed, absorbable suture. An air leak test is then performed to ensure a watertight closure. If the rectum does not seem to be salvageable, resection of the disease rectum followed by colo-anal anastomosis has been reported as a possible alternative.[43]

If the prostate is *in situ* and the fistula is small, one can attempt a primary closure. In situations whereby there is fistulization into prostate with radionecrosis, primary closure may be impossible. Salvage prostatectomy is often necessary to remove the necrotic tissue to allow for watertight closure. Bladder advancement flaps and complex urethral advancement techniques (as described above) may provide distal advancement of the bladder neck to allow for anastomosis to the urethral stump. If possible, a circumferential anastomosis is performed. Otherwise, an augmented anastomotic urethroplasty may be performed with buccal mucosa graft. One must be cognizant that urethral dissection will increase the risk of urethral erosion after AUS placement.[16]

If the fistula is distal, a gracilis flap may be harvested and tunneled into the pelvis and fixed in place between the rectum and the urinary anastomosis which has been shown to be effective with little morbidity[44]; however, this does add an additional surgical site and incision. Alternatively, an omental or rectus flap may be more practical. Omentum is in abundant supply and will reach into the pelvis with mobilization. In proximal and/or large fistulas, a rectus abdominis flap is a useful technique to provide an interposing layer between the bladder and rectum (**Figure 5**). Robotic harvest has eliminated the need for a large midline incision from xiphoid to pubis. Furthermore, the anterior rectus sheath is left intact, reducing the risk of incisional hernia. The robot is redocked contralateral to the rectus to be harvested. If there is a colostomy, the robotic arms should be carefully positioned to avoid injury. The posterior rectus sheath is incised at the level of the inferior epigastric artery taking care not to injure the pedicle. The posterior sheath incision is then advanced to the

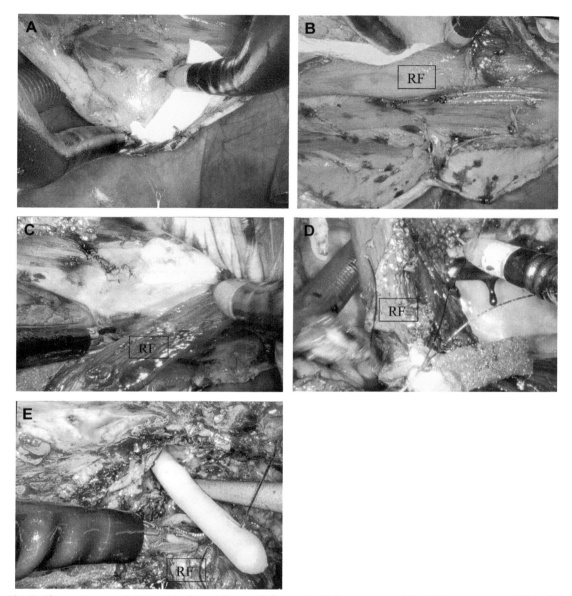

Fig. 5. The peritoneum is incised in the midline and dissected off the posterior side of the rectus muscle (A). The rectus muscle is dissected off the anterior fascia (B) to the aponeurosis laterally and cephalad to the xiphoid process at which point the muscle is transected (C) and dissection carried caudad to the inferior epigastrics maintaining a pedicle in the form of a pulsating perforator. The anterior and posterior fascia are sutured together to avoid Spigelian hernia (D). The flap is then passed posterior to the bladder and affixed using running 3-0 stratafix suture (F). RF = rectus flap.

costal margin. The rectus flap is then dissected circumferentially, and a Penrose drain is passed around it to aid in retraction. Circumferential dissection is then carried superiorly to the level of the costal margin. Close attention is required to the tendinous inscriptions to avoid the violation of the anterior sheath. Bipolar cautery is used to control perforating vessels. The rectus muscle is then amputated at the costal margin and 2 holding stitches are placed with 2 long tails for each suture. The Carter-Thomason suture device is then passed through the lateral perineum, entering the pelvis between the rectum and urethra whereby a single suture is grasped and externalized. The other tail is passed separately and the 2 tails are tied over a xeroform bolster to fix the rectus flap as far distally as possible. This is conducted on the left and right sides of the perineum. The posterior rectus sheath is then anastomosed to the anterior sheath to reduce the risk of intra-abdominal adhesions.

Another promising technique is robotic transanal minimally invasive surgery (TAMIS) for use in cases of simple RUF whereby the interposition of remote tissue is not necessary. An Access Channel is placed across the anus and affixed to the patient. Trocars are preloaded onto the GelSeal Cap, which is then attached to the Access Channel. With the robot now docked, the fistula is circumscribed sharply, and a full-thickness rectal flap is developed. A plane is then developed between the prostate and rectum. The urethra is closed with absorbable suture. A biologic material such as alloderm can be placed over the closed urethra. The rectum is then closed over the mesh with absorbable suture.[45]

SUMMARY

As robotic proficiency becomes more widespread, analogs and extensions of open procedures and operative maneuvers, previously perceived as technically challenging, will become more commonplace. Robotic-assisted procedures carry putative advantages in terms of anastomotic patency, identification and preservation of blood supply, and reduced perioperative morbidity. The role of the reconstructive expert who can leverage both robotic and traditional techniques in the management of complex upper and lower urinary tract pathology will be at the forefront of multidisciplinary management.

CLINICS CARE POINTS

- In cases of complete obliteration of the urethral lumen or bladder neck, the utilization of transrectal ultrasonography and/or flexible cystoscopy concomitantly with a robotic approach can aid in circumferential dissection and excision of the fibrotic tissue.
- For stenoses spanning the membranous urethra, combined robotic-perineal dissection to mobilize the distal urethra may be required.
- Buccal graft may be utilized during robotic repair of posterior urethral strictures and bladder neck pathology when there is presence of a fistula or long strictures (>2cm). The decision of transvesical versus transabdominal approach is dependent on bladder capacity, concern for abdominal adhesions, and whether a flap interposition may be needed.

- Tanagho flap is chosen when there is insufficient healthy bladder neck tissue for anastomosis.
- In cases where ureteral excision is non-mandatory, a side-to-side non-transecting distal ureteral reimplant is efficient and effective.
- In cases of rectourethral fistula where a prostate remains in situ, if the fistula is small a primary closure may be attempted, otherwise a salvage prostatectomy ought to be performed.
- In cases of a distal rectourethral fistula, gracilis, rectus, or omentum may be used as a flap. With proximal/large fistulas, a rectus flap is the best choice. Leaving the anterior sheath intact when harvesting rectus reduces the risk of hernia.

DISCLOSURE

The authors have nothing to disclose.

REFERENCES

1. Babbar P, et al. Robot-assisted ureteral reconstruction - current status and future directions. Urol Ann 2018;10(1):7–14.
2. Covas Moschovas M, Bhat S, Onol F, et al. Early outcomes of single-port robot-assisted radical prostatectomy: lessons learned from the learning-curve experience: Early outcomes of SP RARP. BJU Int 2020. https://doi.org/10.1111/bju.15158.
3. Covas Moschovas M, Bhat S, Rogers T, et al. Technical Modifications Necessary to Implement the da Vinci Single-port Robotic System. Eur Urol 2020; 78:415–23.
4. Abaza R, Murphy C, Bsatee A, et al. Single-port Robotic Surgery Allows Same-day Discharge in Majority of Cases. Urology 2020;148:159–65.
5. Dy GW, Jun MS, Blasdel G, et al. Outcomes of Gender Affirming Peritoneal Flap Vaginoplasty Using the Da Vinci Single Port Versus Xi Robotic Systems. Eur Urol 2021;79(5):676–83.
6. Lenfant L, Kim S, Aminsharifi A, et al. Floating docking technique: a simple modification to improve the working space of the instruments during single-port robotic surgery. World J Urol 2021;39(4): 1299–305.
7. Kaouk J, Aminsharifi A, Sawczyn G, et al. Single-Port Robotic Urological Surgery Using Purpose-Built Single-Port Surgical System: Single-Institutional Experience With the First 100 Cases. Urology 2020;140: 77–84.
8. Steinberg RL, Johnson BA, Meskawi M, et al. Magnet-Assisted Robotic Prostatectomy Using the da

Vinci SP Robot: An Initial Case Series. J Endourol 2019;33:829–34.

9. Wilson M, Badani K. Competing Robotic Systems. Urol Clin North Am 2021;48:147–50.

10. Amanov E, Ropella DS, Nimmagadda N, et al. Transurethral Anastomosis After Transurethral Radical Prostatectomy: A Phantom Study on Intraluminal Suturing With Concentric Tube Robots. IEEE Trans Med Robot Bionics 2020;2:578–81.

11. Elliott SP, et al. Incidence of urethral stricture after primary treatment for prostate cancer: data From CaPSURE. J Urol 2007;178(2):529–34 [discussion: 534].

12. Stanford JL, et al. Urinary and sexual function after radical prostatectomy for clinically localized prostate cancer: the Prostate Cancer Outcomes Study. JAMA 2000;283(3):354–60.

13. Elliott DS, Boone TB. Combined stent and artificial urinary sphincter for management of severe recurrent bladder neck contracture and stress incontinence after prostatectomy: a long-term evaluation. J Urol 2001;165(2):413–5.

14. Brede C, Angermeier K, Wood H. Continence outcomes after treatment of recalcitrant postprostatectomy bladder neck contracture and review of the literature. Urology 2014;83(3):648–52.

15. Nikolavsky D, Blakely SA, Hadley DA, et al. Open reconstruction of recurrent vesicourethral anastomotic stricture after radical prostatectomy. Int Urol Nephrol 2014;46:2147–52.

16. McKibben MJ, Shakir N, Fuchs JS, et al. Erosion rates of 3.5-cm artificial urinary sphincter cuffs are similar to larger cuffs. BJU Int 2019;123:335–41.

17. Keihani S, Chandrapal JC, Peterson AC, et al. Outcomes of Urethroplasty to Treat Urethral Strictures Arising From Artificial Urinary Sphincter Erosions and Rates of Subsequent Device Replacement. Urology 2017;107:239–45.

18. Granieri MA, Weinberg AC, Sun JY, et al. Robotic Y-V Plasty for Recalcitrant Bladder Neck Contracture. Urology 2018;117:163–5.

19. Boswell TC, Hebert KJ, Tollefson MK, et al. Robotic urethral reconstruction: redefining the paradigm of posterior urethroplasty. Transl Androl Urol 2020;9: 121–31.

20. Liu W, Shakir N, Zhao LC. Single-Port Robotic Posterior Urethroplasty Using Buccal Mucosa Grafts: Technique and Outcomes. Urology 2021. https://doi.org/10.1016/j.urology.2021.07.049.

21. Gallagher PV, et al. Tanagho bladder neck reconstruction in the treatment of adult incontinence. J Urol 1995;153(5):1451–4.

22. Whitson JM, et al. Mechanism of continence after repair of posterior urethral disruption: evidence of rhabdosphincter activity. J Urol 2008;179(3):1035–9.

23. Kirshenbaum EJ, Zhao LC, Myers JB, et al. Patency and Incontinence Rates After Robotic Bladder Neck Reconstruction for Vesicourethral Anastomotic Stenosis and Recalcitrant Bladder Neck Contractures: The Trauma and Urologic Reconstructive Network of Surgeons Experience. Urology 2018;118:227–33.

24. Parekh DJ, Reis IM, Castle EP, et al. Robot-assisted radical cystectomy versus open radical cystectomy in patients with bladder cancer (RAZOR): an open-label, randomised, phase 3, non-inferiority trial. Lancet Lond Engl 2018;391:2525–36.

25. Murthy PB, Bryk DJ, Lee BH, et al. Robotic radical cystectomy with intracorporeal urinary diversion: beyond the initial experience. Transl Androl Urol 2020;9:942–8.

26. Hussein AA, May PR, Jing Z, et al. Outcomes of Intracorporeal Urinary Diversion after Robot-Assisted Radical Cystectomy: Results from the International Robotic Cystectomy Consortium. J Urol 2018;199: 1302–11.

27. Ericson KJ, Thomas LJ, Zhang JH, et al. Uretero-Enteric Anastomotic Stricture Following Radical Cystectomy: A Comparison of Open, Robotic Extracorporeal, and Robotic Intracorporeal Approaches. Urology 2020;144:130–5.

28. Hussein AA, Elsayed AS, Aldhaam NA, et al. A comparative propensity score-matched analysis of perioperative outcomes of intracorporeal vs extracorporeal urinary diversion after robot-assisted radical cystectomy: results from the International Robotic Cystectomy Consortium. BJU Int 2020;126: 265–72.

29. Rocco B, Luciani LG, Collins J, et al. Posterior reconstruction during robotic-assisted radical cystectomy with intracorporeal orthotopic ileal neobladder: description and outcomes of a simple step. J Robot Surg 2020. https://doi.org/10.1007/s11701-020-01108-0.

30. Kaouk J, Garisto J, Eltemamy M, et al. Single-port Robotic Intracorporeal Ileal Conduit Urinary Diversion During Radical Cystectomy Using the SP Surgical System: Step-by-step Technique. Urology 2019; 130:196–200.

31. Grilo N, Chartier-Kastler E, Grande P, et al. Robot-assisted Supratrigonal Cystectomy and Augmentation Cystoplasty with Totally Intracorporeal Reconstruction in Neurourological Patients: Technique Description and Preliminary Results. Eur Urol 2020; 79(6):858–65.

32. Xu AJ, Shakir NA, Jun MS, et al. Robotic Assisted Repair of Post-Ileal Conduit Parastomal Hernia: Technique and Outcomes. Urology 2021;158: 232–6. https://doi.org/10.1016/j.urology.2021.08.030.

33. Nakada SY, Best SL. Management of upper urinary tract obstruction. In: Wein AJ, Kavoussi LR, Partin AW, et al, editors. Campbell-Walsh urology. 11th edition. Philadelphia: Elsevier; 2016. p. 1135.

34. Patil NN, Mottrie A, Sundaram B, et al. Robotic-assisted laparoscopic ureteral reimplantation with psoas hitch: a multi-institutional, multinational evaluation. Urology 2008;72(1):47–50.

35. Passoni N, Peters CA. Robotic Ureteral Reimplantation. J Endourol 2020;34(S1):S31–4.

36. Kozinn SI, Canes D, Sorcini A, et al. Robotic versus open distal ureteral reconstruction and reimplantation for benign stricture disease. J Endourol 2012; 26(2):147–51.

37. Schimpf MO, Wagner JR. Robot-assisted laparoscopic Boari flap ureteral reimplantation. J Endourol 2008;22(12):2691–4.

38. JU Stolzenburg, Rai BP, Do M, et al. Robot-assisted technique for Boari flap ureteric reimplantation: replicating the techniques of open surgery in robotics. BJU Int 2016;118:482–4.

39. Slawin J, Patel NH, Lee Z, et al. Ureteral Reimplantation via Robotic Nontransecting Side-to-Side Anastomosis for Distal Ureteral Stricture. J Endourol 2020;34(8):836–9.

40. Choi JH, Jeon BG, Choi S-G, et al. Rectourethral Fistula: Systemic Review of and Experiences With Various Surgical Treatment Methods. Ann Coloproctol 2014;30(1):35–41.

41. Chen S, Gao R, Li H, et al. Management of acquired rectourethral fistulas in adults. Asian J Urol 2018; 5(3):149–54.

42. Bukowski TP, Chakrabarty A, Powell IJ, et al. Acquired Rectourethral Fistula: Methods of Repair. J Urol 1995;153(3):730–3.

43. Netsch C, Bach T, Gross E, et al. Rectourethral Fistula After High-intensity Focused Ultrasound Therapy for Prostate Cancer and Its Surgical Management. Urology 2011;77(4):999–1004.

44. Zmora O, Potenti FM, Wexner SD, et al. Gracilis Muscle Transposition for Iatrogenic Rectourethral Fistula. Ann Surg 2003;237(4):483–7.

45. Robotic TAMIS for Local Repair of Acquired Rectovaginal and Rectourethral Fistulae. Available at: https://www.youtube.com/watch?v=eIsrFVE8TBI. Accessed February 29, 2020.

Neurogenic Bladder: Assessment and Operative Management

Molly E. DeWitt-Foy, MD*, Sean P. Elliott, MD, MS

KEYWORDS

- Neurogenic bladder • Catheterizable channel • Bladder augmentation

KEY POINTS

- A phenotype-based approach to neurogenic bladder (NGB) gives structure and clarity to a complex issue. We describe common presentations, anatomy, and surgical management of adults with spinal cord injury (SCI), spina bifida (SB), cerebral palsy (CP), and multiple sclerosis (MS).
- Surgical management of NGB requires a holistic approach with the consideration of social support, body habitus, and extremity function.
- Postoperative complications are common and follow-up is lifelong.

INTRODUCTION

Neurogenic bladder (NGB) is defined as bladder dysfunction in the setting of a neurologic disorder. Some prefer the term neurogenic lower urinary tract dysfunction because it better incorporates problems like an open bladder neck or detrusor-sphincter dyssynergia but we will use NGB throughout this article. Etiology can be congenital, as in spina bifida (SB), or acquired, as in spinal cord injury (SCI). When strategizing a patient-centered treatment plan, a thorough assessment of the patient's mobility, dexterity, intellectual capacity, and social support is as important as an understanding of bladder function.

Nature of the Problem/Diagnosis

Though many pathologic states can result in NGB, we find it helpful to categorize NGB into the most common phenotypes, namely SCI, SB, cerebral palsy (CP), and multiple sclerosis (MS) **Table 1**.

Spinal cord injury

Nearly 300,000 people in the United States (US) are living with SCI.[1] Most were able-bodied, independent adults before an acute neurologic injury, and are often highly motivated to regain this independence. Patients enter a period of spinal shock immediately following injury, after which a relatively predictable, fixed lesion will develop.[2] In addition to contributing to bladder dysfunction, the level of lesion will dictate extremity function, an important consideration when determining plans for bladder management.

Spina bifida: The incidence of SB in the US is 3 in 10,000 live births, with 75% of people with SB now living to adulthood.[3] It is a congenital defect characterized by incomplete closure of the vertebral column. The most common type of SB is myelomeningocele, in which the spinal cord and meninges are exposed.[4] Hydrocephalus is found in 60% to 80% of people with SB[3] and often results in cognitive and executive dysfunction. Motor and cognitive function can vary widely, with a majority of adult patients with suprasacral SB being dependent on wheelchairs for mobility[5].

Cerebral palsy

CP is a syndrome resulting from perinatal brain injury with a US incidence of 3 per 1000 live births.[6] Causes include hypoxia, jaundice, infection, or trauma. The spectrum of disease is broad, with

University of Minnesota, 420 Delaware St SE, Minneapolis, MN 55455, USA
* Corresponding author.
E-mail addresses: dewit195@umn.edu; mdewittfoy@gmail.com
Twitter: @mdewittfoy (M.E.D.-F.)

Urol Clin N Am 49 (2022) 519–532
https://doi.org/10.1016/j.ucl.2022.04.010
0094-0143/22/© 2022 Elsevier Inc. All rights reserved.

Table 1
Common phenotypes of neurogenic bladder: these descriptions are generalizations of the most common presentation of each phenotype

Phenotype	Typical Body Habitus	Common urodynamic Findings	Extremity Function	Other Considerations
Spinal cord injury	Men > women Normal BMI	NDO Tonic EUS DSD	Muscle spasticity and weakness below the level of lesion	Lesions above T6 associated with autonomic dysreflexia
Spina bifida	Central adiposity Thick-walled bladder	Variable NDO Open bladder neck or DSD	Intact upper extremity function Often require wheelchair by adulthood	Hydrocephalus may result in limits on executive function
Cerebral palsy	Lower than average BMI	Large capacity bladder Myotonic failure Pseudodyssynergia	Contractures, spasticity	Myotonic failure can mask NDO
Multiple sclerosis	Normal BMI	NDO +/-DSD, areflexia	Motor function declines with age	Often progressive disease

Abbreviations: DSD, detrusor sphincter dyssynergia; EUS, external urethral sphincter; NDO, eurogenic detrusor overactivity.

roughly half of individuals experiencing intellectual disability.[7] Muscle spasticity is a characterizing feature and often includes the external urethral sphincter (EUS). This pseudodyssynergia may not become bothersome until early adulthood. Patients with less severe diseases may void volitionally and complain of urgency or obstructive symptoms. For patients who void into diapers, many will "flood," or hold urine for a long period of time and void large volumes once or twice a day. It is uncommon for patients with CP to require regular catheterization, and catheterization is often difficult given sphincter spasticity. Malnutrition, epilepsy, visual and hearing impairments, reflux, and constipation are common comorbidities.[8]

Multiple sclerosis

MS is a chronic acquired syndrome caused by the demyelination of neurons in the brain and spinal cord. Age of onset is most common in the fourth decade of life and the condition is often progressive in nature. Women are affected at nearly three times the rate as men, and US prevalence is approximately one million. Fifty to 90% of patients have urinary symptoms, the most common of which is neurogenic detrusor overactivity (NDO). Upper tract deterioration is relatively rare.[9]

Anatomy

Detailed anatomic and physiologic discussion of the bladder is beyond the scope of this article. We will instead focus on anatomic considerations by phenotype as well as important neurologic landmarks.

CHARACTERISTIC ANATOMY BY PHENOTYPE – *here we focus on typical body habitus, urodynamic findings, and extremity function because they are all important considerations in surgical planning.*

- Spinal cord injury:
  - *Body habitus:* Men are more likely to suffer SCI than women, with 70% of traumatic SCI occurring in men.[10] Patients with SCI, on average, have lower body mass index (BMI) than the general population.[11]
  - *Urodynamic findings/bladder function:* The majority of patients have suprasacral lesions, resulting in NDO and detrusor sphincter dyssynergia (DSD) with a tonic EUS. Those with sacral lesions have a flaccid bladder and an open sphincter. Initially, the bladder will be of normal thickness. Bladder size is roughly normal, at least early on in the course of their disease. This generalization does not hold true for those who have been managed with an indwelling catheter for decades - these bladders tend to be poorly compliant and small in capacity.
  - *Extremity function:* In addition to contributing to bladder dysfunction, the level of lesion will dictate extremity function, an important consideration when determining plans for bladder management

- Spina bifida
  - *Body habitus:* Adults with SB are more likely to have increased central adiposity than the general population.[12] By adulthood, bladders are often thick-walled and inflamed, and/or have been previously augmented. The appendix is rarely available for use by adulthood.
  - *Urodynamic findings/bladder function:* Urodynamics may demonstrate detrusor over- or underactivity with a fixed, open bladder neck or a dyssynergic sphincter.[13]
  - *Extremity function:* Depending on the level of pathology, patients may depend on wheelchairs for ambulation. For female patients in particular this can make urethral self-catheterization very difficult, even though upper extremity function is generally intact.
- Cerebral palsy:
  - *Body habitus:* People with CP are more likely to be underweight than the general population, and may require tube feedings for adequate nutrition[14]
  - *Urodynamic findings/bladder function:* Because CP is a suprapontine injury, children with CP exhibit the NDO characteristic of an upper motor neuron bladder. By adulthood, the pseudodyssynergia has worsened and complicates the picture. Some people have NDO with pseudodyssynergia while others have a large capacity, poorly contractile bladder from years of overdistension. However, their underlying bladder remains an upper motor neuron bladder; the NDO is simply masked by myotonic failure. The NDO often returns after the chronic obstruction is relieved[8]
  - *Extremity function:* Contractures are common in the more advanced cases of CP; lower extremity contractures may make urethral access difficult, especially in women. Selfcatheterization may be limited by upper extremity dexterity and pseudodyssynergia.
- Multiple Sclerosis
  - *Body habitus:* Even among patients with MS with severe disability, the rates of obesity are lower than in the general population. [11,15]
  - *Urodynamic findings/bladder function:* The most common urodynamic finding is NDO. Detrusor external sphincter synergia can also occur, as can, less frequently, detrusor areflexia. Urodynamic findings can be difficult to predict and are often not directly related to the level of the lesion or even symptomatology.[16]

Table 2
Level of lesion

Level of Lesion	UDS Findings	Implicated Anatomy
Suprapontine	NDO Sphincter function intact	Loss of tonic inhibition of PMC– > uninhibited bladder
Pons to T6	NDO Internal and external sphincter dyssynergia (after the resolution of spinal shock) Autonomic dysreflexia	Reorganization of synaptic connections in spinal cord. Afferents more sensitive to low bladder pressures. Disruption of preganglionic sympathetic neurons
T6 to S2	NDO Internal sphincter synergy and external sphincter dyssynergia (after the resolution of spinal shock)	Reorganization of synaptic connections in spinal cord. Afferents more sensitive to low bladder pressures
S2 to S4 WITHOUT damage to pudendal/Onuf's nucleus	Detrusor areflexia Hypertonic external sphincter	Parasympathetic damage. Bladder pressure remains low, protects upper tracts
S2 to S4 WITH damage to pudendal/Onuf's nucleus	Detrusor areflexia Flaccid sphincter	Loss of somatic control of external sphincter from Onuf damage
Peripheral Nerves	Detrusor underactivity Poor sensation of filling Usually tonic sphincter	Capacious bladder + intact sympathetic nervous system – > overflow incontinence

Abbreviations: NDO, neurogenic detrusor overactivity; PMC, pontine micturition center

- *Extremity function:* The majority of patients with MS will have limitations in upper extremity function with a decline in motor function with an increase in age[17]

Level of the Lesion

Nerves involved in bladder storage and emptying

Hypogastric Nerve: Activation of the sympathetic nervous system via the hypogastric nerve causes bladder relaxation and tonic contraction of the outlet, allowing for bladder storage. The hypogastric nerve originates from vertebral levels T10-L2.

Pelvic Nerve: the parasympathetic nervous system, by way of the pelvic nerve, causes detrusor contraction and internal sphincter relaxation necessary for bladder emptying. This nerve originates in the sacral spinal cord and passes through the pelvic plexus.

Pudendal Nerve: the pudendal nerve arises from S2-4 and contains afferent and efferent axons. It provides somatic innervation of the EUS, allowing for the voluntary control of urinary control.

Patients with suprapontine lesions tend to have NDO with synergic sphincters. Adults with CP are an exception to this rule, where urinary retention and/or infrequent large volume voids are the norm[18] (RA Goldfarb). Reasons for this are described above in the urodynamic findings section.

Spinal cord lesions between the pons and T6 may result in NDO and DSD involving the internal and EUS. Autonomic dysreflexia may also be present.

Lesions between T6 and S2 tend to cause DO and DSD. Autonomic dysreflexia is not present.

Sacral nerve root lesions classically cause detrusor areflexia with variable effects on the sphincter depending on the involvement of Onuf's nucleus **Table 2**.

Preoperative/preprocedure Planning

Preoperative evaluation should include complete physical examination, with a focus on cognitive function, upper extremity dexterity, abdominal adiposity, prior surgical incisions, bowel management, mobility status, and reflexes. Stoma marking should be conducted for all patients prior to continent or incontinent diversion.

History should focus on social support, particularly for patients with cognitive impairment. Urodynamics are almost always obtained, with a focus on capacity, compliance, status of the bladder outlet, DO, and DSD. Voiding diary and pad weights are often useful, particularly when the clinical history does not match urodynamic findings.

Prior to surgical intervention, we check a urine culture on all patients. Cross sectional imaging is recommended for patients with unclear operative history.

- SCI: Though roughly half of the people with SCI are using clean intermittent catheterization (CIC) for bladder management on initial discharge from rehabilitation facilities,[19] 50% of these will have an indwelling or condom catheter 5 years later. Suprapubic tube is preferable to indwelling urethral foley given the risk of urethral erosion and other complications.[20] A catherizable channel may be a good option for patients with upper extremity function or excellent social support. This is particularly true for women, as channels permit micturition without transfer out of a wheelchair. Ileal conduit should be a last resort in most patients, though it is a reasonable option for those with a hostile bladder who do not have the dexterity or social support to catheterize or those who have failed a suprapubic tube (eg, due to stones, recurrent infection or upper tract deterioration).

- Spina bifida: Ventriculoperitoneal (VP) shunts, particularly when revised, can cause significant bowel adhesions. Appendicovesicostomy is rarely possible in the adult with spina bifida, due to small contracted bladder, thick abdominal wall, and, often, prior use of the appendix for a Mitrofanoff or antegrade continence enema (ACE) or just a short appendix *in situ*. The small contracted bladder increases the distance to the abdominal wall, often necessitating a channel longer than 10 cm if one is to have an adequate 4 cm tunnel. A chronically inflamed bladder is characteristic of adult SB and is quite different from the recently spinal cord injured patient; this makes tunneling a detrusor flap valve challenging. We prefer a continent cutaneous catheterizable ileocecocystoplasty (CCIC) in this population, as it puts the ileocecal valve at the dome of the augment, allowing for a shorter channel and avoids tunneling a channel in the bladder. A full description of the CCIC is included later in discussion.

- Cerebral palsy: Infrequent, large volume voids ("floods") due to pseuodysynergia and chronic retention are problematic because they exceed the capacity of the incontinence brief and saturate bedding or clothing. Flooding may be well managed with regular botulinum neurotoxin (BoNT) to the EUS. In our experience, this allows for more frequent voids and decreases flooding. We usually avoid urethral CIC because the pseudodysynergia makes this challenging and painful. Other options include suprapubic tube and catheterizable channel. Patients with CP who undergo catheterizable channel creation, particularly those who are not on CIC prior to surgery, are at risk for *de novo* DO postoperatively (see discussion in urodynamics section).[21] For these patients, we recommend the consideration of prophylactic bladder augmentation, or initiation of CIC followed by another urodynamics some months later. Unlike in SB, appendicovesicostomy is usually feasible in adults with CP. Many people with CP (and some with SCI) have subcutaneous baclofen pumps - these may dictate stoma placement but should not interfere with the majority of surgical decision-making.

- Multiple Sclerosis: Catheterizable channel creation is rarely the operation of choice in those with MS, given the progressive nature of the disease. We tend to start with anticholinergics before moving to BoNT for NDO management. Incomplete emptying is first managed with timed voiding sometimes combined with sphincter BoNT, then CIC, then SPT.
- Failure to store
  - Bladder: Failure to store from bladder pathology (eg, NDO) is initially managed with anticholinergics, followed by intravesical BoNT. For those who fail BoNT and/or oral anticholinergics, we offer augmentation cystoplasty. Indications to move forward with augmentation include poor compliance, small capacity, recalcitrant leakage from NDO, with or without upper tract involvement as evidenced by hydronephrosis or vesicoureteral reflux. Preservation of upper tract function and maintenance of a good quality of life are the main goals of any reconstruction.
  - Outlet: Neurologic conditions that cause NGB can also result in stress urinary incontinence from intrinsic sphincter deficiency (ISD). This "lower motor neuron" pathology results from deinnervation of the sphincter through damage to peripheral nerves, and can be seen in SB, SCI with cauda equina syndrome, or can be the sequela of surgical detethering. Chronic indwelling urethral catheters can also cause such severe atrophy/erosion of the sphincter as to cause ISD. Urodynamics will demonstrate stress incontinence with a low valsalva leak point pressure, and concurrent fluoroscopy will show an open bladder neck. This can be

managed with urethral or bladder neck sling or bladder neck artificial urinary sphincter (AUS). While we occasionally use urethral bulking in poor operative candidates, we usually avoid this as it only offers temporary relief. Bulbar urethral AUS is avoided, due to a higher risk of erosion for patients who may use wheelchairs or rely on intermittent catheterization.[22] even bladder neck AUS has a high revision rate, with 48% of patients requiring revision, removal, or replacement, and an average lifespan of 6 years in neurogenic populations. Concomitant AUS and augmentation cystoplasty appears to be safe, with no increased risk of device infection.[23] Neurogenic patients who undergo bladder neck procedures without augmentation, particularly those who void spontaneously, should be monitored regularly for compliance changes to ensure the increase in urethral tone does not lead to upper tract deterioration.

Slings in patients with NGB offer the advantage of a significantly lower revision rate than AUS, but do generally necessitate the utilization of intermittent self cath.[22] Bladder neck slings are typically selected when the patient is already undergoing an abdominal operation (eg, augmentation cystoplasty) and are always fascial slings. Urethral slings in women are conducted transvaginally with rectus fascia or fascia lata. We prefer fascia lata because it is easier to harvest in obese patients and because many in our population have poor rectus fascia. In men who require a urethral sling, the Advance (AdVance, American Medical Systems, Minnesota, USA) synthetic sling is an option. In women, a preoperative vaginal exam is narrow introitus, such as can occur with vaginal atrophy, can make a transvaginal sling procedure much more difficult.

Bladder neck closure (BNC) is typically a last resort procedure, and best used in patients with severe incontinence who are not candidates for sling or AUS[24] (Gor 2017). The ideal BNC patient is a woman with a widely patulous urethra resulting from long-term indwelling urethral catheter. Urinary diversion can be managed with suprapubic catheter or with catheterizable channel plus or minus augmentation cystoplasty. The obvious disadvantage of BNC is that urethra is no longer an option for catheter placement when access to suprapubic cystotomy or catheterizable channel is lost.

- Failure to empty
  - Bladder: Atonic bladder can be managed with Crede or valsalva voiding, CIC per

urethra or catheterizable channel, or suprapubic tube. Valsalva or Crede voiding is safest and most effective in patients with some element of external sphincter denervation or incompetence. Sphincterotomy is associated with a 68% risk of recurrent urinary tract infection (UTI), recurrent DSD, or hydronephrosis and we do not offer it.[25] External compression of the bladder with Crede will trigger a reflexive increase in outlet resistance in patients with an intact arc, which can result in upper tract deterioration over time. Poor compliance or high detrusor leak point pressure is a contraindication to valsalva or Crede voiding.[26]

- Outlet: PseudoDSD, as seen in patients with CP, can be well managed with urethral sphincter BoNT.

Prep & Patient Positioning

Though recent data have recommended against bowel preparation for neurologically intact patients prior to urinary diversion,[27] the NGB/bowel population often requires a different approach. We order a bowel preparation preoperatively for those undergoing diversion or augmentation with colon, or those with multiple prior abdominal surgeries. For patients who are on bowel regimens at home, we increase their normal regimens for 1 week, then start a Go-Lytely prep for 2 days prior to surgery.

Most patients are placed in the supine position, with the abdomen prepped from the xiphoid to the genitalia, including the urethra so a catheter can be placed on the field.

Procedural approach

We focus here on surgical options that allow the patient to remain continent and do not involve removal of the bladder.

- Catheterizable channels: In general, for patients without prior abdominal surgery and without excessive central adiposity we start with a Pfannenstiel incision. If the appendix is present, patent, and reaches from the bladder to the umbilicus, we proceed with appendicovesicostomy (and ileal augmentation, if indicated). If the appendix is inadequate a single Monti channel is performed (and ileal augmentation, if indicated); because a single Monti is short, this requires a good capacity bladder. If a single Monti will not suffice, we move forward with CCIC, as described later in discussion. We usually avoid spiral or double Monti due to high stenosis rates.[28] For patients who require augmentation but are able

to catheterize via urethra, ileal augmentation without catheterizable channel is preferred (**Fig. 1**).

- Continence mechanism
  - Tunneled catheterizable channels: detrusor flaps are developed and closed over a portion of the channel. As the bladder fills, the pressure on the channel increases, preventing leakage. We prefer an extra-vesical tunnel because the chronically inflamed bladder characteristic of many adult patients with decades of NGB can complicate intra-vesical techniques.
    - Appendicovesicostomy (Mitrofanoff): Incision:
      - Robotic assisted has been described but most have abandoned this in the adult population
      - Pfannenstiel incision: default open approach as this may minimize the risk of parastomal and ventral hernia
      - Midline incision: from umbilicus to pubis. This is preferred for obese patients or those with prior midline incisions or concern for significant bowel adhesions. Take care to leave adequate fascia around the umbilicus to avoid injuring the channel during closure.

    Steps:
    - The appendix is identified and measured to ensure adequate length. In adults, 10 cm is often required in order to create a sufficient tunnel and reach the umbilicus. Some tricks for a shorter appendix include hitching the bladder dome to the abdominal wall as close to the umbilicus as possible, or, in thin patients, bringing the appendix to the right lower quadrant. Use of a retrocecal appendix is generally not advised.
    - The cecum is mobilized and the appendix transected with a cuff of cecum.
    - The distal tip of the appendix is removed and the lumen is calibrated to ensure patency.
    - The bladder is filled and 4 cm long detrusor flaps developed off the mucosa
    - A small hole is made in the bladder mucosa and the distal tip of the appendix is anastomosed to the mucosa using interrupted absorbable sutures.

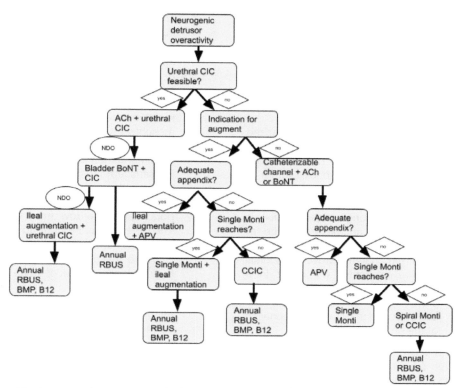

Fig. 1. Algorithmic approach to neurogenic detrusor overactivity.*Abbreviations:* APV, appendicovesicostomy or Mitrofanoff; BMP, basic metabolic panel; BoNT, botulinum neurotoxin; CCIC, continent catheterizable ileal ceco-cystoplasty; CIC, clean intermittent catheterization; NDO, neurogenic detrusor overactivity; RBUS = renal bladder ultrasound.

- The detrusor is closed over-top of the appendix with interrupted absorbable sutures.
- The proximal (cecal) end is brought to the umbilicus and the stoma matured. The channel should be straight and taught but off tension, such that catheterization is easy.

- An indwelling 14F foley is left in the channel.
- Modifications include tunneling the appendix into the tinea of a colonic augment
- Reconfigured ileum (Yang-Monti) **Fig. 2**: Indications: if the appendix is unavailable or inadequate

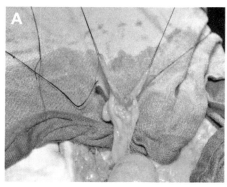
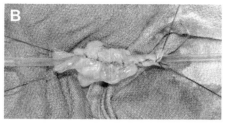

Fig. 2. (*A*) Detubularized 2 cm segment of ileum - note that mesentery is at the center of the bowel segment indicating that the detubularizing incision was made directly antimeseterically. (*B*) Appearance of channel following second suture line. Catheter in image is 14F.

Incision: Midline or pfannenstiel

Steps:

- Two centimeters of ileum are isolated and bowel continuity restored. If an augmentation cystoplasty is performed concurrently, the two segments can be harvested from adjacent ileum.
- The 2 cm segment is detubularized and then retubularized transversely over a 14F straight catheter using two layers of absorbable suture in an interrupted fashion or with multiple short runs.
- If the initial longitudinal incision is made directly antimesenteric the resulting mesentery will be in the middle of the channel. Moving the initial incision off-center will result in a mesentery closer to the distal or proximal end of the channel which can help with maturation or tunneling of the channel, respectively.

A single Monti usually yields a channel of 6 cm. Variations on this theme can yield increased length: a "double Monti," using two side-by-side segments or a "spiral Monti" where a 3.5 cm segment is transected partially in the center with two strips parallel to the mesentery on either side.[29]

- Staple-tapered ileum: the ileum can be tapered over a catheter using a GIA stapler as a separate procedure in the same fashion described in the CCIC section later in discussion but without the cecal augment. We have found this technique limited by the mesentery and have generally avoided it. The axial blood supply of the mesentery dictates an arc-shaped tract of the channel, resulting in a longer and more redundant tract that can be difficult to catheterize.
- Nipple valves: nipple valves achieve continence through circumferential backing of the bladder end of the channel.
- Intussuscepted ileum:
  - Steps:
    - 10 to 12 cm of ileum is harvested and an intussuscepted nipple valve created on the bladder end.
    - If conducted in conjunction with a bladder augmentation, the channel ileum is left intact while the remaining distal bowel is detubularized and used for the augment. If conducted as a separate procedure the bladder end of the ileum is

anastomosed to the bladder mucosa using an intravesical approach. This can also be conducted via an extravesical approach.

- A 5 cm long mesenteric window is created near the middle of the length of bowel, such that 2.5 cm of mesentery remains on the bladder side and 4.5 cm of mesentery remains on the umbilicus side.
- Two Allis clamps are passed into the proximal lumen and used to grasp and intussuscept the ileal wall.
- The resulting nipple is stabilized with two rows of staples from the inside of the pouch and one row from the outside. The other end is brought up through the umbilicus and the stoma matured.[30] Because these staples can be exposed to urine there is a risk of stone formation.

- Ileocecal valve:
  - Surgical technique for tapering of the terminal ileum and reinforcement of the IC valve will be described later in discussion in the CCIC section.

- Augmentation
  - Ileocystoplasty:
    - Incision:
      - Pfannenstiel incision
      - Midline incision from umbilicus to pubis. Favored in patients with prior midline incisions or with significant abdominal adiposity or concern for bowel adhesions.
    - Steps:
      - The cecum is identified and 25 to 30 cm of terminal ileum are harvested, starting at least 15 cm from the ileocecal valve.
      - Bowel continuity is restored and placed cephalad to the harvested segment.
      - Harvested bowel is detubularized using an antimesenteric incision
      - The bowel is reconfigured in an S-shaped patch - initially with Babcock clamps and then with a series of absorbable running sutures.
      - A sagittal cystotomy is used to open the bladder widely, from trigone to bladder neck.
      - Orient the augment segment so that it will reach the anterior and posterior apices. Adjacent absorbable monofilament sutures are placed on the posterior apex of the bladder and then passed through the augment
      - The posterior sides are closed using running absorbable suture. The

anterior wall is parachuted down and closed in the same fashion.

- Before the completion of the closure a 20F suprapubic tube is passed through the abdominal wall and into the native bladder or augment, with a purse-string suture around the cystotomy/enterotomy
- Suprapubic and urethral or channel catheters are left for 1 month (see "Catheter management" in the "Recovery and Rehabilitation" section)

- Sigmoid augment
  - Incision: lower midline
  - Steps:
    - The sigmoid is mobilized and 30 cm of bowel is harvested
    - Bowel continuity is restored
    - The sigmoid is opened along the anterior tenia and reconfigured in a U shape. Because the sigmoid is larger in diameter than the ileum, an S configuration is not required.
    - The posterior inner walls of the U are reapproximated using a running absorbable suture
    - The bladder is open widely using a sagittal cystotomy
    - The bowel patch is then anastomosed to the bladder as described above
    - A suprapubic catheter is placed as described above (for the ileal augmentation).
    - A second foley is left in the urethra or catheterizable channel if one is made
- CCIC: https://www.youtube.com/watch?v=8GMvuasLECl
  - Indications: The continent catheterizable ileal cecocystoplasty (CCIC) is an excellent option for patients who require augmentation with concomitant channel creation in whom an appendiceal or single Monti channel is not an option. In particular, we find this works well for patients with thick abdominal walls and small, contracted bladders, in cases where a single Monti is unlikely to reach the umbilicus. The adult spina bifida patient or one with a chronic suprapubic tube are examples of patients in whom a tunneled channel would be more challenging and the CCIC is preferable.
  - Incision:
    - We favor a combined open and laparoscopic approach as described later in discussion [31]

- Alternatively, a midline laparotomy is used, with the incision extending cephalad enough to mobilize the hepatic flexure.
- Steps:
  - A Pfannenstiel incision is made and a hand assistant port is placed.
  - Additional laparoscopic ports are placed: a 10 mm camera port through the umbilicus can be repurposed later for the stoma site; a 5 mm subxiphoid incision post can be repurposed later for the drain.
  - The ascending colon is mobilized with a hand-assist laparoscopic technique until the first stage of the duodenum is easily visualized in order to ensure the ileocolonic anastomosis will be off-tension. We tried doing this mobilization with pure laparoscopic methods but found that the chronically distended colon from neurogenic bowel made retraction challenging.
  - The hand-assist port is removed and the augmentation cystoplasty and creation of the catheterizable channel are conducted through the Pfannenstiel incision.
  - 10 cm of cecum and 10 cm of terminal ileum are harvested and an ileocolic anastomosis is fashioned.
  - An antimesenteric incision is made to detubularize the cecal portion (**Figs. 3**A and **4**).
  - The ileum is tapered over a 14F catheter with a stapler - we use a GIA 100 to avoid overlapping staple lines (see **Fig. 3**B)
  - The continence mechanism created by the ileocecal valve is reinforced using a series of interrupted monofilament, absorbable sutures (see **Fig. 3**A).
  - The cecal augment is then anastomosed to the native bladder which has been widely opened through a sagittal cystotomy from trigone to anterior bladder neck. We do not reconfigure the cecum into a U-shape because it is already a nice square shape after detubularization.
  - A 20F foley is placed as a suprapubic tube before the completion of the anastomosis as described above (for the ileal augmentation).
- Bladder outlet procedures:
  - Bladder neck artificial urinary sphincter https://www.youtube.com/watch?v=j7DWKnbzXHg
    - Indications: Bladder neck AUS can be employed in patients who void

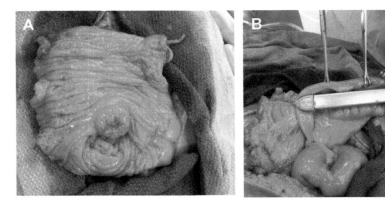

Fig. 3. (*A*) Ileocecal valve as seen from the interior of the detubularized cecum. (*B*) Staple tapering of the terminal ileum.

spontaneously or in those who catheterize intermittently. Adequate dexterity is required for cuff cycling.

- Incision: If no prior augment then robotic transperitoneal or Pfannenstiel extraperitoneal approach. If prior augment then midline laparotomy.
- Steps for robotic approach:
  - A posterior peritoneal incision is made and a plane between the bladder and rectum is developed until the vasa (in a man) and the bladder neck are identified
  - The space of retzius is developed

- The anterior and posterior planes are connected. A cystoscope can help avoid a cystotomy at this point.
- The bladder neck is measured
- The measuring device is exchanged for the cuff and a pressure regulating balloon is placed in the space of retzius
- The peritoneum is closed to restore the space of Retzius
- The pump is tunneled into the hemiscrotum or labia majora
- if using robotic approach the tubing is capped and connections are made extracorporally
- Bladder neck sling:

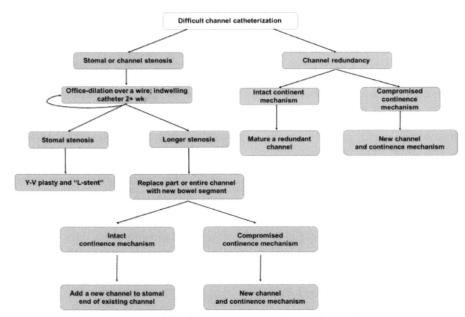

Fig. 4. Stepwise approach in managing difficult to catharize continent channels.

- Autologous fascia (rectus or fascia lata) sling can be placed around the bladder neck in men or women through an abdominal approach. Lithotomy positioning is important so that a sponge stick or finger can be placed in the rectum (in men) vagina to avoid injury during the posterior dissection. When extra tight closure is needed, the arms of the sling can be crossed anteriorly to give nearly circumferential compression.
- Pubovaginal sling
  - Steps:
    - A midline anterior vaginal incision is made and dissection continued on each side of the urethra toward the inferior pubic rami.
    - A 2 × 6 cm graft of fascia lata is harvested from the lateral thigh and 0 permanent monofilament suture placed on either end of the graft
    - The endopelvic fascia is punctured with scissors or a clamp
    - A small transverse suprapubic incision is made and dissection continued down to the rectus fascia
    - A curved suture passer (Raz) is used to puncture the rectus fascia and tunnel down to the periurethral incision taking care to stay close to the pubis so as not to injure the bladder.
    - The sling suture is threaded onto the suture passer and pulled to the abdominal incision
    - The suture is tightened and tied down
    - Cystoscopy is performed to ensure adequate coaptation of the urethra and evaluate for bladder injury
- Advance sling
  - Steps: A synthetic transobturator perineal sling (AdVance, American Medical Systems, Minnesota, USA) is placed in the standard fashion as described by the manufacturer.
    - A midline perineal incision is made and the urethra exposed
    - A suture is placed in the corpus spongiosum at the distal end of the perineal body insertion
    - Bilateral stab incisions are made in the skin 1 finger's breadth inferior to the insertion of the adductor longus tendon and just lateral to the ischiopubic ramus
    - From the perineal incision the inferior pubic ramus is identified
    - The AMS helical trocar is passed from the stab incision to the perineal

incision, through the superior aspect of the obturator foramen, maintaining a 45° angle of the helix
- The sling is attached to the trocar and the course of the trocar is reversed. This step is repeated on the contralateral side
- The mesh is secured to the corpus spongiosum and the excess sling is trimmed
- Bladder neck closure https://auau.auanet.org/content/v2-08-transvaginal-bladder-neck-closure-devastated-female-urethra
  - In women:
    - In women we approach the urethra transvaginally unless bladder neck closure is being performed as a part of a larger abdominal operation
    - Transvaginal:
      - The urethra is mobilized circumferentially. We continue mobilization 2 cm past the bladder neck.
      - The urethra is transected and the bladder neck is closed in layers with interrupted absorbable sutures
      - The closure is reinforced with a Martius flap
    - Transabdominal:
      - Pfannenstiel incision and lithotomy positioning
      - With a finger in the vagina, dissect between the urethra and the vagina with a right angle, feeling the Foley balloon to identify the bladder neck.
      - Divide the urethra at the bladder neck
      - Place ureteral catheters in both ureters
      - Mobilize the bladder cephalad off the vagina for 2 cm (behind the trigone)
      - Close the bladder neck in layers
      - Place an omental flap between the bladder neck and urethra if available[32]
  - In men:
    - In men a perineal approach with the closure of the bulbar urethra has been described[33]
    - More commonly the bladder neck in men is closed through an abdominal incision with steps similar to those described above for the transabdominal approach in women, except that the dissection is between the bladder neck and rectum instead of bladder neck and vagina.[33]

Recovery & Rehabilitation (Including postprocedure Care)

Diet

Though enhanced recovery after surgery (ERAS) protocols have demonstrated good success in decreasing length of stay and time to the consumption of regular diet in neurologically intact adults,[27] we tend to take a slower approach to feeding in patients with neurogenic bowel, given the high rate of ileus in this population.[34] We do administer Entereg (Alvimopan) pre and postoperatively per protocol for patients who do not have contraindications.

Mobility

All patients who are not ambulatory are given a Dolphin, or pulsatile, mattress for postoperative recovery to reduce the risk of pressure ulcers. Patients are encouraged to get back to their baseline ambulatory status with the help of physical therapy consult. Importantly, we do not restrict weight-bearing or even though significant abdominal straining occurs with these activities. Our reasoning is that if we restrict weight-bearing or then we commit the patient to a Hoyer lift and that has tremendous implications for their discharge status. They may not be able to go home or may have few choices in the type of rehabilitation facility that will accept them.

Catheter management

We leave a suprapubic tube and a urethral or channel catheter for 1 month. We do not perform a cystogram. Patients are instructed to irrigate both catheters twice daily. At the postoperative appointment, we fill the bladder and then cap the suprapubic tube. We then remove the channel or urethral catheter and have the patient attempt catheterization. If this is successful all tubes are removed. Antibiotics are given at the time of catheter removal.

Irrigation

In the immediate postoperative period, while both catheters are in place, we recommend patients with bladder augments irrigate both catheters twice daily. After catheter removal, we recommend once daily irrigation with tap water. Tap water is a safe, cheap, convenient, and environmentally friendly alternative to bottles of sterile saline.[34]

Follow-up

We perform a renal-bladder ultrasound on all patients with NGB on an annual basis. Basic metabolic panel and vitamin B12 levels are drawn for

those with urinary tract reconstruction with small bowel.

Management

Outcomes

The risk of complications has been quoted at >90% for patients with SB following laparotomy.[35] Most common complications include ileus, pressure ulcer, urinary tract infection, and wound infection.

Channel complications
- Long-term complications of catheterizable channel occur in 25% to 30%, including stomal stenosis, prolapse, channel incontinence, or diverticula.[36]
- Stomal or channel stenosis can be initially managed with dilation over a wire and leaving an indwelling catheter for 2 weeks. Persistent stomal stenosis can be temporized with an L-stent[37] or surgically repaired with Y-V plasty or mobilizing and rematuring the stoma. Longer segments of narrowing will more often require harvesting new bowel to replace or add to the initial channel.[38]

  Difficulty catheterizing can also result from a channel that is too long - redundancy can be corrected by dissecting out the distal channel and rematuring the stoma such that the channel is more taught.
- Incontinent channels should be evaluated with urodynamics, as leaking may be the result of a continence mechanism and/or the NGB. If the incontinence is a channel, or "stress," incontinence, therapeutic options include the injection of bulking agents, retunneling, or creation of a new channel. Bulking agents can provide temporary relief - with success rates quoted at 50% to 86%[39,40]

Augment complications
- Complications of bladder augmentation include perforation, bladder calculi, metabolic derangements, recurrent infections, ileus/bowel obstruction, renal deterioration, incontinence, bowel complications, and malignancy.
- Perforation is a rare (8.6%) but potentially catastrophic complication and is typically manifested with abdominal tenderness and distension. Diagnosis is made with cystogram and management in most cases is with exploration and primary repair.[41]
- Many complications of augmentation are the result of mucus production from the detubularized bowel and can be prevented by regular vigorous irrigation of the bladder. Husmann has described a reduction in symptomatic

UTIs and bladder calculi with regular irrigation using$\geq$240 mL.[42] We recommend the same quantity of tap water. For the ~15% of patients who require surgical intervention for bladder stones, we prefer initial management with percutaneous over open approach.

SUMMARY

In summary, surgical management of NGB requires a holistic, patient-centered approach. An understanding of the most common neurologic phenotypes can be helpful to guide decision making.

DISCLOSURE

Sean P Elliott disclosure: Urotronic LLC, investigator; Percuvision, shareholder; Boston Scientific, consultant.

REFERENCES

1. National Spinal Cord Injury Statistical Center. Spinal cord injury (SCI) facts and figures at a glance 2018. Available at: https://www.nscisc.uab.edu/Public/Facts%20and%20Figures%20-%202018.pdf. Accessed December 12, 2021.
2. Taweel WA, Seyam R. Neurogenic bladder in spinal cord injury patients. Res Rep Urol 2015;7:85–99.
3. Mukherjee S, Pasulka J. Care for adults with spina bifida: current state and future directions. Top Spinal Cord Inj Rehabil 2017;23(2):155–67.
4. Snow-Lisy DC, Yerkes EB, Cheng EY. Update on urological management of spina bifida from prenatal diagnosis to adulthood. J Urol 2015;194:288–96.
5. Dicianno BE, Karmarkar A, Houtrow A, et al. Factors associated with mobility outcomes in a national spina bifida patient registry. Am J Phys Med Rehabil 2015;94(12):1015–25.
6. Christensen D, Van Naarden Braun K, Doernberg NS, et al. Prevalence of cerebral palsy, co-occurring autism spectrum disorders, and motor functioning - autism and developmental disabilities monitoring network, USA, 2008. Dev Med Child Neurol 2014;56(1):59–65.
7. Reid SM, Meehan EM, Arnup SJ, et al. Intellectual disability in cerebral palsy: a population-based retrospective study. Dev Med Child Neurol 2018; 60(7):687–94.
8. Pariser JJ, Elliott SP. In: Stoffel JT, Dray EV, editors. Ch 11: cerebral palsy in "urological care for patients with progressive neurological conditions. Switzerland AG: Springer Nature; 2020. p. 95–104.
9. Kowalik CG, Wein AJ, Dmochowski RR. Neuromuscular dysfunction of the lower urinary tract. Campbell Walsh Urol 12th Edition 2021;111:2600–36.

10. Bryce TH, Vincent H, Escalon MX. Spinal cord injury. Braddom's Phys Med Rehabil,49;2021: 1049–1100.e6
11. Alschuler KN, Gibbons LE, Rosenberg DE, et al. BMI and waist circumference in persons aging with muscular dystrophy, multiple sclerosis, post-polio syndrome, and spinal cord injury. Disabil Health J 2012;5(3):177–84.
12. Liu JS, Dong C, Vo AX, et al. Obesity and anthropometry in spina bifida: What is the best measure. J Spinal Cord Med 2018;41(1):55–62.
13. Panicker JN, Fowler CJ, Kessler T. Lower urinary tract dysfunction in the neurological patient: clinical assessment and management. Lancet: Neurourology 2015;14(7):710–32.
14. Perenc L, Przysada G, Tzerciak J. Cerebral palsy in children as a risk factor for malnutrition. Ann Nutr Metab 2015;66:224–32.
15. Pinhas-Hamiel O, Livne M, Harari G, et al. Prevalence of overweight, obesity, and metabolic syndrome components in multiple sclerosis patients with significant disability. Eur J Neurol 2015;22(9): 1275–9.
16. Stoffel JT. Contemporary management of the neurogenic bladder for multiple sclerosis patients. Urol Clin North Am 2010;37(4):547–57.
17. Roy S, Frndak S, Drake AS, et al. Differential effects of aging on motor and cognitive function in multiple sclerosis. Mult Scler 2017;23(10).
18. Goldfarb RA, Pisansky A, Fleck J, et al. Neurogenic lower urinary tract dysfunction in adults with cerebral palsy: outcomes following a conservative management approach. J Urol 2016;195(4):1009–13.
19. Cameron AP, Wallner LP, Tate DG, et al. Bladder management after spinal cord injury in the United States 1972-2005. J Urol 2010;184(1):213–7.
20. Romo PGB, Smith CP, Cox A, et al. Non-surgical urologic management of neurogenic bladder after spinal cord injury. World J Urol 2018;36:1555–68. https://doi.org/10.1007/s00345-018-2419-z. Available at.
21. Narayan VM, Pariser JJ, Gor RA, et al. Bladder changes after catheterizable channel creation in adults with cerebral palsy who are in chronic urinary retention. Neurourol Urodyn 2019;38(1):165–70.
22. Myers JB, Mayer EN, Lenherr S. Management options for sphincteric deficiency in adults with neurogenic bladder. Transl Androl Urol 2016;5(1).
23. Viers BR, Elliott DS, Kramer SA. Simultatious augmentation cystoplasty and cuff only artificial urinary sphincter in children and young adults with neurogenic urinary incontinence. J Urol 2014; 191(4):1104–8.
24. Gor RA, Elliott SP. Surgical management of neurogenic lower urinary tract dysfunction. Urol Clin North Am 2017;44(3):475–90.
25. Pan D, Troy A, Rogerson J, et al. Long-term outcomes of external sphincterotomy in a spinal injured

population. J Urol 2009;181(2):705–9. Epub 2008 Dec 16. PMID: 19091341.

26. Boone TB, Stewart JN, Martinez LM. Chapter 127: additional therapies for storage and emptying failure. Campbell-Walsh Urol 2021;12th:2889–904. e4.

27. Azhar RA, Bochner B, Catto J, et al. Enhanced recovery after urological surgery: a contemporary systematic review of outcomes, key elements, and research needs. Eur Urol 2016;70(1):176–87.

28. Szymanski KM, Whittam B, Misseri R, et al. Long-term outcomes of catheterizable continent urinary channels: What do you use, where you put it, and does it matter? J Pediatr Urol 2015;11(4):210.e1–7. Epub 2015 May 30. PMID: 26071074.

29. Levy ME, Elliott SP. Reconstructive techniques for creation of catheterizable channels: tunneled and nipple valve channels. Transl Androl Urol 2016; 5(1):136–44.

30. Thuroff JW, Riedmiller H, Fisch M, et al. Surgery illustrated - surgical atlas mainz Pouch continent cutaneous diversion. BJU Int 2010;1830–54.

31. Stout TE, Roth JD, Gor RA, et al. Technique and outcomes of hand-assist laparoscopic continent cutaneous ileocecocystoplasty. Urology 2021;152: 200.

32. Higuchi T, Yamaguchi Y, Wood HM, et al. 238: Transperineal closure of the male urethra in the setting of suprapubic diversion - an alternative management for urinary incontinence. J Urol 2012;187(4S):e98.

33. Kavanaugh A, Afshar K, Scott H, et al. Bladder neck closure in conjunction with enterocystoplasty and mitrofanoff diversion for complex incontinence: closing the door for good. J Urol 2012;188:1561–6.

34. Birkhauser FD, Zehnder P, Roth B, et al. Irrigation of continent catheterizable ileal pouches: tap water can replace sterile solutions because it is safe, easy, and economical. Eur Urol 2011;59(4):518–23.

35. Loftus CJ, Moore DC, Cohn JA, et al. Postoperative Complications of Patients With Spina Bifida Undergoing Urologic Laparotomy: A Multi-institutional Analysis. Urology 2017;108:233–6. Epub 2017 Jun 21. PMID: 28647562.

36. Hampson LA, Baradaran N, Elliott SP. Long-term complications of continent catheterizable channels: a problem for transitional urologists. Transl Androl Urol 2018;7(4):558–66.

37. Mickelson JJ, Yerkes EB, Meyer T, et al. L stent for stomal stenosis in catheterizable channels. J Urol 2009;182:1786–91. https://doi.org/10.1016/j.juro.2009.02.068. Available at.

38. Pagliara TJ, Gor RA, Liberman D, et al. Outcomes of revision surgery for difficult to catheterize continent channels in a multi-institutional cohort of adults. Can Urol Assoc J 2018;12(3):E126–31.

39. Venugopal S, Mangera A, Molokwu C, et al. Injection of Leaking Mitrofanoff Channel with Bulking Agent: A Minimally Invasive Technique Videourology 2014; 28(6). https://doi.org/10.1089/vid.2014.0020.

40. Roth CC, Donovan BO, Tonkin JB, et al. Endoscopic injection of submucosal bulking agents for the management of incontinent catheterizable channels. J Pediatr Urol 2009;5:265–8.

41. Metcalfe PD, Cain MP, Kaefer M, et al. What is the need for additional bladder surgery after bladder augmentation in childhood? J Urol 2006;176(4S):1801–5.

42. Husmann DA. Long-term complications following bladder augmentations in patients with spina bifida: bladder calculi, perforation of the augmented bladder and upper tract deterioration. Transl Androl Urol 2016;5(1):3–11.

Patient Selection and Outcomes of Urinary Diversion

Kevin J. Hebert, MD, Rano Matta, MD, MSc, MASc, Jeremy B. Myers, MD*

KEYWORDS

- Urinary diversion • Ileal conduit • Preoperative conditioning • Risk assessment
- Intraoperative complication

KEY POINTS

- Preoperative albumin is an important component of nutritional screening and preoperative risk stratification.
- In patients with a history of pelvic radiation, transverse colon is an alternative that is outside of the pelvic radiation field.
- Malnutrition and low albumin may increase the risk of anastomotic leak and in high-risk anastomoses. In a colonic or ileocecal anastomosis in a patient with malnutrition, a proximal fecal diversion may be wise.

INTRODUCTION

Urinary diversions are an integral component of extirpative pelvic surgery, neurogenic bladder management, and urinary reconstruction. Yet appropriate diversion selection and patient optimization by the urologic surgeon can be difficult to navigate given varying surgical indications, baseline patient characteristics, and postoperative expectations. In this article, we aim to provide a comprehensive review covering preoperative optimization, perioperative considerations, and postoperative expectations associated with urinary diversion selection.

URINARY DIVERSION OVERVIEW

Developing a full understanding of the types of urinary diversions is integral to adequately counsel patients preoperatively. Although many variations exist, urinary diversions can be divided into two broad categories: conduits and continent reservoirs.

Conduits

Ileal conduit

The ileal conduit (IC) is the most common form of urinary diversion due to the availability of ileum, surgeon comfort, and decreased operative time compared with other forms of diversion.[1,2] Relative contraindications include a history of inflammatory small bowel disease, extensive prior small bowel resection, and prior abdominal/pelvic radiation. The operative principles include (1) preoperative stoma marking, (2) conduit segment identification, (3) ileoileostomy, (4) ureteroenteric anastomosis, and (5) urostomy creation (**Fig. 1**A–E).

Colon conduit

Colon segments (transverse and sigmoid) are less frequently used for urinary diversion because of higher complication rates and less familiarity of the surgical technique. However, colon conduits afford unique advantages over ileum. First, functional loss of ileum in the setting of inflammatory bowel disease or prior small bowel resections

Genitourinary Injury and Reconstructive Urology, Department of Surgery (Urology), University of Utah, 30 North 1900 East, Room # 3B420, Salt Lake City, UT 84132, USA
* Corresponding author.
E-mail address: Jeremy.myers@hsc.utah.edu

Urol Clin N Am 49 (2022) 533–551
https://doi.org/10.1016/j.ucl.2022.04.011

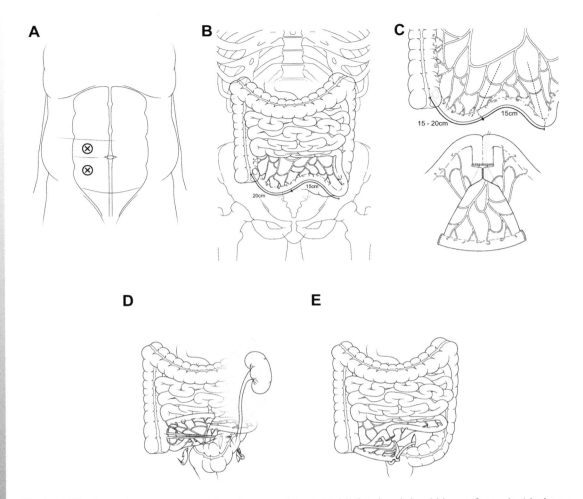

Fig. 1. (*A*) The importance of preoperative stoma marking is highlighted and should be performed with the patient in a seated position. Bilateral stoma sites should be marked in a visible location for the patient while avoiding skin folds. The sites should be mid-rectus to decrease the risk of parastomal hernia. (*B*) After identifying the terminal ileum, a 20 cm segment is measured proximally and serves as the distal limb of the future ileoileostomy. A second 15 to 20 cm segment proximal to this will become the IC. (*C*) The IC segment is based on a robust vascular pedicle identified through transillumination of the mesentery. The bowel is transected with a stapling device and the mesentery is divided with a sealing device. The conduit is placed below the ileoileostomy which is performed in a hand-sewn or stapled fashion. Last, the mesenteric defect is closed to prevent internal hernia. (*D*) The kidney and ureter are shown posterior to the descending colon. The left ureter is tunneled under the sigmoid colon mesentery caudal to the inferior mesenteric artery to allow a tension-free ureteroenteric anastomosis to the IC. If ureteral length is an issue, the inferior mesenteric artery may be ligated to improve mobility of the ureter. (*E*) The IC is shown below the ileoileostomy following bilateral ureteroenteric anastomosis which can be performed in a Bricker fashion (as shown) or via the Wallace approach.

may render use of ileum not possible for diversion or increase the risk of short-gut. Prior abdominal or pelvic radiation can result in poor tissue quality. Conversely, transverse colon is often outside of the radiation field in this setting and is a good alternative bowel segment. Proximal ureteral strictures or distal radiation injury to the ureters can require proximal transection of the ureter, making a ureteroenteric anastomosis difficult or impossible when performing an IC. The use of transverse colon in

this setting allows anastomosis of the conduit to either renal pelvis directly without having to tunnel the conduit under the mesentery.

Sigmoid colon can also be used in specific circumstances. When an abdominopelvic or low anterior resection is being performed, a segment of sigmoid colon proximal to the resection can be used for colon conduit creation with an end colostomy performed proximal to this utilizing the ascending or transverse colon. The benefit for the patient is avoidance of the perioperative morbidity of a bowel anastomosis.

When a patient requires urinary diversion in the setting of having a prior colostomy, a colon switch is advantageous. In this setting, the prior colostomy is converted into a colon conduit urinary diversion by transecting the colostomy at the desired urinary conduit length. A ureteroenteric anastomosis is performed to the new colon conduit, and a new colostomy site is matured in a different location using the colon proximal to the site of transection (**Fig. 2**A–E). This also allows the patient to avoid the perioperative morbidity associated with a bowel anastomosis.

When performing a colon conduit urinary diversion, there are several unique operative considerations including the larger, but less frequent vascular arcades (**Fig. 3**) when compared with blood supply to the ileum. Likewise, with the decreased number of vascular arcades, there is a significant dependency of arterial flow on the arc of Drummond. Watershed areas include the distal two-third of the transverse colon which is the boundary of the superior mesenteric and inferior mesenteric arteries and the sigmoid colon which is the boundary of the inferior mesenteric artery and hypogastric artery. When transverse colon is used, complete mobilization of the ascending/descending colon and release of the omentum from the transverse colon is integral to ensure a tension-free bowel anastomosis (**Fig. 4**A–D).

Continent Diversions

Orthotopic neobladder

The orthotopic neobladder has been increasing utilization over the past two decades and provides unique benefits to the appropriately selected patient.[1,3,4] The ability to avoid a urostomy appliance and store urine can hold significant value from a quality-of-life perspective. However, this must be balanced with the high rates of urinary incontinence and urinary retention most frequently seen in the female population.[5] Thus, it is integral to ensure patients understand these risks and are both willing and able to catheterize via the urethra if necessary postoperatively. Relative contraindications include preoperative eGlomerular filtration rate (GFR) <40,[6] prior radiation therapy, and inflammatory small bowel disease. However, positive urethral margin and urethral stricture disease are the only absolute contraindications. Although multiple variations of the neobladder exist, the basic principles include the (1) isolation of ~60 cm of bowel 20 cm proximal to the terminal ileum, (2) hand-sewn or stapled ileoileostomy, and (3) folding of the 60 cm bowel segment while in some iterations of the neobladder preserving a 10 to 15 cm afferent limb to reduce reflux (**Fig. 5**A–C).

Continent catheterizable pouches

The Indiana pouch (right colon pouch) is the most commonly used continent catheterizable pouch with slight variations including the Florida and Miami pouch. The use of terminal ileum as a catheterizable channel with a plicating ileocecal valve provides a continence mechanism with low rates of postoperative incontinence.[7–11] Alternative intestinal segments for channel creation include the appendix and Yang-Monti ileal channel. Limitations include a steep learning curve, lack of surgeon experience, and high rates of revision surgery.[11] However, the Indiana pouch provides an alternative for patients seeking a continent reservoir who are not candidates for orthotopic neobladder or who are unwilling to accept the potential risk of incontinence or need for urethral catheterization associated with the orthotopic neobladder. Surgical principles include (1) isolation of 25 cm of cecum/ascending colon with 12 cm of terminal ileum; (2) ileocolonic hand-sewn or stapled anastomosis; (3) creating a defunctionalized spherical reservoir, efferent channel creation; (4) plicating the ileocecal valve; (5) tapering the ileal channel; and (6) ensuring ability to catheterize the pouch (**Fig. 6**A, B).

PREOPERATIVE OPTIMIZATION
Preoperative Evaluation and Optimization

Standard preoperative assessment for patients undergoing urinary diversion includes a review of the patient's non-modifiable and modifiable characteristics. Non-modifiable factors include age, some comorbidities, surgical history, and prior cancer therapies including radiation. Modifiable factors include underlying cardiovascular or respiratory comorbidities and metabolic derangements due to underlying chronic kidney disease or diabetes.

Frailty Assessment

Besides standard preoperative assessment, there has been growing evidence to support the evaluation and improvement of physiologic reserves, including patient nutrition and functional capacity before surgery. This includes evaluation of a patient's "frailty," namely their ability to cope with stressors resulting in disability, increased health care utilization, and mortality. Frailty is associated with morbidity and mortality following urologic surgery,[12] and preoperative frailty assessment

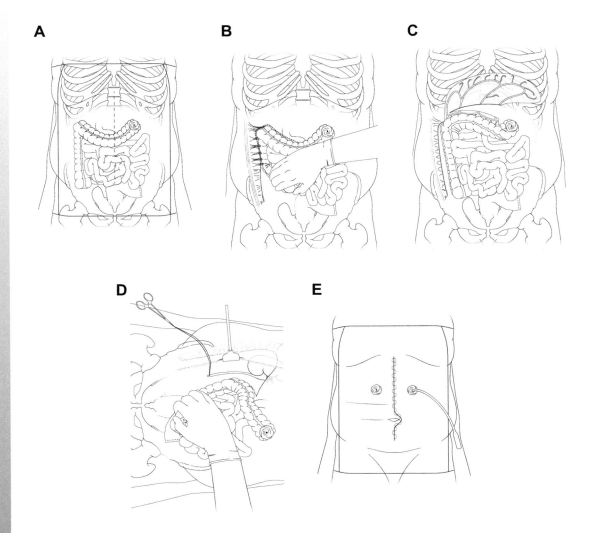

Fig. 2. (*A*) Patients with a prior end colostomy as shown are candidates for a colon switch urinary diversion. In this setting, the transverse colon and existing end colostomy are repurposed into a colon conduit, although the ascending colon proximal to this is refashioned into an end colostomy. (*B*) The right colon and cecum are mobilized in standard fashion up to the hepatic flexure. At the level of the transverse colon, the omentum is mobilized to completely free the remaining attachments. (*C*) The omentum is completely mobilized from the transverse colon using a sealing device. (*D*) The colon is positioned to determine the best location for transection. If inadequate ureteral length is present due to stricture or radiation injury, the colon can be directly anastomosed to the renal pelvis. The colon is transected using a stapling device, and a ureterocolonic anastomosis is performed in standard fashion. (*E*) The prior colostomy is now a urostomy in the left upper quadrant with a new end colostomy in the right upper quadrant.

enables a more accurate measurement of operative risk.[13]

Prehabilitation

There has been a clinical impetus to intervene for frailty in the perioperative setting to improve patient outcomes. This is termed "prehabilitation," which is a multimodal approach to evaluating and improving a patient's condition with the aim of reducing the incidence and severity of perioperative and postoperative impairments.

For patients undergoing urinary diversion, nutrition is an important component to consider. Patients undergoing urinary diversion are often elderly and may have poor nutritional status due to comorbidities and decreased oral intake. Patients with a history of cancer or active malignancy may experience tumor- or treatment-induced anorexia and catabolic tumor effects. Poor

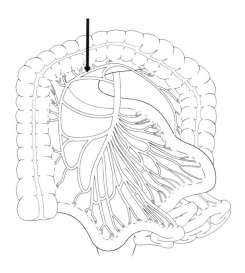

Fig. 3. Key differences in bowel vascular are highlighted with smaller and more frequent vessels noted in the ileum compared with larger and less frequent vessels in the large bowel which depends heavily on the artery of Drummond (*arrow*). The less frequent vessels in the large bowel allow deeper transection of the mesentery for improved mobility.

nutritional status will lead to sarcopenia, which is a predictor of increased morbidity,[14] longer hospital stay,[15] and decreased cancer specific and overall survival in patients with bladder cancer undergoing radical cystectomy (RC).[16] In addition, urinary diversion and the postoperative recovery can further deplete the nutritional stores for a patient. Mathur and colleagues evaluated patients undergoing RC and found that patients experienced a 7% loss in body protein during the first 2 weeks postoperatively, and they only regained 63% of this by 6 weeks.[17] A significant attention has been given to the importance of preoperative albumin as a surrogate of preoperative nutrition and predictor of postoperative morbidity. Patients with hypoalbuminemia (<3.5 g/dL) before RC have worse survival.[18,19] In patients undergoing colorectal surgery, hypoalbuminemia is associated with increased major and minor postoperative complications including postoperative ileus and anastomotic leak (AL). The American Society for Parenteral and Enteral Nutrition's Clinical Guidelines recommends not using albumin alone.[20] The American College of Surgeons (ACS) recommends using additional screening tools in addition to albumin, including a four-question nutrition risk assessment.[21] Such tools can identify malnourished patients who require

further evaluation and treatment by a dietician during the perioperative period. For patients undergoing urinary diversion, there is still limited evidence supporting preoperative oral nutrition support. In a randomized trial of 61 patients receive either multivitamins or enriched oral nutrition supplement 4 weeks pre-RC and post-RC, the intervention group was protected against the development of postoperative sarcopenia.[22] However, there was no effect on postoperative complications. Surgery disrupts cell-mediated immunity and the balance of T-helper1/T-helper2 cells, resulting in exaggerated adaptive immune suppression and inflammatory response. Perioperative immune-nutrition (IN) is a dietary supplement that is thought to modulate the immune system perturbations during surgical stress. The most studied nutrients are glutamine, arginine, and omega-3 fatty acids. In gastrointestinal cancers, there have been several postoperative benefits identified in patients receiving perioperative immunonutrition, including decreased postoperative infection and AL.[23] However, there has been a limited evidence of IN benefits after RC. Hamilton-Reeves et al. evaluated the postoperative effects of IN with arginine or standard oral nutritional supplements for 5 days before and 5 days after RC in 29 patients.[24] They observed no difference in 30-day postoperative morbidity, although IN lowered the infection rate at 90 days. In contrast, Lyon and colleagues found no difference in postoperative complications when comparing 40 patients that received IN versus 104 patients from a historical control cohort receiving RC.[25] A recent Cochrane review of all the studies evaluating perioperative nutrition surrounding RC concluded that there was limited low-quality evidence for a benefit of perioperative nutrition interventions.[26]

Exercise and preoperative physical conditioning are also thought to be beneficial after urinary diversion. Poor cardiopulmonary reserve has been shown to be a significant predictor of prolong length of stay and 90-day complications after RC.[27,28] A systematic review of exercise programs implemented before intrabdominal surgery found they can decrease incidence of postoperative complications.[29] Exercise programs alone before RC have demonstrated improvement in functional capacity, although have not been shown to change postoperative outcomes.[30]

Multimodal preoperative conditioning programs combine exercise training, nutritional therapy, and psychological interventions. Such a multimodal strategy, Strong for Surgery, has also been promoted by the ACS for colorectal surgery.[21] The evidence for such an approach is limited. A recent randomized clinical trial of multimodal

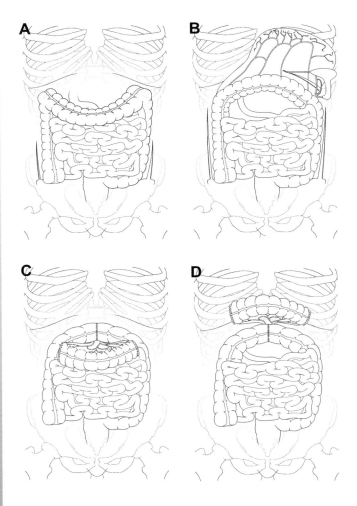

Fig. 4. (*A*) The ascending and descending colon are completely mobilized including the cecum and distal ileum to allow a tension-free bowel anastomosis. (*B*) After mobilizing the colon bilaterally, the omentum is dissected of the transverse colon which maximizes mobility of the colon conduit as well as a tension-free bowel anastomosis. (*C*) The colon conduit can be dropped below the bowel anastomosis (shown here) or raised above the bowel anastomosis (shown in Fig. 4D). If dropped below the anastomosis as shown here, the ureter must be tunneled through the mesentery to reach the conduit. (*D*) The conduit is shown above the bowel anastomosis. This approach allows direct anastomosis to the renal pelvis in the setting of proximal ureteral stricture or radiation injury without having to tunnel the ureter or conduit through the mesentery.

prehabilitation compared with postoperative rehabilitation in patients undergoing RC found that there was an earlier recovery of postoperative walking ability, although no difference after 8 weeks. Moreover, there was no difference in 30-day complications, length of stay, hospital readmissions, or emergency department visits.[31]

KEY POINTS PREOPERATIVE OPTIMIZATION

- Does the patient have any modifiable risk factors that can be improved before surgery?
- If possible, a frailty assessment should be performed in the preoperative setting
- Preoperative albumin is an important component of nutritional screening and preoperative risk stratification
- Consider consultation with dietician for patients at risk of malnutrition

PERIOPERATIVE CONSIDERATIONS
Irradiated Bowel Segments

Urinary diversion after radiation therapy involves significantly higher rates of complications when compared with RC in radiation naïve patients.[20,32] While IC urinary diversion is the standard approach in most cases,[32,33] ileum may not be suitable if it was in the irradiated field. There has been long-term experience with transverse colon conduits, which have proven to be a safe option in patients receiving large doses of pelvic radiation,[34] as the transverse colon is typically outside the radiation field.

Among patients receiving continent urinary diversion, use of the ileocecal reservoir (Mainz I) in irradiated patients has been associated with a high rate of serious complications when compared with nonirradiated patients, including failure of continence mechanism, ureteral complications,

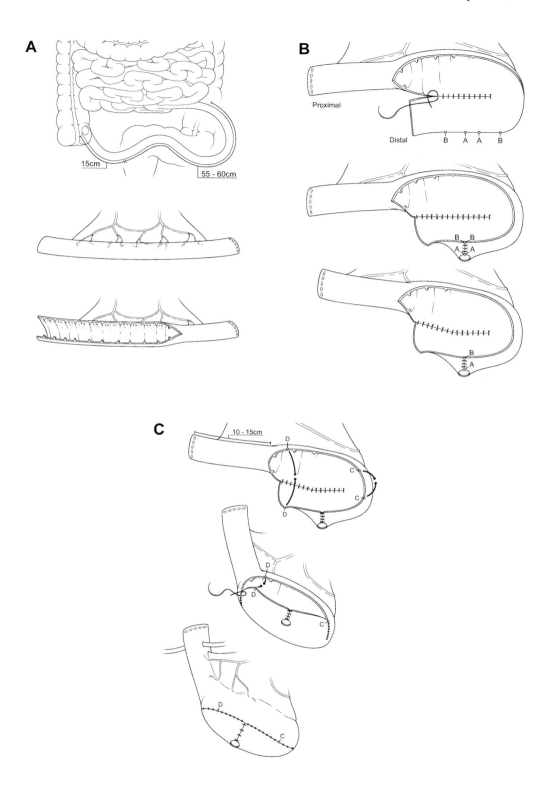

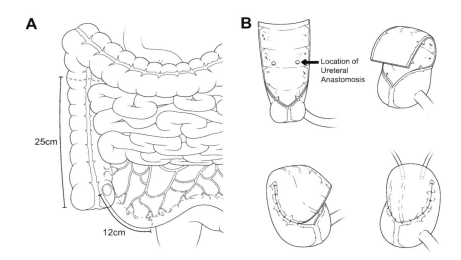

Fig. 6. (*A*) 25 cm segment of ascending colon and cecum is mobilized including a 12 cm segment of terminal ileum. (*B*) The ascending colon and cecum are detubularized on the antimesenteric surface, 1 cm lateral the free taenia (*upper left*). The after performing the ureterocolonic anastomosis, the colon is folded craniocaudally (*upper right*). The suture line is then completed laterally to medially from each side as shown. The channel is plicated and tapered in standard fashion.

and stomal complications.[35] In contrast, in our analysis of 53 patients undergoing a right colon pouch (ie, Indiana pouch), there was an increased risk of readmission associated with higher body mass index (BMI) (mean 30.7 vs 25.9, $P = 0.012$) and prior abdominal surgery (83.3% vs 55.2%, $P = 0.029$).[11] A history of radiation was not associated with major complications, 90-day readmission, or major reoperation. Others have reported the similar results, for instance, Salom and colleagues found no increase in complications after right colon pouch creation in patients who received pelvic radiation.[36] In contrast, when we looked at patients undergoing all types of urinary diversion, who had true radiation injury stemming from the treatment of gynecologic cancer, we found a rate of bowel or urinary fistula of 20%.[37]

In addition, Wilkin and colleagues found that the right colon pouch (ie, Indiana pouch) has an increased risk of ureteral complications, incontinence, and renal insufficiency in radiated patients compared with nonradiated patients.[38] This is likely related to radiation damage of the distal ureteral blood supply and ileocecal valve. Despite contradictory evidence, many reconstructive surgeons are cautious about offering continent diversion after abdominal radiation. In our practice, we offer right colon pouch urinary diversions to patients with localized radiation therapy, such as prostate cancer treatment; however, we are very cautious about offering this when a patient has a history of radiation injury and more diffuse radiation treatment fields that could have affected the small bowel, such as treatment for gynecologic

Fig. 5. (*A*) ~60 cm segment of ileum is isolated 15 to 20 cm proximal to the terminal ileum. The distal segment is opened on the antimesenteric border. In some neobladders, the proximal 10 to 15 cm is not detubularized (shown here) and serves as an afferent limb to which the ureteral anastomosis is performed. (*B*) The proximal limb is folded across the detubularized segment creating a "J" configuration. The backwall (*top*) is then completed in a running, locking fashion. As this suture line will be obscured by the mesentery, it is imperative to ensure this is performed in a watertight fashion. The dependent portion of the neobladder is determined by pulling the bowel to the previously transected urethra. A neourethra for the future anastomosis is created over a 24 French sound (*middle*). The front wall of the neobladder is then run away from the neourethra in a perpendicular fashion (*bottom*). (*C*) Once the front wall is partially completed, the neourethra to urethra anastomosis is performed in a running or interrupted fashion over a catheter (*top*). A key step is to perform part of the front wall suture line (A to B) prior to performing the urethral anastomosis as this can be difficult to reach under the pubic bone. The neobladder is then folded cranio-caudally (D to D and C to C). The front wall is then completed with the resulting the resulting "T" configuration (*bottom*). Before completion of the front wall, the ureteroenteric anastomosis is performed in standard fashion.

malignancy. In addition, it is important to recognize that there may be a difference in patients what have had radiation and those with a true radiation injury. There may be something very different in somatic health, or the genetic milieu of patients that have sustained a high-grade radiation injury that put them at higher risk for bowel or urinary complications compared with patients that have just had radiation but not sustained an injury. The knowledge gaps surrounding radiation therapy and postoperative risks highlight the importance of preoperative discussion of all urinary diversion options and the patient acknowledging that intraoperative evaluation may necessitate alternative decisions.

The transverse ascending colon or transverse descending colon pouches (Mainz III), although rare, may have relatively low rates of complications, with the efferent segment created from a tapered segment of bowel. Leissner and colleagues found that among a small cohort of 36 patients, only two experienced incontinence, which was resolved with creation of a new efferent segment, and no patients experienced ureteral complications.[39] The benefit of using transverse colon for both continent and non-continent urinary diversion is its proximity to the proximal ureter where it can be attached up to the renal pelvis while also providing a choice of lateral abdominal location of the stoma.

Obesity and stomas
Stomal complications after creation of urinary diversion include stomal stenosis, parastomal hernia, and stomal prolapse. Obesity has been shown to be a significant predictor of stomal complications. Among patients undergoing IC diversion, patients who experienced stomal complications had a significantly higher BMI (26.5 vs 30.8 kg/m2; $P = 0.012$).[40]

Conduit stoma maturation can be difficult due to thick abdominal wall, bulky mesentery, or poor bowel compliance due to radiation. Several techniques to creating a stoma in an obese patient have been described: using a Turnbull (loop) stoma[41,42] (**Fig. 7**), performing panniculectomy at the time of IC diversion,[42,43] and creating a non-everted stoma.[44] Miller and colleagues found that using a non-everted stoma maturation technique in a cohort with a mean BMI of 30.2 provided a good stoma protuberance in 83% of patients with few stoma complications.[44]

Ureteral Considerations

Before urinary diversion, it is important to consider the condition of the ureters as this may affect the type of diversion and selection of bowel segment.

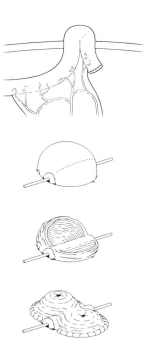

Fig. 7. A loop of ileum at the most mobile point of mesenteric tethering is pulled through the rectus muscle and stoma site in standard fashion. A window is created on the mesenteric side of the ileum with blunt dissection to allow the placement of a rod. The bowel is opened perpendicular to the length of the bowel. The bowel mucosa is approximated to the skin with interrupted absorbable sutures. The rod can be removed on postoperative day 10 to 14.

In patients with radiation damage or other inflammatory conditions, patients may have distal ureteric strictures, which can make ureteral mobilization and ureteroenteric anastomosis difficult. As stated above, one option is to use a longer ileal segment or transverse colon conduit to allow for limited ureteral mobilization and anastomosis directly to the renal pelvis.[34] This is also a feasible approach for patients with a preexisting history of renal stones who may need stone intervention in the future.

Bowel Prep

Ileal anastomosis
A recent metanalysis evaluated randomized studies of limited versus complete bowel prep for ileal anastomoses during RC.[45] Six studies were analyzed and most compared a limited bowel prep or no bowel prep to complete bowel prep with antibiotics and oral laxatives. Although there was a lot of heterogeneity between these studies almost all of the complete bowel prep arms involved oral laxatives and oral antibiotics, the

limited bowel prep or no bowel prep arms did not involve intensive mechanical prep or oral antibiotic administration. The authors of this metanalysis found lessened time to postoperative flatus and bowel movement in the limited bowel prep patients. In addition, there was no difference in AL, mortality, or overall complications in patients with limited bowel prep compared with a complete bowel prep. Likewise, there were slightly higher rates of fever and wound complications in the pooled analysis of patients undergoing a complete bowel prep. The study represents level 1 evidence that at least complete bowel prep that is antibiotic and mechanical is not needed before RC for a planned ileal anastomosis.

Enhanced recovery after surgery (ERAS) pathways have increasingly been adopted throughout the world and have been shown to decrease the length of stay and complications. A key element to most ERAS protocols is omitting bowel preparation when there is a planned ileal anastomosis. In fact, omitting a bowel preparation is one element of ERAS that has been adopted most readily by surgeons performing cystectomy with bowel urinary diversion.[46]

Ileocolic or colon anastomoses

The need for bowel prep for colonic anastomosis has been debated over the last decade. Two recent studies of the National Surgical Quality Improvement Program (NSQIP) showed advantage to antibiotic-based bowel preparation for elective colon surgery.[47,48] Authors found that compared with no bowel preparation, mechanical preparation with or without antibiotics was associated with a lower ileus rate, decreased surgical site infection, lower rates of readmission, and when antibiotics were used in the bowel preparation a lower AL rate. However, at least in one of the studies, those patients in the no bowel preparation group did have higher rates of adverse characteristics, such as steroid use and disseminated cancer.[47]

In contrast, a recent well-designed randomized study was reported in the Lancet, and the authors found in patients undergoing elective colectomy randomized to either no bowel preparation or to a mechanical, antibiotic-based preparation there were no differences in surgical site infections, AL, or other quality measures.[49] The debate about bowel preparation for colectomy no doubt will take some time to resolve; however, during urinary diversion when colon or ileocolic segments are used, it can be challenging to control bowel contamination compared with colectomy. For instance, in creation of a right colon pouch, approximately 25 cm of right colon is opened

longitudinally. A bowel preparation allows irrigation of the segment before opening it and minimizes contamination of the abdomen with stool. Thus, from a practical standpoint, it is our opinion that to complete a urinary diversion, utilizing a colon or ileocolic segment without gross contamination of the abdomen that a full antibiotic-based bowel prep is essential to minimizing complication.

KEY POINTS PERIOPERATIVE CONSIDERATIONS

- In patients with a history of pelvic radiation, transverse colon is an alternative that is outside of the pelvic radiation field. This is also useful in the case of long ureteral strictures.
- Obesity is a predictor of stomal complications.
- Turnbull stomas or flat stomas maneuvers may be used when obesity-related issues prevent maturation of a standard urostomy.
- For routine cystectomy with a planned small bowel anastomosis, no bowel preparation is necessary

POSTOPERATIVE EXPECTATIONS
Bowel Anastomotic Leak Rates and Risk Factors

Ileocolic and colonic leak rates

AL rates after right hemicolectomy and ileocolic anastomoses were recently reported in a large prospective observational study from the European Society of Coloproctology.[50] AL occurred in 7.4% and was in line with other large prospective recent studies.[51,52] AL increased the risk of death from 1.6% to > 10% when present. In this study, 12% of patients did undergo right colectomy for urgent or emergency indications; however, in an adjusted analysis, this did not predict a higher rate of AL. In fact, there were no patient factors that were associated with the increased risk of AL; the increased risk of AL was only associated with surgical factors including stapled versus hand-sewn anastomosis, open surgery versus laparoscopic surgery, and operative time. Hand-sewn anastomoses have been consistently identified in recent studies as being associated with the decreased risk of AL.[46,50,51] This is inconsistent with a Cochrane review on the topic[53]; however, authors note that the recommendations for stapled anastomoses from the Cochrane review were made based on four randomized studies all before 1995, and 75% of the studies were done by the same center. In our hands, we prefer a hand-sewn, two-layer anastomosis for ileocolic and colonic anastomoses and believe this technique offers greater safety compared with stapled anastomosis.

There is limited data in urologic surgery for ileocolic AL. An ileocolic anastomosis is created after right colon pouch or continent cutaneous ileoce-cocystoplasty (CCIC). In one multi-institutional retrospective study, the confirmed AL rate was 3.5%,[54] however, there were four other intrabdominal abscesses requiring drainage or exploration; some if not all should be classified as occult bowel leak, bringing the possible bowel leak rate to 7% which is more in line with series of right colectomy in the general surgery literature. In a recent scoping review of the literature on right colon pouch, the confirmed AL was between 1% and 6%, but there were many deep incisional or organ space infections that were no doubt very heterogenous in their definition and ranged from 4% to 33%.[55] These findings are in line with our series of right colon pouch where the confirmed leak rate was 3.7%, but again there were another 5.6% of patients with deep abscess that was drained postoperatively.[11]

Small bowel anastomotic leak after radical cystectomy

Most of the bowel complications after urinary diversion occur at a small bowel anastomosis, given that almost all patients undergo an IC or neobladder made out of small bowel. Analogous operations with small bowel anastomoses are not as common in general surgery other than in the setting of Crohn's disease or trauma. Therefore, there are no as well-defined morbidity and mortality within the literature. Small bowel AL is likely not as devastating as leaks involving the large bowel but are certain to increase morbidity and mortality. A recent systematic review of perioperative morbidity and mortality reported that the pooled AL rate after RC was only 1.1% in greater than 3000 evaluable patients.[56]

Risk factors for anastomotic leak

Low albumin and malnutrition are one of the leading risk factors for AL defined with the literature and across many different types of bowel anastomoses. Low albumin and malnutrition are not addressed specifically in the urologic literature regarding the risk of AL; however, as reviewed elsewhere in this article, low albumin has been demonstrated in large studies of patients undergoing RC to be associated with increased perioperative complications including death as well as worse disease-free survival.[18,19] Thresholds defining low albumin in these studies were < 3.5 g/dL and < 4 g/dL.

In studies of ileocolic or colonic anastomoses, within the general surgical or gynecologic literature, low preoperative albumin has been linked to the increased risk of AL. In one study of colorectal anastomoses after pelvic exenteration, every 1 gm/dl increased serum albumin was associated with a 62% decreased risk of AL.[57,58] Despite this association, surgeons in this collaborative study did not choose to perform a protective proximal fecal diversion for malnutrition and low albumin and instead chose based on other factors such as multiple bowel resections, hemorrhage, and prior chemotherapy use.[58] In an analysis of the NSQIP database, again low albumin (<4.0 g/dL) had an associated increase in the risk of colorectal AL by 32%.[59] Other factors in this study, as well as other studies, associated with increased risk of AL were age, history of radiation, chronic steroid use, and smoking.

Early Complications

Urinary diversions are associated with significant early (30 days) and late (>30 days) morbidity with up to an 82% reported overall 90-day complication rate.[60] Although most complications are low grade (Clavien I–II), nearly one-third of patients will experience a Clavien IIIa–V complication with readmission rates ranging between 8.6% and 31%.[61,62] Although early complications following urinary diversion have been well described in the literature, there is less robust evidence regarding long-term outcomes and morbidity associated with urinary diversion.

Late Complications

Compared with early complications, late complications more frequently involve small bowel obstruction, development of renal dysfunction, chronic infections (urinary tract infections/pyelonephritis), urolithiasis, and structural-related complications (stomal stenosis, ureteral stricture disease, parastomal hernia/conduit stenosis). Understanding the temporal associations of theses complications is imperative for appropriate survivorship follow-up.

Bowel

Although anastomotic bowel leak and ileus are of significant concern in the early postoperative period, bowel-related late complications are a frequent source of morbidity. In a large single-institution cohort of 1057 patients undergoing RC with ileal or colon conduit diversion, the most frequent source of late morbidity was bowel-related complications (20.3%).[63] Bowel obstruction is the most common morbidity occurring in

16.0% but only required surgical intervention in 7.1% at a median follow-up of 15.5 years.[63] Although, these findings were isolated to patients undergoing going ileal/colon conduit diversion, similar rates of late small bowel obstruction have been reported following continent diversion. In 1565 patients undergoing urinary diversion with 20% representing a diversion other than IC, the 5-year risk of small bowel obstruction was 12.5% with no difference in the rate of small bowel obstruction noted between diversion types.[64]

In addition to small bowel obstruction, intraabdominal abscess formation and enteric fistula development occurred at 3.6% (median 0.9 years) and 2.7% (median 1.9 years), respectively.[63] The similar rates of enteric fistula development (3.2%) were reported when including IC, continent diversion, and other forms of urinary diversion.[64]

Renal

Deterioration of renal function following urinary diversion is common due to bowel mucosa absorption of urine, increased urine dwell time, metabolic changes, and poor drainage. These concerns and preoperative renal function often direct the type of urinary diversion offered to patients. However, high rates of baseline comorbidities in this patient population and the multifactorial nature of renal function decline in the postoperative period have made this difficult to study. Furthermore, varying definitions of renal function decline and the unknown clinical significance of these outcomes make interpretation of these data difficult.

Shimko and colleagues reported renal function-related complications in 20.2% of patients at a median 2.2 years after surgery.[63] The authors point out the high rates of preexisting renal dysfunction in this population as 6.9% of their cohort had a preoperative creatinine of 2.0 mg/dL or higher. However, 19.0% of patients without a history of renal dysfunction went on to develop chronic kidney disease (defined >2.0 mg/dL) with 2.5% going on to renal replacement therapy.[63] Renal failure was noted in 4.04%, 3.57%, and 7.45% of patients undergoing IC, continent diversion, and other diversion, respectively.[64] However, the definition of renal failure was not provided by the authors. These studies are limited in their assessment of renal function following urinary diversion as they inadequately control for comorbidities and normal age-related changes that frequently contribute to progressive loss of renal function.

A more granular assessment of renal function following IC diversion and continent diversion in 1383 patients with preoperative chronic kidney disease stages 2 and 3a was performed by Gershman and colleagues[65] In patients presenting with Chronic kidney disease (CKD) stage 2, a 10 point or greater decline in renal function was noted in 40% and 81% of patients at 1 and 10 years follow-up, respectively. Interestingly, patients presenting with CKD state 3a displayed less decline in renal function with 22% and 70% of patients experiencing a 10 point or greater decline at 1 and 10 years follow-up, respectively.[65] Although progressive decline in renal function was reported, urinary diversion choice (incontinent vs continent) was not associated with loss of renal function.[64] Faraj and colleagues also noted the progressive loss of renal function in 563 patients undergoing IC and neobladder urinary diversion with mean eGFR reduction at 5 years of 14% and 17%, respectively.[66] Time from surgery may also impact the rate of loss of renal function. In a study of 1631 patients undergoing urinary diversion, patients receiving continent diversions had a higher median eGFR preoperatively.[67] When followed postoperatively, this difference was maintained for 7 years at which point no statistical difference in median renal function was noted.[67] By 10-year follow-up, the risk of renal function decline was 71% and 74% in those electing for continent versus incontinent diversion, respectively.[67] However, these findings should be interpreted in the context of age-associated declines in renal function of 1 mL/min/m^2 per year starting in the third decade of life.[68]

Studies to date have not shown a difference in postoperative renal function based on diversion choice. However, the literature reinforces the importance of long-term cancer survivorship follow-up due to the high rate of progressive renal dysfunction and the multifactorial contribution of many modifiable risk factors such as recurrent infection, hypertension, hydronephrosis, and ureteroenteric anastomotic stricture.[67]

Diversion complications

Structural-related morbidity following conduit diversions leads to significant quality-of-life issues for patients. Poor urostomy location, body habitus, and parastomal hernia formation can lead to chronic urine leakage and skin changes. Parastomal hernia development is the most common structural complication occurring in 13.9% to 28.1% of patients at a median 2.3 years postoperatively.[40,63,69–71] Studies assessing the incidence of parastomal hernia following colon conduit are very limited with a single study reporting a rate of 2.4%.[72] Compared with parastomal hernia, stomal stenosis following IC diversion occurs at lower frequency with a reported rate of 2.1%.[63] It is imperative to recognize that although patients may be asymptomatic with stoma-related conditions, progressive loss of renal function can occur due to obstructive uropathy.

Catheterizable continent reservoirs present with frequent structural-related complications. Cutaneous stenosis (6%), channel stricture (6%), stomal prolapse (5%), and leakage (9%) are frequently reported and are often sources of operative revision in up to 22.7% of ileal channels and 17.2% of appendiceal channels.[7,73] In a multicenter review of 114 adult patients undergoing CCIC, 20.2% required catheter channel revision within 90 days of surgery.[54] O'Conner and colleagues reported stomal complications in adults with continent catheterizable channels in 165 patients with a median age of 42 years and median follow-up of 60 months.[7] The 55% of patients had difficulty catheterizing. Of those with ileal channels 22.7% developed channel stenosis while 17.2% with appendiceal channels developed stenosis.[7] Revision surgery was common, with 41% undergoing superficial channel revision and 38.7% undergoing complete channel replacement.[7] The continent catheterizable colon pouch is undoubtedly an excellent urinary diversion in appropriately selected patients. However, its higher morbidity and reoperation rates reinforce the importance of adequate preoperative counseling.

In attempt to mitigate postoperative structural complications, we have found the following intraoperative maneuvers helpful. We routinely reinforce the ileocecal valve by intussuscepting the channel into cecum using buttressing sutures placed through windows of Deaver.[74] Plicating sutures over the anterior surface of this portion of the channel serve to improve continence by increasing pressure on the channel as the pouch fills. Progressively tightened imbricating stitches are placed near the ileocecal valve to help funnel the catheter to the ileocecal valve. After placing theses sutures, the channel is catheterized to ensure patency, and appropriate resistance is present at the plicated valve. We refer to this technique as the Utah-Anti-incontinence Reinforced Channel Hitch. In addition, channel redundancy should be resected and the channel should be tailored to the patient's body habitus. When the channel is localized at the umbilicus, a parastomal hernia is common unless the channel is brought through the rectus just to the right and lateral to the umbilical stalk. Last, we take care to bring the ileocolic bowel anastomosis medially and fix this in place; this maneuver prevents the bowel anastomosis from slipping lateral to the pouch, which seems to be its natural tendency, and the maneuver also prevents small bowel from traveling outside the natural "bowel" of the large bowel mesentery. Similarly, we take care to close windows that are created posterior to the pouch by reconstructing the incision in the posterior right peritoneum, as well as shutting down all potential windows, such as the window between the course of the catheterizable channel and the abdominal wall, which could lead to an internal small bowel herniation, obstruction, or strangulation.

Urolithiasis

Urolithiasis is a common source of morbidity following urinary diversion surgery and occurs more frequently in continent diversions due to the increased urine dwell time. Rates of stone disease following urinary conduit diversion range from 4.6% to 15.3% and occur with increased frequency in the upper tracts (13.3%) compared with the conduit (4.5%).[63,64,75] Rates of stone formation in the continent diversions occur in 8.9% to 10.4%.[64,76,77]

Ureteral stricture

Ureteroenteric stricture following urinary diversion has been well documented with reported rates ranging between 4.2% and 19% with a median time to presentation ranging from 5.3 to 7.5 months.[78–82] The most likely etiology for stricture development is ischemia and tissue manipulation which is supported by higher rates of left-sided strictures as more extensive mobilization is necessary to tunnel the ureter under the colonic mesentery and a greater length of ureter is needed with a higher likelihood of distal ureteric ischemia. Stratifying stricture incidence by laterality shows the percentage of left-sided involvement ranging from 63.8% to 70.0%.[82,83] When assessing for potential ureteroenteric stricture disease, it is imperative to consider malignant obstruction which typically presents later (32.4 months).[82] However, late benign stricture development is not uncommon, occurring in up to 5% of patients 10 years after diversion again highlighting the importance of sustained survivorship follow-up.[84] Given the implications for loss of renal function, infection, sepsis, and inability to perform upper tract surveillance, there has been a significant interest in risk factor identification for ureteroenteric anastomotic strictures.

Patient-specific risk factors have been assessed in retrospective series with urine leak, urinary tract infection, Clavien III or greater postoperative complication, and high BMI inferring the greater risk of postoperative stricture formation.[78,79,85,86] The assessment of 2888 patients with a prior history of RC also showed American society of Anesthiologists score > 2, LN positive disease, and prior abdominal surgery to increase risk of Ureter-oenteric (UE) stricture occurrence.[79] Last, Hautmann and colleagues reported preoperative ureteral dilation increased UE stricture rates with up to 19.3% going on to develop stricture disease within 10 years compared with 6.4% in those without preoperative dilation.[87]

Risk factors related to the operative approach have also been studied including anastomosis type (Wallace/Bricker [**Fig. 8**A, B], running vs interrupted suture, suture type) without clear differences in risk.[88] As most strictures are thought to be related to ischemia, the impact of length of ureteral resection before anastomosis was reviewed by Richards and colleagues but was not found to decrease UE stricture rates postoperatively.[86] The effect of robotic-assisted RC has also been evaluated but has been difficult to assess due to the high rates of extracorporeal urinary diversion. In a study of 478 patients undergoing open RC (375) and robotic RC with extracorporeal diversion (103), no difference in postoperative UE stricture rates was noted, 8.5% versus 12.6%, respectively.[80] These findings were reinforced by Ericson and colleagues who compared UE stricture rates between open RC (279 patients), robotic RC with extracorporeal diversion (382 patients), and robotic RC with intracorporeal diversion (307 patients) with reported UE stricture rates of 9.3%, 11.3%, and 13%, respectively.[89] It is often argued that the steep learning curve of intracorporeal urinary diversion artificially increases the rates of UE stricture. This viewpoint is logical and is supported in a subgroup analysis of the first 75 intracorporal diversions compared with the last 232

diversions as a drop in stricture incidence from 17.5% to 4.9% was noted, respectively.[89] The relative high rates of UE stricture formation have produced further interest in intraoperative measures that may decrease postoperative UE stricture rates.

Near-infrared fluorescence imaging (NIFI) for real-time assessment of tissue perfusion has been used in colorectal surgery with reduction in ischemia-related complications.[90] As this technology is available for both open and robotic applications, there has been a significant interest in the utility of this technology in the assessment of ureteral perfusion. Following intravenous indocyanine green injection, a near-infrared laser is used to assess for perfusion which is displayed on the surgeon console. Perfusion is then assessed based on the degree of enhancement. (**Fig. 9**) Shen assessed the impact of NIFI before UE anastomosis and found 34.4% of distal ureters showed decreased perfusion.[91] Although 7.5% of patients developed strictures when NIFI was not used, 0 of 97 patients went on to develop a stricture when NIFI was used.[91] Similar findings were noted by Ahmadi and colleagues with 0/47 patients developing strictures with NIFI use in the robotic setting compared with 14 of 132 (10.6%) without NIFI utilization.[92] The only other available study showed more modest results in open urinary diversion with 3.2% stricture rate with use of NIFI compared with 16.7% without use of NIFI.[93] These data should be viewed with healthy skepticism until larger, multi-institutional studies are peer-reviewed with similar findings. However, this technique holds significant promise as stricture reduction would significantly

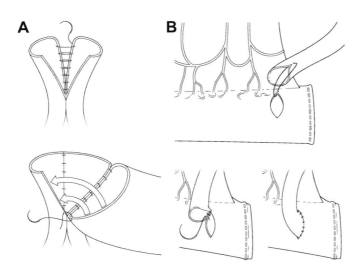

Fig. 8. (*A*) The Wallace anastomosis allows both ureters to be anastomosed to the urinary diversion. The medial aspect of each ureter is sutured together using fine absorbable suture. The backwall of the ureter is then sutured to the bowel. The anastomosis is completed by suturing the front wall in a similar fashion. This can often be performed at the butt end of the conduit to eliminate a suture line as shown. (*B*) The Bricker anastomosis is performed by anastomosing each ureter to the diversion independently. The site of anastomosis should be staggered along the length of the diversion to improve blood supply to the anastomosis.

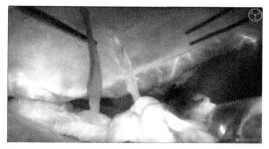

Fig. 9. After administration of indocyanine green, vascular perfusion can be assessed using near-infrared light. In this image, the right ureter displays good perfusion as indicated by increased enhancement. This is compared to the left distal ureter which shows poor enhancement and thus poor perfusion.

reduce postoperative morbidity and health care utilization.

KEY POINTS POSTOPERATIVE EXPECTATIONS

- Small bowel anastomoses are low risk for anastomotic leak.
- Ileocolic and colonic bowel anastomoses have higher anastomotic leak rates and when leaks occur the morbidity and mortality is high.
- Malnutrition and low albumin may increase the risk of anastomotic leak and in high-risk anastomoses. In a colonic or ileocecal anastomosis in a patient with malnutrition, a proximal fecal diversion may be wise.
- The most common late complications are bowel related followed by loss of renal function.
- Benign ureteral strictures most commonly present within 1 year of surgery.
- Evolving technology like near-infrared fluorescent imaging may reduce ureteroenteric strictures but requires additional multi-institutional studies.

SUMMARY

Urinary diversions will continue to be associated with significant morbidity despite a wide range of diversion options because of the comorbid patient population, poor baseline nutritional and functional status, and the frequent need of a bowel anastomosis which increases both early and late morbidity. However, careful preoperative planning and risk stratification can moderate perioperative risks. Evolving technology including NIFI is promising but requires higher volume studies to support their use.

DISCLOSURE

The authors have no conflicts of interest or pertinent disclosures to related to this article.

CLINICS CARE POINTS

- Ileocolic and colonic bowel anastomoses have higher anastomotic leak rates and when leaks occur the morbidity and mortality is high.
- The most common late complications are bowel related followed by loss of renal function.
- Benign ureteral strictures most commonly present within 1 year of surgery.

REFERENCES

1. Almassi N, Bochner BH. Ileal conduit or orthotopic neobladder: selection and contemporary patterns of use. Curr Opin Urol 2020;30(3):415–20.
2. Maurice MJ, Kim SP, Abouassaly R. Socioeconomic status is associated with urinary diversion utilization after radical cystectomy for bladder cancer. Int Urol Nephrol 2017;49(1):77–82.
3. Kim SP, Shah ND, Weight CJ, et al. Population-based trends in urinary diversion among patients undergoing radical cystectomy for bladder cancer. BJU Int 2013;112(4):478–84.
4. Roghmann F, Becker A, Trinh QD, et al. Updated assessment of neobladder utilization and morbidity according to urinary diversion after radical cystectomy: a contemporary US-population-based cohort. Can Urol Assoc J 2013;7(9–10):E552–60.
5. Smith AB, Crowell K, Woods ME, et al. Functional outcomes following radical cystectomy in women with bladder cancer: a systematic review. Eur Urol Focus 2017;3(1):136–43.

6. Sperling CD, Lee DJ, Aggarwal S. Urinary diversion: core curriculum 2021. Am J Kidney Dis 2021;78(2): 293–304.

7. O'Connor EM, Foley C, Taylor C, et al. Appendix or ileum-which is the best material for mitrofanoff channel formation in adults? J Urol 2019;202(4): 757–62.

8. Carroll PR, Presti JC Jr, McAninch JW, et al. Functional characteristics of the continent ileocecal urinary reservoir: mechanisms of urinary continence. J Urol 1989;142(4):1032–6.

9. Bihrle R. The Indiana pouch continent urinary reservoir. Urol Clin North Am 1997;24(4):773–9.

10. Rowland RG. Present experience with the Indiana pouch. World J Urol 1996;14(2):92–8.

11. Myers JB, Martin C, Cheng PJ, et al. Outcomes of right colon continent urinary pouch using standardized reporting methods. Neurourol Urodyn 2019; 38(5):1290–7.

12. Suskind AM, Walter LC, Jin C, et al. Impact of frailty on complications in patients undergoing common urological procedures: a study from the American college of surgeons national surgical quality improvement database. BJU Int 2016;117(5):836–42.

13. Hall DE, Arya S, Schmid KK, et al. Association of a Frailty Screening Initiative With Postoperative Survival at 30, 180, and 365 Days. JAMA Surg 2017; 152(3):233–40.

14. Smith AB, Deal AM, Yu H, et al. Sarcopenia as a predictor of complications and survival following radical cystectomy. J Urol 2014;191(6):1714–20.

15. Saitoh-Maeda Y, Kawahara T, Miyoshi Y, et al. A low psoas muscle volume correlates with a longer hospitalization after radical cystectomy. BMC Urol 2017; 17(1):87.

16. Psutka SP, Carrasco A, Schmit GD, et al. Sarcopenia in patients with bladder cancer undergoing radical cystectomy: impact on cancer-specific and all-cause mortality. Cancer 2014;120(18):2910–8.

17. Mathur S, Plank LD, Hill AG, et al. Changes in body composition, muscle function and energy expenditure after radical cystectomy. BJU Int 2008;101(8): 973–7. discussion 977.

18. Djaladat H, Bruins HM, Miranda G, et al. The association of preoperative serum albumin level and American society of anesthesiologists (ASA) score on early complications and survival of patients undergoing radical cystectomy for urothelial bladder cancer. BJU Int 2014;113(6):887–93.

19. Garg T, Chen LY, Kim PH, et al. Preoperative serum albumin is associated with mortality and complications after radical cystectomy. BJU Int 2014;113(6): 918–23.

20. Gontero P, Pisano F, Palou J, et al. Complication rate after cystectomy following pelvic radiotherapy: an international, multicenter, retrospective series of 682 cases. World J Urol 2020;38(8):1959–68.

21. Surgeons ACo. Optimizing nutrition prior to surgery. Available at: http://www.facs.org/quality-programs/strong-for-surgery/clinicians/nutrition. Accessed Dec 13, 2021.

22. Ritch CR, Cookson MS, Clark PE, et al. Perioperative oral nutrition supplementation reduces prevalence of sarcopenia following radical cystectomy: results of a prospective randomized controlled trial. J Urol 2019;201(3):470–7.

23. Yu K, Zheng X, Wang G, et al. Immunonutrition vs standard nutrition for cancer patients: a systematic review and meta-analysis (Part 1). JPEN J Parenter Enteral Nutr 2020;44(5):742–67.

24. Hamilton-Reeves JM, Stanley A, Bechtel MD, et al. Perioperative immunonutrition modulates inflammatory response after radical cystectomy: results of a pilot randomized controlled clinical trial. J Urol 2018;200(2):292–301.

25. Lyon TD, Turner IIR, McBride D, et al. Preoperative immunonutrition prior to radical cystectomy: a pilot study. Can J Urol 2017;24(4):8895–901.

26. Burden S, Billson HA, Lal S, et al. Perioperative nutrition for the treatment of bladder cancer by radical cystectomy. Cochrane Database Syst Rev 2019; 5(5):Cd010127.

27. Prentis JM, Trenell MI, Vasdev N, et al. Impaired cardiopulmonary reserve in an elderly population is related to postoperative morbidity and length of hospital stay after radical cystectomy. BJU Int 2013; 112(2):E13–9.

28. Tolchard S, Angell J, Pyke M, et al. Cardiopulmonary reserve as determined by cardiopulmonary exercise testing correlates with length of stay and predicts complications after radical cystectomy. BJU Int 2015;115(4):554–61.

29. Moran J, Guinan E, McCormick P, et al. The ability of prehabilitation to influence postoperative outcome after intra-abdominal operation: A systematic review and meta-analysis. Surgery 2016; 160(5):1189–201.

30. Jensen BT, Laustsen S, Jensen JB, et al. Exercise-based pre-habilitation is feasible and effective in radical cystectomy pathways-secondary results from a randomized controlled trial. Support Care Cancer 2016;24(8):3325–31.

31. Minnella EM, Carli F, Kassouf W. Role of prehabilitation following major uro-oncologic surgery: a narrative review. World J Urol 2020. https://doi.org/10.1007/s00345-020-03505-4.

32. Bassett MR, Santiago-Lastra Y, Stoffel JT, et al. Urinary diversion for severe urinary adverse events of prostate radiation: results from a multi-institutional study. J Urol 2017;197(3 Pt 1):744–50.

33. Chang SS, Alberts GL, Smith JA Jr, et al. Ileal conduit urinary diversion in patients with previous history of abdominal/pelvic irradiation. World J Urol 2004;22(4):272–6.

34. Beckley S, Wajsman Z, Pontes JE, et al. Transverse colon conduit: a method of urinary diversion after pelvic irradiation. J Urol 1982;128(3):464–8.

35. Wammack R, Wricke C, Hohenfellner R. Long-term results of ileocecal continent urinary diversion in patients treated with and without previous pelvic irradiation. J Urol 2002;167(5):2058–62.

36. Salom EM, Mendez LE, Schey D, et al. Continent ileocolonic urinary reservoir (Miami pouch): the University of Miami experience over 15 years. Am J Obstet Gynecol 2004;190(4):994–1003.

37. Smith D, Albersheim J, Moses R, et al. Outcomes of urinary diversion for late adverse effects of gynecologic radiotherapy. Urology 2020;144:214–9.

38. Wilkin M, Horwitz G, Seetharam A, et al. Long-term complications associated with the Indiana pouch urinary diversion in patients with recurrent gynecologic cancers after high-dose radiation. Urol Oncol 2005;23(1):12–5.

39. Leissner J, Black P, Fisch M, et al. Colon pouch (Mainz pouch III) for continent urinary diversion after pelvic irradiation. Urology 2000;56(5):798–802.

40. Kouba E, Sands M, Lentz A, et al. Incidence and risk factors of stomal complications in patients undergoing cystectomy with ileal conduit urinary diversion for bladder cancer. J Urol 2007;178(3 Pt 1):950–4.

41. Bloom DA, Lieskovsky G, Rainwater G, et al. The Turnbull loop stoma. J Urol 1983;129(4):715–8.

42. Klein FA, Herr HW, Sogani PC, et al. Panniculectomy in conjunction with radical cystectomy in the obese patient. Surg Gynecol Obstet 1983;156(1):31–3.

43. Hugar LA, Turner RM, Gusenoff JA, et al. Panniculectomy and Cystectomy: An Approach to the Morbidly Obese Patient. Case Rep Urol 2016;2016: 6980843.

44. Miller DT, Maganty A, Theisen KM, et al. Novel creation of a noneverted stoma during ileal conduit urinary diversion: Technique and Short-term Outcomes. Urology 2020;146:260–4.

45. Feng D, Li X, Liu S, et al. A comparison between limited bowel preparation and comprehensive bowel preparation in radical cystectomy with ileal urinary diversion: a systematic review and meta-analysis of randomized controlled trials. Int Urol Nephrol 2020;52(11):2005–14.

46. Gustafsson P, Jestin P, Gunnarsson U, et al. Higher frequency of anastomotic leakage with stapled compared to hand-sewn ileocolic anastomosis in a large population-based study. World J Surg 2015; 39(7):1834–9.

47. Kiran RP, Murray AC, Chiuzan C, et al. Combined preoperative mechanical bowel preparation with oral antibiotics significantly reduces surgical site infection, anastomotic leak, and ileus after colorectal surgery. Ann Surg 2015;262(3):416–25. ; discussion 423-5.

48. Morris MS, Graham LA, Chu DI, et al. Oral Antibiotic bowel preparation significantly reduces surgical site infection rates and readmission rates in elective colorectal surgery. Ann Surg 2015;261(6):1034–40.

49. Koskenvuo L, Lehtonen T, Koskensalo S, et al. Mechanical and oral antibiotic bowel preparation versus no bowel preparation for elective colectomy (MOBILE): a multicentre, randomised, parallel, single-blinded trial. Lancet 2019;394(10201):840–8.

50. European Society of Coloproctology Collaborating G. Predictors for anastomotic leak, postoperative complications, and mortality after right colectomy for cancer: results from an international snapshot audit. Dis Colon Rectum 2020;63(5):606–18.

51. Frasson M, Granero-Castro P, Ramos Rodriguez JL, et al. Risk factors for anastomotic leak and postoperative morbidity and mortality after elective right colectomy for cancer: results from a prospective, multicentric study of 1102 patients. Int J Colorectal Dis 2016;31(1):105–14.

52. Bakker IS, Grossmann I, Henneman D, et al. Risk factors for anastomotic leakage and leak-related mortality after colonic cancer surgery in a nationwide audit. Br J Surg 2014;101(4):424–32. ; discussion 432.

53. Choy PY, Bissett IP, Docherty JG, et al. Stapled versus handsewn methods for ileocolic anastomoses. Cochrane Database Syst Rev 2011;9: CD004320.

54. Cheng PJ, Keihani S, Roth JD, et al. Contemporary multicenter outcomes of continent cutaneous ileococystoplasty in the adult population over a 10-year period: A Neurogenic Bladder Research Group study. Neurourol Urodyn 2020;39(6):1771–80.

55. Myers JB, Lenherr SM. Perioperative and long-term surgical complications for the Indiana pouch and similar continent catheterizable urinary diversions. Curr Opin Urol 2016;26(4):376–82.

56. Maibom SL, Joensen UN, Poulsen AM, et al. Short-term morbidity and mortality following radical cystectomy: a systematic review. BMJ Open 2021; 11(4):e043266.

57. Lago V, Fotopoulou C, Chiantera V, et al. Risk factors for anastomotic leakage after colorectal resection in ovarian cancer surgery: A multi-centre study. Gynecol Oncol 2019;153(3):549–54.

58. Lago V, Fotopoulou C, Chiantera V, et al. Indications and practice of diverting ileostomy after colorectal resection and anastomosis in ovarian cancer cytoreduction. Gynecol Oncol 2020;158(3):603–7.

59. Parthasarathy M, Greensmith M, Bowers D, et al. Risk factors for anastomotic leakage after colorectal resection: a retrospective analysis of 17 518 patients. Colorectal Dis 2017;19(3):288–98.

60. Furrer MA, Huesler J, Fellmann A, et al. The comprehensive complication index CCI: a proposed modification to optimize short-term complication reporting

after cystectomy and urinary diversion. Urol Oncol 2019;37(4):291.e9–18.

61. Gore JL, Lai J, Gilbert SM. Readmissions in the postoperative period following urinary diversion. World J Urol 2011;29(1):79–84.

62. Harraz AM, Osman Y, El-Halwagy S, et al. Risk factors of hospital readmission after radical cystectomy and urinary diversion: analysis of a large contemporary series. BJU Int 2015;115(1):94–100.

63. Shimko MS, Tollefson MK, Umbreit EC, et al. Long-term complications of conduit urinary diversion. J Urol 2011;185(2):562–7.

64. Gilbert SM, Lai J, Saigal CS, et al. Downstream complications following urinary diversion. J Urol 2013;190(3):916–22.

65. Gershman B, Eisenberg MS, Thompson RH, et al. Comparative impact of continent and incontinent urinary diversion on long-term renal function after radical cystectomy in patients with preoperative chronic kidney disease 2 and chronic kidney disease 3a. Int J Urol 2015;22(7):651–6.

66. Faraj KS, Mi L, Eversman S, et al. The effect of urinary diversion on long-term kidney function after cystectomy. Urol Oncol 2020;38(10):796. e15–21.

67. Eisenberg MS, Thompson RH, Frank I, et al. Long-term renal function outcomes after radical cystectomy. J Urol 2014;191(3):619–25.

68. Waas T, Schulz A, Lotz J, et al. Distribution of estimated glomerular filtration rate and determinants of its age dependent loss in a German population-based study. Sci Rep 2021;11(1):10165.

69. Movassaghi K, Shah SH, Cai J, et al. Incisional and parastomal hernia following radical cystectomy and urinary diversion: the university of southern California experience. J Urol 2016;196(3):777–81.

70. Narang SK, Alam NN, Campain NJ, et al. Parastomal hernia following cystectomy and ileal conduit urinary diversion: a systematic review. Hernia 2017;21(2):163–75.

71. Su JS, Hoy NY, Fafaj A, et al. The European Hernia Society classification applied to the rare cases of parastomal hernia after ileal conduit urinary diversion: a retrospective cohort of 96 patients. Hernia 2021;25(1):125–31.

72. Alemozaffar M, Nam CS, Said MA, et al. Avoiding the need for bowel anastomosis during pelvic exenteration-urinary sigmoid or descending colon conduit-short and long term complications. Urology 2019;129:228–33.

73. Welk BK, Afshar K, Rapoport D, et al. Complications of the catheterizable channel following continent urinary diversion: their nature and timing. J Urol 2008;180(4 Suppl):1856–60.

74. Stein JP, Skinner DG. Surgical atlas: the orthotopic T-pouch ileal neobladder. BJU Int 2006;98(2):469–82.

75. Turk TM, Koleski FC, Albala DM. Incidence of urolithiasis in cystectomy patients after intestinal conduit or continent urinary diversion. World J Urol 1999;17(5):305–7.

76. Ali-el-Dein B, Shaaban AA, Abu-Eideh RH, et al. Surgical complications following radical cystectomy and orthotopic neobladders in women. J Urol 2008;180(1):206–10. discussion 210.

77. Holmes DG, Thrasher JB, Park GY, et al. Long-term complications related to the modified Indiana pouch. Urology 2002;60(4):603–6.

78. Ahmed YE, Hussein AA, May PR, et al. Natural history, predictors and management of ureteroenteric strictures after robot assisted radical cystectomy. J Urol 2017;198(3):567–74.

79. Amin KA, Vertosick EA, Stearns G, et al. Predictors of benign ureteroenteric anastomotic strictures after radical cystectomy and urinary diversion. Urology 2020;144:225–9.

80. Anderson CB, Morgan TM, Kappa S, et al. Ureteroenteric anastomotic strictures after radical cystectomy-does operative approach matter? J Urol 2013;189(2):541–7.

81. Tal R, Sivan B, Kedar D, et al. Management of benign ureteral strictures following radical cystectomy and urinary diversion for bladder cancer. J Urol 2007;178(2):538–42.

82. Westerman ME, Parker WP, Viers BR, et al. Malignant ureteroenteric anastomotic stricture following radical cystectomy with urinary diversion: patterns, risk factors, and outcomes. Urol Oncol 2016;34(11):485.e1–6.

83. Nassar OA, Alsafa ME. Experience with ureteroenteric strictures after radical cystectomy and diversion: open surgical revision. Urol Aug 2011;78(2):459–65.

84. Yang DY, Boorjian SA, Westerman MB, et al. Persistent, long-term risk for ureteroenteric anastomotic stricture formation: the case for long term follow-up. Transl Androl Urol 2020;9(1):142–50.

85. Faraj KS, Rose KM, Navaratnam AK, et al. Effect of intracorporeal urinary diversion on the incidence of benign ureteroenteric stricture after cystectomy. Int J Urol 2021;28(5):593–7.

86. Richards KA, Cohn JA, Large MC, et al. The effect of length of ureteral resection on benign ureterointestinal stricture rate in ileal conduit or ileal neobladder urinary diversion following radical cystectomy. Urol Oncol 2015;33(2):65.e1–8.

87. Hautmann RE, de Petriconi R, Kahlmeyer A, et al. Preoperatively dilated ureters are a specific risk factor for the development of ureteroenteric strictures after open radical cystectomy and ileal neobladder. J Urol 2017;198(5):1098–106.

88. Benson CR, Ajay D, Barrett-Harlow BL, et al. Ureteroenteric anastomosis in orthotopic neobladder

creation: do urinary tract infections impact stricture rate? World J Urol 2021;39(4):1171–6.

89. Ericson KJ, Thomas LJ, Zhang JH, et al. Uretero-enteric anastomotic stricture following radical cystectomy: a comparison of open, robotic extracorporeal, and robotic intracorporeal approaches. Urology 2020;144:130–5.

90. Chan DKH, Lee SKF, Ang JJ. Indocyanine green fluorescence angiography decreases the risk of colorectal anastomotic leakage: systematic review and meta-analysis. Surgery 2020;168(6):1128–37.

91. Shen JK, Jamnagerwalla J, Yuh BE, et al. Real-time indocyanine green angiography with the SPY fluorescence imaging platform decreases benign ureteroenteric strictures in urinary diversions performed during radical cystectomy. Ther Adv Urol 2019;11. 1756287219839631.

92. Ahmadi N, Ashrafi AN, Hartman N, et al. Use of indocyanine green to minimise uretero-enteric strictures after robotic radical cystectomy. BJU Int 2019;124(2):302–7.

93. Doshi CP, Wozniak A, Quek ML. Near-infrared fluorescence imaging of ureters with intravenous indocyanine green during radical cystectomy to prevent ureteroenteric anastomotic strictures. Urology 2020;144:220–4.

Complex Lower Genitourinary Fistula Repair
Rectourethral Fistula and Puboprostatic Fistula

Jack G. Campbell, MD, Alex J. Vanni, MD*

KEYWORDS

- Rectourethral fistula • Puboprostatic fistula • Radiation damage • Prostate cancer survivorship

KEY POINTS

- There is a significant difference in nonirradiated and irradiated/ablative RUF both in outcomes and complications.
- For complex RUF repair, interposition of healthy muscle is critical.
- RUF repair is best performed at high-volume referral centers.
- In order to be a candidate for PPF repair without extirpation, patients need adequate bladder capacity, compliance, and free of urethral stricture disease.

RECTOURETHRAL FISTULA
Introduction

Rectourethral fistula (RUF) is a rare but potentially devastating complication most commonly resulting from the treatment of pelvic cancer (typically prostate or anorectal), although inflammatory bowel disease, pelvic trauma, iatrogenic injury, and infectious complications may also result in RUF. Historically, the most common etiology of RUF was radical prostatectomy, with rates ranging from 1% to 2% in open prostatectomy series.[1] However, the incidence of surgical RUF is decreasing with less than 1% of robotic radical prostatectomies resulting in RUF.[2,3] In patients undergoing radical prostatectomy, previous pelvic radiation, rectal surgery, and transurethral resection of the prostate increase the risk of a rectal injury and potential RUF.[1]

The incidence of RUF appears to be increasing due to the increased incidence of radiation and other ablative therapies. A review from Duke University identified a 3.8% history of radiation in patients with RUF prior to 1998 (315 total patients) compared to 52.6% (350 total patients) from 1998 to 2012.[4] The risk of RUF in external beam radiation therapy (EBRT) monotherapy, brachytherapy monotherapy, and EBRT + brachytherapy are well under less than 1%, 0.2%, and 2.9%, respectively,[5] and while data are more limited, appear to be less than 1% for both primary cryosurgical ablation and primary high intensity focused ultrasound.[6,7]

Nature of the Problem

RUF has long-term implications on urinary, bowel, and sexual function leading to significant impairments in a patient's quality of life. Patients typically present with pneumaturia, fecaluria, and urinary tract infection, but not uncommonly also develop pelvic abscesses requiring drainage and sepsis. Patients with radiation RUF also commonly have

Division of Urology, Lahey Hospital and Medical Center, 41 Burlington Mall Road, Burlington, MA 01805, USA
* Corresponding author.
E-mail address: Alex.j.vanni@lahey.org

Urol Clin N Am 49 (2022) 553–565
https://doi.org/10.1016/j.ucl.2022.04.012
0094-0143/22/© 2022 Elsevier Inc. All rights reserved.

severe pelvic/perineal pain that can at times severely impact physical activity.

RUF is a challenging surgical entity because the pathology occurs in an inaccessible space deep into both the urinary and anal sphincters with proximity to erectile anatomy. Due to aberrant wound healing from a combination of fixed postsurgical tissue, prior radiation or ablative therapy, urinoma, infections, and drains, the tissue quality and wound healing are often poor. Additionally, concurrent pathology is often present including stricture of the urethra or rectum, urinary or fecal incontinence, and rectal dysfunction.

Anatomy

Most postprostatectomy RUF are located at the prior vesicourethral anastomosis; however, fistula location is variable in cases where the prostate remains in situ. The plane of dissection through a transperineal approach will move in a direction where the anus/rectum and external anal sphincter are posterior while the superficial transverse perineal muscle, perineal body, and bulbospongiosus muscle are anterior. The urinary sphincter should remain anterior during dissection and the rectum posterior. Thorough dissection will encounter the levator ani muscles moving deep as well as the inferior surface of peritoneum once dissection has been carried cephalad to the bladder floor.

PREOPERATIVE/PREPROCEDURE PLANNING
Exam Under Anesthesia

All patients evaluated for RUF repair undergo exam under anesthesia using an interdisciplinary approach with both urology and colorectal surgery. Retrograde urethrography is performed before placing the patient into dorsal lithotomy position, not only for assessing the presence of a RUF, but also to evaluate for stricture disease or any secondary fistula. Careful cystourethroscopy is then performed assessing the size of the fistula, quality of the tissue, presence of foreign bodies such as suture, stones, surgical clips and staples, or brachytherapy seeds, coaptation of the urethral sphincter, status of the bladder neck, presence of urethral stricture disease, bladder capacity, proximity of the ureteral orifices to the bladder neck, and for the presence of radiation cystitis. If the prostate remains in situ, evaluation for necrosis, which tends to appear as white, fluffy tissue, is important as it impacts the type of reconstruction that we ultimately may decide upon.

Colorectal surgery then performs flexible sigmoidoscopy to evaluate the rectal side of the fistula evaluating size, tissue quality, distance from the anal sphincter, quality of the anal

sphincter, and foreign bodies. All foreign bodies should be removed from both the urinary or gastrointestinal tract at this time, when feasible. In cases of a large defect, concurrent cystoscopy and sigmoidoscopy are not necessary; however, in cases of a small fistula or if there is a question of a healed fistula, simultaneous endoscopy is helpful. In some cases, a wire can be passed from one side to the other to define the fistula. If not already present, a suprapubic is placed percutaneously.

Patient Selection

Patient selection is paramount for successful RUF repair and in setting patient expectations. A key component of patient selection is the findings of our multi-disciplinary EUA discussed above. **Fig. 1** displays the authors' algorithmic approach to RUF. In contrast to other authors, fistula size is not an explicit component of the management pathway. While it is taken into account, our experience is that size does not preclude successful reconstruction if the principles of tension-free closure and interposition of healthy muscle are performed **Fig. 1**.

PREOPERATIVE PLANNING
Hyperbaric Oxygen Therapy

Multiple series have observed lower success rates of RUF repair in irradiated/ablative compared to nonirradiated RUF,[4,8–10] and thus preoperative optimization is especially important in irradiated/ablative RUF. Hyperbaric oxygen has been shown to stimulate angiogenesis, reduce the mechanical effects of fibrosis, and mobilize local stem cells.[11] While benefits have not been directly evaluated in RUF, both a recent randomized controlled trial[12] and meta-analysis[13] have demonstrated benefits in hemorrhagic cystitis. Of note, Oscarsson and colleagues (2019) did observe grade 1 to 2 adverse events related to sight and hearing in 41% of patients; however, all changes were transient.[12] As the physiologic benefits of hyperbaric oxygen in healing should translate to RUF, our institution hyperbaric oxygen therapy is recommended preoperatively for all patients with radiation/ablative fistulas.

Bowel Diversion

The rate of preoperative fecal diversion is reported to be anywhere from 57% to 100%,[14,15] and some surgeons do not feel it is necessary, even in some cases of irradiated/ablative fistulas.[16] Other authors will perform fecal diversion at the time of repair.[9,17] At our institution, preoperative fecal

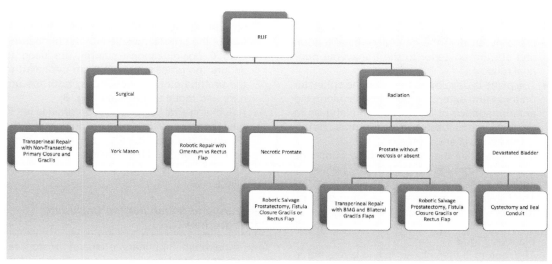

Fig. 1. Surgical approach to rectourethral fistula repair (RUF).

diversion is performed for all patients with irradiated/ablative fistulas, and recommended for surgical RUF in order to maximize chances for RUF surgical closure. If fecal diversion has not been performed prior to referral, loop colostomy is preferred to loop ileostomy given superior nutritional and fluid status.

Nutrition

Given the risk of chronic infection and decreased mobility, patients with RUF may be predisposed to nutritional deficiency. Therefore, a multidisciplinary approach between urology, colorectal, referring providers, and dieticians may be necessary. Farrell and colleagues (2021) identified hypoalbuminemia in 25/126 (20%) of patients who underwent surgery for RUF in the National Surgical Quality Improvement Program (NSQIP) database and observed that hypoalbuminemia was associated with increased odds of a 30-day complication (OR 2.49, 95% CI 1.06–5.86, $P = .036$).[18] Assessing the nutritional status of patients preoperatively helps with patient counseling regarding the risk of postoperative complication, and provides an opportunity to improve nutritional status prior to reconstruction.

SURGICAL APPROACH
Prep and Patient Positioning

The patient is placed in dorsolithotomy position using Yellofin stirrups. While most rectoureteral fistula repairs can be completed in approximately 4 hours, some may extend much longer, so meticulous attention must be paid to adequate angulation of padding of the lower limbs to prevent neuropraxia or compartment syndrome. Tape is used to secure the patient to the table, allowing for safe Trendelenberg positioning, if necessary. The perineum, genitals, suprapubic region, and both medial thighs are then shaved, and ChloraPrep is used to prep these areas entirely, taking care to include both medial thighs extending to the medial popliteal fossa bilaterally in case bilateral gracilis flap harvest is necessary.

Procedural Approach

The authors prefer a transperineal approach as this allows the flexibility to reconstruct virtually all types of pathology associated with RUF. As seen in **Fig. 1**, this repair is used for both nonirradiated and irradiated/ablative fistulas, and can be easily combined with other procedures, including buccal mucosa grafting (BMG) for concurrent urethral stricture repair or closure of larger radiation RUF defects, and easily facilitates the use of gracilis muscle interposition flaps to separate suture lines, fill dead space, and provide blood supply to BMG if used. Additionally, in cases with a necrotic prostate in which we advocate performing a robotic salvage prostatectomy, a combined transperineal approach is often required to treat the concomitant transmembranous urethral stricture that is often present.

Rectourethral Fistula Repair

- Cystoscopy is performed and a 5 Fr open-ended ureteral catheter is placed across the fistula

- An inverted U incision is carried from approximately 2 cm inferior to the ischial tuberosities bilaterally up to the pubic symphysis. **Fig. 2**
- Dissection moves deep into the rectourethral plane by dividing the central perineal tendon and staying posterior to the transverse perineal muscles.
- The plane is developed between the sphincter urethrae and external anal sphincter along the anterior surface of the rectum and laterally to the ischiorectal fossa and levator muscles until the fistula is encountered.
- It is imperative that the dissection continues cephalad through the inferior peritoneal surface
- The fistula tract is then exposed and divided, followed by further cephalad dissection to both expose and mobilize the floor of the bladder. **Fig. 3**
- The rectum is then closed in two layers transversely if possible to minimize rectal narrowing. **Fig. 4**
- Closure of the urethral defect depends on size, tissue quality, and mobility, and whether there is a concomitant urethral stricture. Virtually all surgical RUF are smaller (2 cm or less) and closed in a single layer of interrupted 4 to 0 monocryl. Most radiated RUF are avascular, fibrotic, and frequently associated with larger defects (>2 cm). In patients without an obliterative urethral stricture, we use a BMG patch of the urethral defect (4–0 monocryl) to avoid mobilizing the urethra, thereby preserving the external urinary sphincter. **Figs. 5 and 6**

Gracilis Muscle Interposition

- The gracilis muscle is identified proximally at its insertion of the ischiopubic ramus posterior to the adductor longus tendon, and distally with the tendon medial to the easily palpable semitendinosus tendon in the popliteal fossa.
- The medial thigh compartment is opened (this can be 3 small incisions in the medial thigh or 1 long incision), and the gracilis muscle is identified.
- The gracilis muscle receives its blood supply from the medial femoral circumflex artery.
- Proximally, doppler ultrasound aids in the identification of the major pedicle, which is 8 to 10 cm from the pubic bone.
- After confirming the dominant pedicle, circumferential dissection of the gracilis is achieved and the distal tendon is divided. **Fig. 7**
- There are 2–3 minor pedicles that are suture ligated and divided. The gracilis muscle is then mobilized proximally, with care taken to avoid injury to the dominant, proximal pedicle.
- A wide tunnel that can accommodate 3 fingerbreadths is created to allow tension-free rotation of the gracilis muscle into the perineum
- 3 to 0 polydioxanone sutures are used to secure the gracilis muscle 2 cm cephalad to the urethral closure, separating both the urinary and rectal suture lines. **Fig. 8**
- A Jackson-Pratt closed suction drain is left in the perineum with tubing extending out the length of the gracilis harvest site and out superior to the distal thigh incision.
- The perineum and thigh are closed in multiple layers.

Recovery and Rehabilitation (Including PostProcedure Care)

Any impairment in urinary drainage postoperatively can be catastrophic. Hence, the authors prefer double drainage with both urethral catheter and suprapubic tube. Postoperative voiding cystourethrogram (VCUG) is performed at approximately 4 weeks or 6 weeks for surgically induced and radiation-induced fistulas, respectively. Depending on the difficulty of the repair, the suprapubic tube may be left in place after imaging for a capping trial before being removed. Even with the extravasation of contrast on the initial VCUG, there is a high likelihood of spontaneous closure with a catheter in place as long as no contrast enters the rectum. Patience and reassurance are recommended, as the authors have observed closure with conservative management as far as 9 months postoperatively.

At 3 months postoperatively, cystoscopy and retrograde urethrogram are performed. If the urinary system remains closed, the patient is evaluated by colorectal surgery with flexible proctoscopy and a water-soluble contrast enema before being scheduled for fecal undiversion. Subsequent follow-up includes the assessment of incontinence and candidacy for artificial urinary sphincter, which is performed 6 months after fecal undiversion, if necessary.

Management and Outcomes

The complexity and challenge of RUF repair are reflected in the many techniques employed, even within institutions, including the anterior transanorectal, Kraske laterosacral, and posterior transanosphincteric repairs (York-Mason).[19] Sagittal dissection of the York-Mason repair typically allows rectal innervations, urinary continence, and potency to be preserved, and careful recreation of the sphincter and rectal wall results in no risk

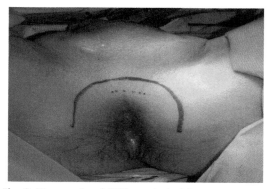

Fig. 2. Transperineal RUF repair; incision.

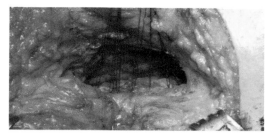

Fig. 4. Primary transverse closure of the rectal defect; second layer.

of fecal incontinence.[20] Success rates with a York-Mason repair are consistently reported to be 80% to 90% or above,[4,20,21] however, this is predominantly in simple, nonirradiated /ablative fistulas. Hanna and colleagues (2014) observed a 100% success rate with nonirradiated RUF using a York-Mason repair; however, the success decreased to 50% in irradative/ablative fistulas.[4] Interposition of healthy muscle is generally not feasible with a York-Mason repair, which is not only restricts its use to the more-simple, nonirradiated RUF but also limits intraoperative decision-making. This repair also has been demonstrated to be less successful in patients with prior attempted RUF repair.[22] Nonetheless, in carefully selected patients it remains an important option, and there may be a future role for a minimally invasive modification of the York-Mason as robotic transanal minimally invasive surgery (TAMIS) has been described to fix two small, nonirradiated fistulas.[23]

Over the last two decades, a transperineal (sphincter-sparing) approach has emerged as the dominant technique, with one systematic review observing that it represents 66% of all RUF repair.[24] The transperineal repair is attractive for multiple reasons, including avoidance of both the urinary and anal sphincters, use of a nontransecting technique that may be beneficial in patients who need a future artificial urinary sphincter (AUS), ease of using a gracilis or other muscle interposition flap, and ability to treat concomitant urethral strictures. Regarding the latter, urethral stricture or bladder neck contracture is present in 14%-43% of RUF,[10,25] so the ability to fix urethral stricture is important. The wide exposure with a transperineal repair facilitates the use of BMG in cases of a larger fistula incompatible with primary repair. **Box 1** displays outcomes data from the transperineal technique, with success rates of 84% to 100%. In studies that reported outcomes separately between nonirradiated and irradiated/ablative fistulas, success was consistently higher in the former group, with the 2 largest series demonstrating surgical RUF closure in 99% to 100% of cases and 86% to 87% in irradiated/ablative RUF.[9,10] **Box 1**.

The first RUF repair using a gracilis muscle for interposition was performed by Dr. Leonard Zinman in 1971; however, this technique would not be published until 1979.[26] As **Box 1** illustrates, gracilis muscle flap has become an essential tool for RUF repair. Gracilis muscle has reliable anatomy that allows efficient harvesting and has a robust blood supply. The benefit of muscle interposition includes separating suture lines, filling dead space, providing blood supply for BMG all with low functional morbidity. It is worth noting that with questionnaire-based review, 43% of patients reported problems related to their gracilis flap.[25]

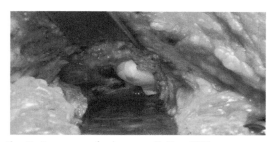

Fig. 3. Exposure of a large radiation RUF.

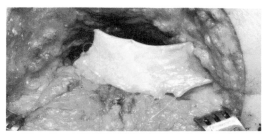

Fig. 5. Parachuting of the buccal mucosa graft (BMG) for closure of large urethral defect.

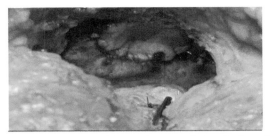

Fig. 6. BMG Sutured into place; Both Urethral and Rectal defects Closed.

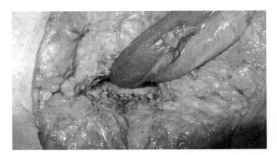

Fig. 8. Final position of the gracilis flap for complete interposition between urinary and rectal defects.

While these were minor, the authors did note that this impacted their future counseling. While some authors have argued that gracilis muscle will not reach past the prostate,[16] we find that with adequate mobilization and a wide tunnel, gracilis muscle can be reliably sutured 2 to 3 cm cephalad to the bladder neck for complete separation of the urinary and rectal closures. The authors have not observed gracilis flap necrosis; however, it was described by Ghoniem and colleagues (2018) in 2 patients,[17] and by Wexner and colleagues (2008) in one patient.[14]

Complications

The incidence of complications after RUF repair depends heavily on the definitions used and length of follow-up. It has been reported to be as low as 11%,[10] however, one series where all patients had irradiated/ablative fistulas observed 24 total complications in 22 patients.[27] Nonetheless, the rate of Clavien-Dindo III adverse events is reported to be low at 10%-22%.[9,15,25] The largest single-institution study evaluated short and long-term outcomes stratified by nonirradiated fistulas and irradiated/ablative fistulas.[9] The rate of 30-day complication rate for Clavien-Dindo grade III or higher was 4% and 8% for nonirradiated and irradiated/ablative fistulas. The 90-day complication rates were 2% and 22% for these groups, respectively; however, most of the complications for

irradiated/ablative patients within 90 days were fistula recurrence.

This stands in stark contrast to complication rates for cystectomy and urinary diversion. Cohn and colleagues (2014) observed a 47% risk of Clavien-Dindo grade III or higher complications within 30 days of undergoing cystectomy and urinary diversion for benign disease.[28] Importantly, they also observed a higher complication rate in patients with fistula compared to neurogenic bladder, and the overall complication rate for patients with irradiated/ablative fistula was 100%. Another study identified a 57% incidence of Clavien-Dindo grade II or higher complications.[29] Despite the high risk of complications, it is important to note that in a study of 19 patients undergoing urinary diversion for radiation-related damage, 95% of patients later reported they wished they had conducted the surgery earlier.[30]

Quality of Life After Rectourethral Fistula Repair

Historically, there has been a paucity of data concerning quality of life (QOL) outcomes in patients who undergo RUF repair; however, studies in the last decade are generally favorable. Hampson and colleagues (2018) evaluated 21 men who had undergone RUF repair with questionnaires, and at a median follow-up of 45 months, 80% of

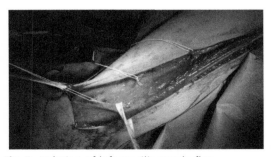

Fig. 7. Isolation of left gracilis muscle flap.

| **Box 1** |
| **Transperineal technique for RUF repair** |

NI: Nonirradiated Fistula

I/A: Irradiated/Ablative Fistula

TP: Transperineal

TA: Transabdominal

*Multi-institutional

ᵃ4 patients were treated with permanent urinary and fecal diversion patients said surgery had positively impacted their life and no patients would have opted for urinary diversion.[25,31] However, 21% did report that they were unable to do the things they wanted in their daily lives. Samplaski and colleagues (2011) also evaluated patients after RUF repair with QOL questionnaires, and while only 3/13 (23%) reported voiding per urethra and being completely continent, only 2/13 (15%) reported that urinary symptoms have a significant impact on their overall life.[32] Importantly, all patients reported minimal or no complaints in the "Embarrassment" domain of the questionnaire which captures unknowing fecal leakage, worry about odor, and feelings of shame. Most recently, Sbizzera and colleagues (2021) found favorable QOL scores using the Urinary Symptom Profile (USP), St Mark's fecal incontinence score, Patient and Observer Scar Assessment Scale (POSAS), and lower extremity functionality score.[15]

It does appear that the rate of incontinence patients report with QOL assessment is greater than reported in previous trials. In the above series, the rate of incontinence ranged 61%-80%,[15,25,32] compared to as low as 31% in another series.[9] The difference in the rates of incontinence in these series may also reflect differences in surgical technique, and one of the reasons we advocate the sphincter sparing transperineal approach. In cases of severe incontinence, artificial urinary sphincter (AUS) does appear to be a safe and effective option with high patient satisfaction rates.[33] The largest series of AUS placement after RUF repair reported AUS placement in 14/98 (14%), including 5 patients with nonirradiated/ablative fistula and 9 patients with irradiated/ablative fistula.[9] Of these 14 patients, there was one erosion and one infection at median follow-up 25 months.

Ultimately, rates of permanent urinary and fecal diversion are highly dependent on patient selection and counseling. A systematic review of 416 total patients, 40% of whom had a history of irradiated/ablative fistula, observed permanent fecal and urinary diversion rates of 10.6% and 8.3%. The rate of fecal undiversion represents another difference between nonirradiated and irradiated/ablative fistulas, and Vanni and colleagues (2010) observed a 3% versus 31% risk of permanent fecal diversion in these groups, respectively (Vanni and colleagues 2010).

SUMMARY

RUF remains a challenging surgical entity due to complex anatomy, risk of injuring important nearby structures, and frequently altered tissue quality

and wound healing. Nonetheless, with appropriate patient selection, adequate tissue interposition, and meticulous surgical technique, most patients can be spared permanent urinary and fecal diversion and expect a positive quality of life.

CLINICS CARE POINTS

- There is a significant difference in nonirradiated and irradiated/ablative RUF both in outcomes and complications.
- Patient selection, counseling, and preoperative optimization are crucial.
- Interdisciplinary evaluation and management are highly recommended.
- For complex RUF repair, interposition of healthy muscle is critical.
- RUF repair is best performed at high-volume referral centers.

PUBOPROSTATIC FISTULA
Introduction

Puboprostatic fistula (PPF) can result from pelvic surgery, radiation, trauma, or infection; however, the vast majority are caused by prostate cancer treatment.[34] Most patients who develop PPF have a history of radiation or ablative therapy, and in some series, the incidence of irradiation/ablation history is 100%.[35–37] Endoscopic therapy after treatment for prostate cancer is another major risk factor for the development of PPF, and is present in 100% of two larger studies.[36,38] Pubic bone pain is often the dominant presenting symptom and is typically exacerbated by ambulation and often debilitating. Additional presenting symptoms can include recurrent urinary tract infections, urosepsis, perineal, scrotal, or thigh abscesses, and chronically draining sinus tracts. Osteoneocrosis of the pubic bone can occur, which without treatment, can lead to osteomyelitis.

Nature of the Problem/Diagnosis

PPF represents an immensely challenging entity for multiple reasons. The pathology exists in the deep pelvis but given the presence of prolonged infection, may spread into adjacent spaces including the medial thighs and presacral space. In fact, Sexton and colleagues (2019) identified some degree of inflammatory myositis in 11/16 (58%) of patients undergoing MRI for PPF evaluation.[39] The center of the pathology is an often necrotic prostate fixed to surrounding structures including the pubic symphysis. Concomitant pathology with the bladder neck, bladder health, urethral stricture disease is common, and the resulting osteomyelitis is difficult to treat. These patients often have significant comorbidities and are significantly deconditioned due to pain and immobility.

Anatomy

PPF extends from the prostate, deep in the male pelvis anteriorly to the pubic symphysis. The superior or more likely inferior pubic ramus can also be involved, and given the proximity of the origin of leg adductors, infections and fistulization to the medial thighs may occur. The space of Retzius cephalad and anterior to the prostate is often significantly fibrotic even if it has not been surgically violated.

PreOperative/PreProcedure Planning

All patients undergo imaging with a VCUG or RUG to initially evaluate the fistula. Cystoscopy is also performed in order to assess for urethral stricture disease, bladder neck function, quality of prostate tissue, and size and health of the bladder. Pelvic MRI is performed on all patients, mainly given the superior evaluation of the prostate anatomy, location of fistula to the symphysis, and bone in cases of osteomyelitis.[40] Acute osteomyelitis is characterized by fluid accumulation within the medulla (instead of fat), resulting in low signal on T1W imaging and high signal on T2W imaging. Intraosseous abscesses may develop which are low signal on T1W images and high signal on T2W imaging. There often is an enhancing peripheral rim on fat suppressed-T1 imaging known as the "penumbra sign." Sinus tracts may develop in acute osteomyelitis as well as periostitis. Chronic osteomyelitis is characterized by the development of a sequestrum, or a separate fragment of necrotic bone surrounded by pus, which has a low signal on both T1 and T2 imaging. Furthermore, MRI also typically can visualize the fistula itself better than CT. MRI demonstrating both PPF and findings of acute osteomyelitis is displayed in **Fig. 9**.

Patients need to be stabilized from an infectious standpoint and this often entails close interdisciplinary care with Infectious Disease specialists. The rate of spontaneous closure is likely quite low; however, some patients can be managed conservatively with a urethral catheter and appropriate antibiotics. Reconstruction should be reserved only for patients with adequate bladder capacity, no urethral stricture disease, relatively vigorous health, and who understand there are significant risks with reconstructive surgery. In patients who are not a candidate for reconstruction, cystectomy and ileal conduit with pubectomy are advised.

Similar to irradiated/ablative RUF, hyperbaric oxygen therapy is recommended to all patients considering reconstruction for PPF, as well as the optimization of nutrition and functional activity.

Prep and Patient Positioning

The patient is placed in dorsolithotomy position using Yellofin stirrups. Meticulous attention is paid to positioning as avoid neuropraxis of the lower limbs. The patient is secured to the table to allow for Trendelenberg positioning, shaved, and ChloraPrep is used to prep the entire abdomen and genitals.

Procedural Approach

The authors perform an open abdominal repair with vertical rectus abdominis muscle flap; however, a robotic approach is also feasible. Hebert and colleagues (2021) described a robotic approach to either PPF repair or urinary diversion using a holmium laser to debride pubic bone.[41] In this small series there was no major complication and no recurrence of osteomyelitis at follow up of 7 to 16 months. Harvest of a rectus flap has been described for use in posterior urethroplasty,[42] as well as after abdominoperineal resection.[43]

- Cystoscopy is performed to identify the location of the urethral defect
- A suprapubic catheter is placed if the patient is not already in place and a urethral catheter is placed for drainage.
- A suprapubic incision is made and dissection carried down into the Space of Retzius
- The anterior rectus sheath is identified and incised with electrocautery
- The anterior sheath is dissected free, allowing the rectus muscle to be encircled posteriorly and divided off the costal margin.
- Dissection is then carried caudal to the deep inferior epigastric artery (DIEA). The DIEA reaches the rectus muscle from an inferolateral path and there is often an area of fat lateral to the rectus muscle identifying that the DIEA is near as dissection is carried caudally.
- The fistulous tract is then dissected out and circumferentially excised
- Osteotomes and Rongeurs are used to debride all necrotic pubic bone until there is healthy bleeding bone.
- Cases of significant bleeding area rare; however, bone wax should be available.

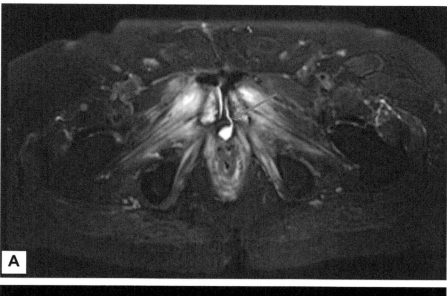

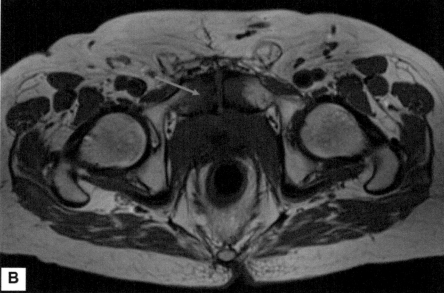

Fig. 9. MRI of PPF and Acute Osteomyelitis. (*A*) T2 image demonstrating fistula extension to pubic symphysis and T2 hyperintensity of the adjacent bone marrow. (*B*) T1 hypointensity of the pubic symphysis consistent with acute osteomyelitis.

- Bone cultures are typically sent for culture.
- The rectus flap is then rotated 180° and interposed between the urinary repair and remaining pubic bone. The rectus can be secured in this location with 2 to 0 polydioxanone suture.
- Once the fistula has been excised down to healthy prostatic urethral tissue, the defect is closed using interrupted monocryl suture either primarily or with a y-v bladder advancement flap. A BMG can be used, if necessary.

- The rectus flap is then rotated posteroinferiorly to cover the urethral closure and fill space in between prostate and pubic symphysis. Polydioxanone suture is used to secure the muscle to the anterior prostate and to close the anterior rectus sheath. **Fig. 10**

Recovery and Rehabilitation (Including PostProcedure Care)

Patients typically stay in the hospital for 1 to 3 days postoperatively and are discharged with both the

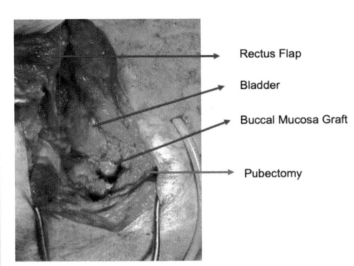

Fig. 10. Exposure of PPF repair.

Rectus Flap

Bladder

Buccal Mucosa Graft

Pubectomy

urethral and suprapubic catheters for drainage. The urethral catheter can be removed at 6 weeks postoperatively, a voiding cystourethrogram (VCUG) is performed via the suprapubic catheter. In some cases, if there is no urinary extravasation the suprapubic catheter may be left for a capping trial; however, in the majority of cases, it is removed in the clinic. Cystoscopy is performed at 3 months postoperatively to ensure urethral patency and fistula closure, with routine measurement of post void residual urine volume and uroflowmetry out to 1 year postoperatively.

Management and Outcomes

Interdisciplinary care is crucial in treating PPF, with a likely combination of urology, infectious disease, plastic surgery, and potentially colorectal surgery.

As these patients may be severely deconditioned with multiple comorbidities, a shared-decision making model is recommended. Some patients may be very poor surgical candidates, so while there is little data supporting spontaneous closure of PPF with urethral catheter maintenance and antibiotic treatment, we have found this to be a successful and acceptable option for some.

Madden-Fuentes et al. (2017) advocate for supratrigonal cystectomy without salvage prostatectomy given the high rate of complication.[34] In their experience, no patients have experienced the recurrence of prostate cancer and the number of patients fit to consider reconstruction is very small. Indeed, of 12 patients presenting to Memorial Sloan Kettering Hospital with PPF after prostate cancer, 10 (83%) went on to cystectomy and urinary diversion.[36]

While reconstruction in this population is difficult, good outcomes in highly selected patients are possible. Kaufman and colleagues (2016) reported outcomes for 4 patients with radiation-induced PPF who were treated with pubic symphysis debridement, fistula closure, and interposition rectus abdominis muscle flap, and found a 100% success rate at a median follow-up of 27 months.[37]

Bugeja and colleagues (2016) reported on 16 patients for urosymphyseal fistulas after prostate cancer treatment, all of whom had received radiotherapy as primary or after prostatectomy, and 3 of whom had also received salvage cryotherapy.[35] Fifteen of these patients underwent surgery, with a total of 7 patients undergoing reconstruction with a combined abdominoperineal approach including excision of the fistula tract, debridement of the pubic symphysis, and omental flap. Salvage prostatectomy was performed in 4 patients, redo vesicourethral anastomosis in 3, and augmentation colocystoplasty in 2. Eight patients were treated with cystectomy or cystoprostatectomy and ileal conduit diversion after excision of the fistula, pubectomy, and omental flap, and overall 13 of 15 (87%) of surgically treated patients were successful.[35]

Regardless of approach, debridement of infected bone is paramount, and bone cultures should always be sent to help guide future antimicrobial therapy. Nose and colleagues (2020) evaluated patients with pubic bone osteomyelitis in prostate cancer survivors with PPF undergoing bone resection and extirpative surgery.[44] In this series 92% of patients had a positive bone culture and the three most common organisms were candida (22%), enterococcus (18%), and pseudomonas (10%), and there was a statistically significant correlation between positive urine and blood cultures.[44] Adequate bone debridement not only allows for infectious control but also is crucial to alleviating pain. Our experience, and those of two separate authors have independently observed a consistent and often immediate relief of pain postoperatively, regardless of whether they were treated with reconstruction or extirpation.[35,45]

SUMMARY

PPF often occurs in debilitated patients with extensive comorbidities. Many patients managed surgically will go on to cystectomy and urinary diversion; however, reconstruction can achieve fistula closure and resolution of pain in highly selected patients. PPF repair should be reserved for highly selected patients at tertiary referral centers.

CLINICS CARE POINTS

- In order to be a candidate for PPF repair without extirpation, patients need adequate bladder capacity, compliance, and free of urethral stricture disease.
- Similar to RUF, interposition of healthy muscle tissue is important to prevent recurrence in avascular, fibrotic, often chronically infected tissue.

DISCLOSURE

Dr A.J. Vanni has the following funding to disclose:

- R21 NIH - Understanding the effects of local and systemic inflammation on the development and treatment of urethral stricture disease
- REW Grant – Investigation into the pathogenesis of urethral lichen sclerosus
- REW Grant – Investigation into the microRNA profile of lichen sclerosis urethral stricture disease
- Ellison Foundation Research Grant – Investigation into the pathophysiology of urethral stricture disease
- Boston Scientific Fellowship Training Grant

None of these sources of funding created a conflict of interest for this publication.

REFERENCES

1. McLaren RH, Barrett DM, Zincke H. Rectal injury occurring at radical retropubic prostatectomy for prostate cancer: etiology and treatment. Urology 1993;42(4):401–5.
2. Igel TC, Barrett DM, Segura JW, et al. Perioperative and postoperative complications from bilateral pelvic lymphadenectomy and radical retropubic prostatectomy. J Urol 1987;137(6):1189–91.
3. Wedmid A, Mendoza P, Sharma S, et al. Rectal injury during robot-assisted radical prostatectomy: incidence and management. J Urol 2011;186(5):1928–33.
4. Hanna JM, Turley R, Castleberry A, et al. Surgical management of complex rectourethral fistulas in irradiated and nonirradiated patients. Dis Colon Rectum 2014;57(9):1105–12.
5. Theodorescu D, Gillenwater JY, Koutrouvelis PG. Prostatourethral-rectal fistula after prostate brachytherapy: Incidence and risk factors. Cancer 2000;89(10):2085–91.
6. Zippe CD. Cryosurgery of the prostate: techniques and pitfalls. Urol Clin 1996;23(1):147–63.
7. Ganzer R, Fritsche HM, Brandtner A, et al. Fourteen-year oncological and functional outcomes of high-intensity focused ultrasound in localized prostate cancer. BJU Int 2013;112(3):322–9.
8. Vanni AJ, Buckley JC, Zinman LN. Management of surgical and radiation induced rectourethral fistulas with an interposition muscle flap and selective buccal mucosal onlay graft. J Urol 2010;184(6):2400–4.
9. Kaufman DA, Zinman LN, Buckley JC, et al. Short- and long-term complications and outcomes of radiation and surgically induced rectourethral fistula repair with buccal mucosa graft and muscle interposition flap. Urology 2016;98:170–5.
10. Harris CR, McAninch JW, Mundy AR, et al. Rectourethral fistulas secondary to prostate cancer treatment: management and outcomes from a multi-institutional combined experience. J Urol 2017;197(1):191–4.
11. Feldmeier JJ. Hyperbaric oxygen therapy and delayed radiation injuries (soft tissue and bony necrosis): 2012 update. Undersea Hyperb Med 2012;39(6):1121.
12. Oscarsson N, Müller B, Rosén A, et al. Radiation-induced cystitis treated with hyperbaric oxygen therapy (RICH-ART): a randomised, controlled, phase 2–3 trial. Lancet Oncol 2019;20(11):1602–14.
13. Cardinal J, Slade A, McFarland M, et al. Scoping review and meta-analysis of hyperbaric oxygen therapy for radiation-induced hemorrhagic cystitis. Curr Urol Rep 2018;19(6):1–8.
14. Wexner SD, Ruiz DE, Genua J, et al. Gracilis muscle interposition for the treatment of rectourethral,

rectovaginal, and pouch-vaginal fistulas: results in 53 patients. Ann Surg 2008;248(1):39–43.

15. Sbizzera M, Morel-Journel N, Ruffion A, et al. Rectourethral Fistula Induced by Localised Prostate Cancer Treatment: Surgical and Functional Outcomes of Transperineal Repair with Gracilis Muscle Flap Interposition. Eur Urol 2022 Mar;81(3):305–12.

16. Bugeja S, Ivaz S, Frost A, et al. Complex fistula disease in the pelvic malignancy cancer survivor who has been treated with radiation. Curr Bladder Dysfunct Rep 2016;11(2):113–9.

17. Ghoniem G, Elmissiry M, Weiss E, et al. Transperineal repair of complex rectourethral fistula using gracilis muscle flap interposition—can urinary and bowel functions be preserved? J Urol 2008;179(5):1882–6.

18. Farrell MR, Tighiouart H, Vanni AJ. Hypoalbuminemia is Associated With Increased 30-Day Complications Following Rectourethral Fistula Repair: A National Surgical Quality Improvement Program Study. Urol Pract 2021;3:10–97.

19. Nyam DC, Pemberton JH. Management of iatrogenic rectourethral fistula. Dis Colon Rectum 1999;42(8):994–7.

20. Hadley DA, Southwick A, Middleton RG. York-Mason procedure for repair of recto-urinary fistulae: a 40-year experience. BJU Int 2012;109(7):1095–8.

21. Garofalo TE, Delaney CP, Jones SM, et al. Rectal advancement flap repair of rectourethral fistula. Dis Colon Rectum 2003;46(6):762–9.

22. Falavolti C, Sergi F, Shehu E, et al. York Mason procedure to repair iatrogenic rectourinary fistula: our experience. World J Surg 2013;37(12):2950–5.

23. Hebert KJ, Naik N, Allawi A, et al. Rectourethral Fistula Repair Using Robotic Transanal Minimally Invasive Surgery (TAMIS) Approach. Urology 2021 Aug;154:338.

24. Hechenbleikner EM, Buckley JC, Wick EC. Acquired rectourethral fistulas in adults: a systematic review of surgical repair techniques and outcomes. Dis Colon Rectum 2013;56(3):374–83.

25. Hampson LA, Muncey W, Sinanan MN, et al. Outcomes and quality of life among men after anal sphincter-sparing transperineal rectourethral fistula repair. Urology 2018;121:175–81.

26. Ryan JA, Beebe HG, Gibbons RP. Gracilis muscle flap for closure of rectourethral fistula. J Urol 1979;122(1):124–5.

27. Lane BR, Stein DE, Remzi FH, et al. Management of radiotherapy induced rectourethral fistula. J Urol 2006;175(4):1382–8.

28. Cohn JA, Large MC, Richards KA, et al. Cystectomy and urinary diversion as management of treatment-refractory benign disease: the impact of preoperative urological conditions on perioperative outcomes. Int J Urol 2014;21(4):382–6.

29. Osborn DJ, Dmochowski RR, Kaufman MR, et al. Cystectomy with urinary diversion for benign disease: indications and outcomes. Urology 2014;83(6):1433–7.

30. Al Awamlh BA, Lee DJ, Nguyen DP, et al. Assessment of the quality-of-life and functional outcomes in patients undergoing cystectomy and urinary diversion for the management of radiation-induced refractory benign disease. Urology 2015;85(2):394–401.

31. Gupta G, Kumar S, Kekre NS, et al. Surgical management of rectourethral fistula. Urology 2008;71(2):267–71.

32. Samplaski MK, Wood HM, Lane BR, et al. Functional and quality-of-life outcomes in patients undergoing transperineal repair with gracilis muscle interposition for complex rectourethral fistula. Urology 2011;77(3):736–41.

33. Selph JP, Madden-Fuentes R, Peterson AC, et al. Long-term artificial urinary sphincter outcomes following a prior rectourethral fistula repair. Urology 2015;86(3):608–12.

34. Madden-Fuentes RJ, Peterson AC. Pubic bone osteomyelitis and pubosymphyseal urinary fistula: a poorly recognized complication in prostate cancer survivors. Oncology 2017;31(3):169–73.

35. Bugeja S, Andrich DE, Mundy AR. Fistulation into the pubic symphysis after treatment of prostate cancer: an important and surgically correctable complication. J Urol 2016;195(2):391–8.

36. Matsushita K, Ginsburg L, Mian BM, et al. Pubovesical fistula: a rare complication after treatment of prostate cancer. Urology 2012;80(2):446–51.

37. Kaufman DA, Browne BM, Zinman LN, et al. Management of radiation anterior prostato-symphyseal fistulas with interposition rectus abdominis muscle flap. Urology 2016;92:122–6.

38. Gupta S, Zura RD, Hendershot EF, et al. Pubic symphysis osteomyelitis in the prostate cancer survivor: clinical presentation, evaluation, and management. Urology 2015;85(3):684–90.

39. Sexton SJ, Lavien G, Said N, et al. Magnetic resonance imaging features of pubic symphysis urinary fistula with pubic bone osteomyelitis in the treated prostate cancer patient. Abdom Radiol 2019;44(4):1453–60.

40. Lee YJ, Sadigh S, Mankad K, et al. The imaging of osteomyelitis. Quant Imaging Med Surg 2016;6(2):184.

41. Hebert KJ, Boswell TC, Bearrick E, et al. Robotic puboprostatic fistula repair with holmium laser pubic debridement. Urology 2022 Feb;160:228.

42. Liu W, Shakir N, Zhao LC. Single-port robotic posterior urethroplasty using buccal mucosa Grafts: technique and outcomes. Urology 2022 Jan;159:214–21.

43. Hammond JB, Howarth AL, Haverland RA, et al. Robotic Harvest of a Rectus Abdominis Muscle Flap

After Abdominoperineal Resection. Dis Colon Rectum 2020;63(9):1334–7.

44. Nosé BD, Boysen WR, Kahokehr AA, et al. Extirpative cultures reveal infectious pubic bone osteomyelitis in prostate cancer survivors with urinary-pubic symphysis fistulae (UPF). Urology 2020;142:221–5.

45. Lavien G, Chery G, Zaid UB, et al. Pubic bone resection provides objective pain control in the prostate cancer survivor with pubic bone osteomyelitis with an associated urinary tract to pubic symphysis fistula. Urology 2017;100:234–9.

Moving?

Make sure your subscription moves with you!

To notify us of your new address, find your **Clinics Account Number** (located on your mailing label above your name), and contact customer service at:

Email: journalscustomerservice-usa@elsevier.com

800-654-2452 (subscribers in the U.S. & Canada)
314-447-8871 (subscribers outside of the U.S. & Canada)

Fax number: 314-447-8029

Elsevier Health Sciences Division
Subscription Customer Service
3251 Riverport Lane
Maryland Heights, MO 63043

Printed and bound by CPI Group (UK) Ltd, Croydon, CR0 4YY

08/05/2025

01864724-0014